THE GREENWOOD ENCYCLOPEDIA OF
LOVE, COURTSHIP,
& Sexuality THROUGH HISTORY

THE GREENWOOD ENCYCLOPEDIA OF LOVE, COURTSHIP, AND SEXUALITY THROUGH HISTORY

The Ancient World, Volume 1
James W. Howell

The Medieval Era, Volume 2
William E. Burns

The Early Modern Period, Volume 3
Victoria L. Mondelli and Cherrie A. Gottsleben, with the assistance of Kristen Pederson Chew

The Colonial and Revolutionary Age, Volume 4
Merril D. Smith

The Nineteenth Century, Volume 5
Susan Mumm

The Modern World, Volume 6
James T. Sears

THE GREENWOOD ENCYCLOPEDIA OF LOVE, COURTSHIP, & *Sexuality* THROUGH HISTORY

THE EARLY MODERN PERIOD
Volume 3

Edited by
VICTORIA L. MONDELLI AND CHERRIE A. GOTTSLEBEN,
with the assistance of
KRISTEN PEDERSON CHEW

GREENWOOD PRESS
Westport, Connecticut • London

Library of Congress Cataloging-in-Publication Data

The Greenwood encyclopedia of love, courtship, and sexuality through history /
volume editors, James W. Howell ... [et al.].
    p. cm.
  Includes bibliographical references and index.
  Contents: v. 1. The ancient world / James W. Howell, editor—v. 2. The medieval era / William E. Burns, editor—v. 3. The early modern period / Victoria L. Mondelli and Cherrie A. Gottsleben, editors—v. 4. The colonial and revolutionary age / Merril D. Smith, editor—v. 5. The nineteenth century / Susan Mumm, editor—v. 6. The modern world / James T. Sears, editor.
  ISBN-13: 978–0–313–33359–0 (set : alk. paper)—ISBN-13: 978–0–313–33583–9 (vol. 1 : alk. paper)—ISBN-13: 978–0–313–33519–8 (vol. 2 : alk. paper)—ISBN-13: 978–0–313–33653–9 (vol. 3 : alk. paper)—ISBN-13: 978–0–313–33360–6 (vol. 4 : alk. paper)—ISBN-13: 978–0–313–33405–4 (vol. 5 : alk. paper)—ISBN-13: 978–0–313–33646–1 (vol. 6 : alk. paper)
  1. Sex—History—Encyclopedias. 2. Love—History—Encyclopedias. 3. Courtship—History—Encyclopedias. I. Howell, James W. II. Title.
  HQ21.G67125 2008
  306.703–dc22   2007023728

British Library Cataloguing in Publication Data is available.

Copyright © 2008 by Victoria L. Mondelli, Cherrie A. Gottsleben, and Kristen Pederson Chew

All rights reserved. No portion of this book may be
reproduced, by any process or technique, without the
express written consent of the publisher.

Library of Congress Catalog Card Number: 2007023728
ISBN-13: 978–0–313–33359–0 (set code)
          978–0–313–33583–9 (Vol. 1)
          978–0–313–33519–8 (Vol. 2)
          978–0–313–33653–9 (Vol. 3)
          978–0–313–33360–6 (Vol. 4)
          978–0–313–33405–4 (Vol. 5)
          978–0–313–33646–1 (Vol. 6)

First published in 2008

Greenwood Press, 88 Post Road West, Westport, CT 06881
An imprint of Greenwood Publishing Group, Inc.
www.greenwood.com

Printed in the United States of America

The paper used in this book complies with the
Permanent Paper Standard issued by the National
Information Standards Organization (Z39.48–1984).

10 9 8 7 6 5 4 3 2 1

Contents

List of Entries   vii

Set Preface   ix

Preface   xi

Acknowledgments   xiii

Introduction   xv

Guide to Related Topics   xxv

Chronology of Selected Events   xxix

The Encyclopedia   1

Selected Bibliography   233

Index   235

About the Editors and Contributors   239

List of Entries

Abortion and Contraception
Actors
Adolescents
Adultery
Africa
Americas (North and South)
Anal Sex
Annulment
Architecture, European
Aretino, Pietro (1492–1556)
Art, European
Asia

Bastardy
Berdache
Bestiality
Betrothal
Boleyn, Anne. *See* Henry VIII
The Book of the Courtier (Baldassare Castiglione, 1528)
Borgia, Lucrezia (1480–1519)
Brothels
Buddhism

Calvin, John (1509–1564)
Caste
Castiglione, Baldassare. *See The Book of the Courtier*
Castillo, Bernal Díaz del. *See* Díaz del Castillo, Bernal
Castration
Celibacy
Chastity
Childbirth
Childhood
Chinese Treasure Fleets
Christianity
Churching

Concubines
Confucianism
Contraception. *See* Abortion and Contraception
Council of Trent. *See* Trent, Council of
Courtesans
The Courtier. *See The Book of the Courtier*
Cross-Dressing
Cupid. *See* Eros

Daoism
D'Aragona, Tullia (c. 1510–1556)
Diane de Poitiers (1499–1566)
Díaz del Castillo, Bernal (c. 1495–1584)
Divorce
Domestic Violence
Dona Marina. *See* La Malinche
Dowry

Elizabeth I, Queen of England (1533–1603)
Eros
Eunuchs
Europe
Exploration and Colonization, European

Fatherhood
The First Blast of the Trumpet Against the Monstrous Regiment of Women (John Knox, 1558)
Fonte, Moderata (1555–1592)
Footbinding
Fornication. *See* Premarital Sex

Forteguerri, Laudomia (1515–c. 1555)
Foundlings and Orphans

Ganymede
Gilles de Rais (c. 1404–1440)

Harem/Seraglio
Henry III, King of France (1551–1589)
Henry VIII, King of England (1491–1547)
Hermaphrodites
Hinduism
Homoeroticism
Homosexuality

Il cortegiano. *See The Book of the Courtier*
Illegitimacy
Impotence
Incest
Incubi/Succubi
Index of Prohibited Books
Infanticide
'Ishq
Islam

Jeanne d'Arc. *See* Joan of Arc
Joan of Arc (c. 1412–1431)
Judaism
Julian of Norwich (1342–c.1416)

Kama Sutra
Knox, John. *See The First Blast of the Trumpet Against the Monstrous Regiment of Women*

LIST OF ENTRIES

La Malinche (c. 1502–c. 1529 or 1551–1552)
Lesbianism
Literacy
Literature, European
Love
Love Sickness
Love Songs
Luther, Martin (1483–1546)

Magic, Love, and Sex
Malinal. *See* La Malinche
The Malleus Maleficarum (Kramer, 1486)
Mandeville, Sir John. *See The Travels of Sir John Mandeville*
Marguerite de Navarre (1492–1549)
Marlowe, Christopher (1564–1593)
Marriage
Masculinity
Masturbation
Medicine
Menstruation
Middle East
Midwives
Mikveh
Mistresses

Motherhood
Mystics

Obstetrical Manuals
Oral Sex
Orphans. *See* Foundlings and Orphans

Pederasty
Penitential Practices
The Perfumed Garden for the Soul's Delectation (al-Nafzawi, Fifteenth Century)
Platonic Love
Polygamy/Polyandry
Pornography
Pozzo, Modesta. *See* Fonte, Moderata
Pregnancy
Premarital Sex
Printing
Prostitution

Raleigh, Sir Walter (1552–1618)
Rape
The Reformation
Remarriage/Widows

Sati
Savonarola, Michele (1390–1462)

Science
Seraglio. *See* Harem/Seraglio
Shakespeare, William (1564–1616)
Sikandar Lodhi (d. 1517)
Slavery
Sodomy. *See* Anal Sex
"The Story of Layla and Majnun" (Ganjavi)
Succubi. *See* Incubi/Succubi
Sufi Romances
Suttee. See Sati

Taoism. *See* Daoism
Theater
The Travels of Sir John Mandeville (c. 1366)
Trent, Council of (1545–1563)
Two-Spirited People. *See* Berdache

Venereal Disease
Villon, François (1431–c. 1463)
Virginity

Widows. *See* Remarriage/Widows
Witches
The Witches' Hammer. See The Malleus Maleficarum

Zinä

Set Preface

Sex and love are part of the very fabric of daily life—universal concepts that permeate every human society and are central to how each society views and understands itself. However, the way sex and love are expressed or perceived varies from culture to culture, and, within a particular society, attitudes toward sex and love evolve over time alongside the culture from which they arose. To capture the multicultural and chronological dimensions of these vital concepts, the six-volume *The Greenwood Encyclopedia of Love, Courtship, and Sexuality through History* explores the array of ideas, attitudes, and practices that have constituted sex and love around the world and across the centuries.

Each volume of alphabetically arranged entries was edited by an expert in the field who has drawn upon the expertise of contributors from many related disciplines to carefully analyze views toward sex and love among many cultures within a specified time period. Students and interested general readers will find in this work a host of current, informative, and engaging entries to help them compare and contrast different perceptions and practices across time and space. Entries cover such topics as customs and practices; institutions; legislation; religious beliefs; art and literature; and important ideas, innovations, and individuals. Users of this encyclopedia will, for instance, be able to learn how marriage in ancient Rome differed from marriage in Victorian England or in colonial America; how prostitution was viewed in medieval Europe and in the contemporaneous Islamic societies of Africa and the Middle East; and how or even if celibacy was practiced in eighteenth-century India, ancient Greece, or early modern Europe.

Edited by James W. Howell, Volume 1, *The Ancient World*, explores love and sexuality in the great societies of Europe, Africa, and Asia in the period before around 300 CE. Entries include Marriage, Homosexuality, Temple Prostitution, and Sex in Art. Volume 2, *The Medieval Era*, by William E. Burns examines sex and love in Europe, East Asia, India, the Middle East, Africa, and pre-Columbian Mesoamerica in the period between around 300 and 1400. Entries in this volume include Arthurian Legend, Concubinage, Eunuchs, Krishna, Seclusion of Women, *Thousand and One Nights*, and Virginity.

Volume 3, *The Early Modern Period*, edited by Victoria L. Mondelli and Cherrie Ann Gottsleben, with the assistance of Kristen Pederson Chew, focuses on sex and love in Europe, India, China, the Middle East, Africa, and the Americas in the fifteenth and sixteenth centuries. Some important entries in this volume are Bastardy, Confucianism, Dowries, Sex Toys, Suttee, and William Shakespeare. Edited by Merril D. Smith,

SET PREFACE

Volume 4, *The Colonial and Revolutionary Age*, looks at love and sexuality in western Europe, eastern Asia, India, the Middle East, Africa, and the Americas in the seventeenth and eighteenth centuries. The volume offers entries such as Bestiality, Castration, Berdache, Harems, Pueblo Indians, and Yoshiwara.

Volume 5, *The Nineteenth Century*, edited by Susan Mumm, explores sex and love in the Victorian period, primarily in Europe and the United States, but also in India, Asia, and the Middle East. Entries in this volume include Birth Control, Courtship, Fetishism, Native Americans, and Ottoman Women. Edited by James T. Sears, Volume 6, *The Modern World*, explores major topics in sex and sexuality from around the world in the twentieth and twenty-first centuries. Entries include AIDS/HIV, Domestic and Relationship Violence, Internet Pornography, Politics and Sex, Premarital Sex, Television, and the Women's Movement.

Each volume is illustrated and several cross-references to entries are provided. The entries conclude with a list of additional information resources, including the most useful books, journal articles, and Web sites currently available. Other important features of the encyclopedia include chronologies of important dates and events; guides to related topics that allow readers to trace broad themes across the entries; bibliographies of important general and standard works; and useful appendices, such as lists of Chinese dynasties and selections of important films and Web sites. Finally, detailed subject indexes help users gain easy access to the wealth of information on sex, love, and culture provided by this encyclopedia.

Preface

The Early Modern Period is the third volume in the six-volume *The Greenwood Encyclopedia of Love, Courtship, and Sexuality through History*, which covers sexual attitudes and practices in many cultures around the world from antiquity to the present. This volume contains over 125 entries on topics relating to human love, courtship, and sexuality in the early modern era, a period defined roughly as the years from 1400 to 1600, or the fifteenth and sixteenth centuries. Topics range from the sexual practices and attitudes prevalent in various world regions and religions to examinations of important institutions, such as marriage and divorce; common social phenomena, such as adultery and bastardy; and specific individuals. Although the main focus of this volume is on Europe, where the Reformation sparked differences in sexual views between Catholics and Protestants, there are numerous articles on other civilizations, including Asia, Africa, the Americas, and the Middle East. This volume is intended as a reference work for the general public, and for students at various levels from high school through college who want to learn about love and sex in various world cultures during the early modern period.

The entries are arranged alphabetically. Each entry begins by describing or defining its topic and its importance to the general themes of early modern love, courtship, and sexuality before proceeding to a general overview of the subject. Since almost 60 authors have contributed to this volume, they sometimes have different perspectives or disagreeing interpretations. Each entry, therefore, concludes with a bibliography of additional sources, including books, articles, and Web sites, where the reader can find more information. Cross-references to other entries in the volume are in bold in text or noted in the "See also" line at the end of the entry, and a Guide to Related Topics will help users to trace broad themes and concepts across the entries quickly and easily. The volume also includes a general bibliography, an introduction providing overall context for the entries, a chronology of significant events of the period, and a detailed subject index. Many entries are also illustrated.

Acknowledgments

Victoria Mondelli wishes to acknowledge the generous assistance of Margaret L. King, PhD, and Cherrie Gottsleben wishes to thank Sharmain van Blommestein, PhD, for her kind assistance. Kristen Chew would like to thank Elizabeth and Tom Cohen and Richard Raiswell for their generous help, and Tori Mondelli, to whom she owes more than she's comfortable thinking about. She would also like to thank John Wagner, senior development editor at Greenwood Press, for his forbearance, his patience in the face of extreme provocation, and his encouragement when things looked dark. If it wasn't for him, this volume wouldn't be here at all.

Introduction

The Early Modern Period, the third volume in *The Greenwood Encyclopedia of Love, Courtship, and Sexuality through History*, provides a view of the world through the lens of sex, love, and culture during the fifteenth and sixteenth centuries (1400–1600). Entries in this volume provide essential historical and literary analyses of important texts, people, and concepts that shaped human sexuality at that time. While the volume has a primarily European focus, many entries deal with ideas, people, and subject matter from the Americas, Africa, Asia, and India.

"The sexual is the idiom which channels and resonates with a multitude of themes,"[1] one scholar has said, and the entries in this volume will provide the reader with multiple entry points into a complicated, many-faceted subject. Gaining an understanding of the dynamics of sex, power, and privilege during this period is best undertaken by consulting a range of original sources that reveal much about early modern cultures. Entries in this volume rely upon the interpretation of legal records, literary works, demographic statistics, diaries, accounts, and a host of other primary documents to present a general introduction to erotic, romantic, and culturally important themes.

Scholars today agree that sex and gender are cultural constructs; that is, societies assign and interpret *the sexual* in relation to their own particular culture and experiences. What is normative and what is deviant is determined by the dominant, or hegemonic, groups operating within a given society, and these culturally constructed concepts typically become reified through law and custom. For example, monogamous, heterosexual marriages were the only sexual unions to enjoy approbation by Church/Temple and State in both early modern Christian and European Jewish cultures, and all other sexual unions were deemed by them to be unchaste, sinful, polluting, or dangerous to the functioning of society. However, it would be a mistake to assume that laws and practices were static, unchanging, and universal even within their cultures of origin. The early modern period was a time of great social upheaval and change throughout much of the world, during which norms of sexual and cultural interaction were redefined by internal and external hegemonic forces: within Europe, for example, the Reformation led to reconsiderations of the nature and need for marriage, while colonialism, conquest, and religious conversion significantly changed the ways in which Native American societies dealt with questions of courtship, male and female societal roles, and definitions of acceptable sexuality. The establishment of Portuguese settlement in West Africa and Asia provided new opportunities for sexual dangers and transgressive unions, as Portuguese traders formed liaisons with nonwhite, non-Christian women. Both Portuguese religious and government officials strove to prevent these racially and religiously "mixed" unions, but their efforts and severe legal punishments failed to dissuade the amorous, who found the de facto spaces in de jure situations. In other arenas, too, we will see that early modern peoples had a more flexible attitude toward sexual practices than the religious and secular laws left behind might suggest.

The rest of this introduction will be spent on major themes that are relevant and provide context for the entries that will follow.

SEXUALITY AND IDENTITY

Early modern European cultures had a different understanding of sexual identity than contemporary Western culture. "Sexual behavior did not represent a sign or marker of a person's sexual identity; it did not indicate or express some more generalized or holistic feature of the person, such as that person's subjectivity, disposition, or character," David M. Halperin says in "Forgetting Foucault: Acts, Identities, and the History of Sexuality."[2] One's position in society, religious affiliation, and gender informed one's "generalized" identity to a much greater extent than one's sexual behavior or identity.

Consequently, the early modern period did not have "homosexuals" and "lesbians," in our modern usage of the terms, nor did people self-identify, as they do now, by their sexual orientation. This does not mean that same-sex desire and intimacy did not occur; expressions of both appear in legal records, literature, and diaries all over the globe, and it was possible for a single individual to participate in both heterosexual and homosexual acts in their own lifetime without contradiction. Diverse cultures had their own interpretative frameworks from which to view and relate to same-sex relations. In Europe, "sodomites" (men who sexually penetrated other men or boys) were legislated against and persecuted because of a deep-seated cultural fear that such actions were contrary to God's will, whereas there was "a *lack* of anxiety" about female-to-female eroticism.[3] Berdaches in North American tribes, on the other hand, blurred the boundaries between male and female by dressing and behaving culturally like women, while still fighting like men.

BODIES AND SOCIETY

For early modern peoples, there were intense spiritual and economic dimensions to the physical body that were key as people passed through major life stages. As historian Mary Fissell explains, "The body is at once both intensely individual and a collective representation, an image of the social world shared by inhabitants. However, these representations are not fixed or stable; they are made and remade in response to specific circumstances and are often contested across multiple realms."[4] For women, the life stages of marriage, childbearing, and widowhood each had their claims on their bodies, although the exact nature of these claims differed around the globe.

Bodies were the texts upon which society wrote its needs, ideals, and desires. Women in particular were vulnerable to the physical manifestations of hegemonic desire. The practice of foot binding in China, where women's feet were broken and bound to create a fetishistic ideal of small, dainty feet, is a particularly vivid example of how ideals of beauty and bodily manipulation had dramatic ramifications for women, their families, and for society. The desired existence of women deliberately made incapable of any physicality beyond mere ornamentation is a reflection of Chinese ideals about the status of women, and the economic desires of the men who supported them in that state.

Beyond the purely metaphorical, bodies could actually be "remade" through writing, as writers used physical descriptions of people to further ideological and colonial desires. How non-Europeans were described by European writers has been documented by

Jennifer L. Morgan in her 2005 article "Male Travelers, Female Bodies, and the Gendering of Racial Ideology." Morgan's study found that in describing African women, "early modern writers focused on their breasts and their reproductive capacities more generally as sites of fascination and markers of primitiveness."[5] She goes on to argue that travel accounts were often the only "linkages" Europeans at home had to the wider world, and such racialized images of women helped "to justify the many faces of European colonialism (economic, political, cultural)."[6] The representation of the body in word and image was powerful indeed.

LOVE AND DESIRE

Love has many dimensions, and early modern people recognized that desire was only one aspect amongst many. From the courtly tradition of medieval Europe, early modern Europeans developed the idea of a kind of "noble" love that expressed intense desire but did not consummate or tarnish the love through sexual contact. This type of chivalric love morphed again into a courtly form of neo-Platonic love, where one would only admire and praise a lady without letting desire turn the pure sentiment into lust. In Book III of Baldassare Castiglione's *Book of the Courtier*, one character attested to the moral nature of love. He rejoiced, "It is impossible for vileness ever again to rule in a man's heart where once the flame of love has entered."[7]

Others grouped love and desire together as a perfect pair in securing a monogamous relationship. The love letters of King Henry VIII of England (r. 1509–1547) to Anne Boleyn when he was wooing her in the late 1520s declared as much: "Assuring you that henceforward my heart shall be dedicated to you alone, with a strong desire that my body could be also thus dedicated."[8] The unfortunate fate of Boleyn, who was executed for treason and adultery in 1536, suggests the flaws inherent in such feverish assurances, or maybe just in those coming from a monarch.

Desire, as Anne Boleyn learned to her sorrow, had its darker, more dangerous, and violent side. Early modern Europeans were warned by the Church of the dangers of unbridled, uncontrolled desire, and it was something to be feared on a societal as well as an individual level. Untrammeled desire could subvert the social order when inappropriate choices of affection caused romances to cross caste, economic, or political lines, as with Romeo and Juliet, or when it drove lovers to murder and criminality. Love sickness was recognized as a type of madness, to be feared while it was simultaneously glorified, as in the great Middle Eastern poem "Leyla and Majnun," where the hero loses his sanity for the sake of the beautiful Leyla. People desperate with desire often turned to black magic, entered into pacts with the Devil, and faced Inquisitional charges of heresy, all for love and sex. As Guido Ruggiero shows in the following passage from *Binding Passions: Tales of Magic, Marriage, and Power at the End of the Renaissance*,

> To understand their world one has to understand this central discourse that built out from a world where the macrocosm suffused the microcosm with power and meaning, metaphors, signs—a world replete with a rich poetics of the everyday that played across the holy and the unholy, space, the home, and the body. . . . In turn it was a world where the Devil was a strong presence. In matters of passion he could be utilized as just another force or worshipped as the true master.[9]

Desire and love moved people to take mortal and eternal risks. In the historical tales of love, magic, and desire, we glimpse why and how such risks seemed worth taking to the impassioned.

SEX AND CONQUEST

The early modern period is sometimes called the Age of Exploration, when European explorers, in search of gold, trade, slaves, and conquest, spread out across the globe. Between 1400 and 1600, Europeans made first contact, or renewed ancient contact, with North and South America; Eastern, Southern, and Western Africa; India; and Asia. In the resulting clash of cultures, many heretofore isolated societies around the globe underwent tremendous cultural transformations and hybridizations. Some cultures shattered as their members were conquered, enslaved, or killed; some absorbed European influences into themselves; and still others, as Japan did in the early 1600s, shut out foreign influences all together.

As Europeans conquered and established trade colonies throughout the world, the coming together of cultures became practical as well as metaphorical. Forced and consensual sex between the Spaniards and Native Americans produced new creole and mestizo cultures in the Americas. In the case of Spanish America, Spanish authority and patriarchy drastically changed indigenous patterns of marriage, sex, and even gender roles.[10] Unable to step outside their own cultural perspective, Spaniards interpreted native sexual practices within their own warrior and Christian codes of behavior. They moved quickly to eradicate males involved in same-sex or gender-blurring activities (*berdaches*), as if they were doing God's work in punishing sodomites, and petitioned the Crown to permit the death sentence for homosexuality.

European attempts to enslave Native Americans ended in disease and death for the enslaved, leaving behind a void and a need for new workers for European interests in North and Central America. Soon, Europeans began to ship African slaves to American soil, marking the start of the Atlantic slave trade and its attendant miseries and profound effects on race relations and the history of Africa and North America to this day. The unequal power relationship between master and slave was upheld in public and private encounters, as owners and their employees treated slaves as their sexual property. Children of slave mothers, no matter the paternity, were legally rendered as slaves. Slave families were often broken up as owners decided to sell children or parents for economic reasons. The existence of mulatto, *mestizo*, and other mixed-race children was sometimes glossed over, and sometimes the children were rejected by both societies. Their existence added to further social destabilization that was mostly felt by the colonized, rather than by the colonizers.

INVENTIONS OF POWER

Tremendous change came not only through the devastating consequences of exploration in the Americas and the advent of the Atlantic slave trade, but also through the development of key European inventions, foremost among them the printing press, with its moveable type, and firearms. As one scholar observes, European inventions brought a host of burdensome challenges for the rest of the globe: "the often violent imposition of European modernity on 'subject peoples' in the form of technology, capitalist labor practices, and the Christian civilizing mission has meant that cultures on the receiving end of such contact have been in a reactive and at times defensive posture with respect to dominant forms of 'global' influence."[11] Firearms gave European conquerors a significant advantage over much of its opposition, enabling them to establish favorable trade terms and control over newly colonized areas more quickly. The printing press, licenses for which were needed, put control of printed information in colonial territories squarely in the hands of the colonizer. As the

Europeans increasingly became literate, indigenous peoples and slaves were rarely instructed in reading or writing, except in the context of missionary efforts.

RELIGIOUS ATTITUDES TOWARD SEX

In an age of belief, where religion infused every aspect of life and religious choices outside the established norm could mean persecution or death, religious beliefs had a profound effect upon the expression and acceptable (and unacceptable) forms of sex, love, and courtship.

For Christians, mainly in Europe but in growing numbers throughout the rest of the world, attitudes toward sex and the body evolved from beliefs inherited from classical antiquity and the medieval period. For many classical Greeks, sexual pleasure was not laudable. In some of their writings, both Plato (428/7–327 BCE) and Aristotle (384–322 BCE) characterized sexual pleasure as unworthy, and categorized it with gluttony. Going even further, Aristotle placed sexual pleasure within the realm of bestial activity. In the *Symposium*, Plato extols the experience of homosexual intimacy, only to condemn it as "unnatural" in his *Laws*. Eventually, he confined sexual activity to the purpose of procreation, or advocated subsuming it into spiritual and intellectual ideals. His theory of a higher, more spiritual, and nonphysical love became a leading idea of the Renaissance. The Greeks and Romans enacted laws with severe penalties to regulate sexual conduct, many of which were biased against women. In the case of adultery, a married woman who committed adultery was given a choice of death, imprisonment, or financial penalty. Overall, marital faithfulness was demanded of wives rather than of husbands. The ancient Greeks also disapproved of rape and incest, but temple prostitution in Athens was commonplace.

As Christianity emerged as a new religion, Platonic views on sex and bodily appetites were combined with Judaism's ritual laws on bodily purity to influence establishment attitudes toward sex and the body. Thus, for the medieval church, sex became synonymous with sinful bodily appetites, and its sinfulness was tied to the female body through the actions of Eve, Adam's seducer and the cause of his fall. Some male writers within the Church represented the man as possessing the higher attributes related to the mind: "[t]hey stressed male as power, judgment, discipline and reason, female as weakness, mercy, lust and unreason."[12] Women were viewed as possessing a more insatiable sexual appetite than men.

The Apostle Paul (10–67 CE), however, presented a different view, in that he understood that both husband and wife were equally subject to sexual desires.

In I Corinthians 7:1–12, he required that a man and woman first obtain permission from his/her spouse before withholding sex for periods of fasting and prayer. However, a man and wife soon had to "come together" again, so that they would not be tempted because of their "incontinency." Although he viewed celibacy as a preferable state, he affirmed the wife's "power" over her husband's body and the husband's "power" over the body of his wife. Husband and wife had a conjugal duty toward each other. The sacredness of sex within marriage solidified the idea that a married couple could indulge in sex for procreation or pleasure, and yet remain chaste as long as they were faithful to each other. Contrary to St. Paul's command, however, the Roman Church was strongly influenced by the work of St. Augustine of Hippo (354–430 CE), who believed that the sexual urge could be controlled, and demanded celibacy of all clergy. Augustine also connected the notion of original sin, the original fall from grace, with human sexuality.[13]

Up until the Reformation, sexuality and religion had an uneasy coexistence. Women were expected to be chaste before marriage, as were men, although the importance of chastity before marriage depended greatly upon social position and economic class. Marriage did not become a sacrament of the Catholic Church until after the Council of Trent (c. 1563), and before that time it was not uncommon for a couple to be considered married in the eyes of their village simply by moving in together, and declaring themselves husband and wife. According to the Church, sexual relations were not permitted during Lent, or on holy days and feast days, and breaches of these rules were cause for confession. The common medieval belief that attributed the inducing of sexual desire to the Devil was still popularly prevalent into the early modern period; other beliefs that credited sexual cravings to astrological influences, namely the planet Venus, were also still circulating with vigor throughout the fifteenth and sixteenth centuries.

In the sixteenth century, when the religious wave of the Protestant Reformation spread out from Germany and across western Europe, the German reformer and theologian Martin Luther (1483–1546) adopted St. Paul's views on marital sex but declared celibacy an affront to God's gift of companionship. Contrary to St. Augustine as well, Luther believed sexual urges to be uncontrollable because they were not voluntary. Sexual urges, he insisted, were a vital part of human nature, and no shame should be imposed upon the fulfilling of those desires especially, since they played a significant part in human health. Marriage, therefore, remedied sexual promiscuity. Both Luther and John Calvin accepted marital sex for the purpose of pleasure as legitimate and without sin. However, while Luther emphatically denounced fornication as evil, Calvin, as indicated in the following passage, thought that sex outside of marriage played a role in Salvation's design:

> The sordid squalor of extramarital sex, particularly with prostitutes [argued Calvin], made manifest the fallen condition of mankind. Prostitution, Calvin believed, was thus a God-given sign of the consequences of sin, and the harlot played a role in the design of salvation, since the spectacle of her depraved life should incite God-fearing Christians to reform their own lives.[14]

Unlike the early modern Catholic clergy, who were moving toward the firmer enforcement of clerical celibacy during this time, the sixteenth-century Reformers honored marriage and marital sex, even for its religious leaders. For them, the body and its sexual needs were natural. As a result, the Reformers refused to accept marriage as a sacrament because of its direct link to sexual activity, and all the natural effects to which the body is subject. In their estimation, no natural part of human beings could be accepted as sacramental, or a part of the grace of God. Since, in addition to procreation, the purpose of marriage was to control sexual lust, it could not be classed with the work of redemption: "All bodies were natural, finite, prone to sin, distant from God. Christ's redeeming act had transcended nature and its proclivity to sin, bringing a redeeming grace that was beyond nature and unavailable through it."[15] With the desacramentalization of marriage by Protestant thinkers, divorce (still rejected by the Roman Catholic Church) became an option in cases of adultery, a husband's impotence, desertion, and a wife's refusal to have sex with her husband. Although Luther allowed these justifications for divorce, he lacked any enthusiasm for breaking the marriage bond. In one instance, he recommended bigamy to a man whose wife refused to render to him sexual satisfaction.[16] Both Martin Bucer (1491–1551), the German Protestant reformer and former member of the Dominican order, and, later, John Milton (1608–1674), English poet and political tract writer, deemed incompatibility a justified reason for divorce.[17]

The Council of Trent, convened by the Catholic Church in 1545 in response to Protestant challenges to its authority, addressed doctrinal reform and dictated the future course of Catholicism. By its conclusion in December 1563, the status quo had been codified, and there was very little dramatic change within canon law on the subject of marriage or in resolving the deep ambivalence within the Church on the subject of the appropriateness of sexual pleasure. Soon after the Council, the work of the Spanish Jesuit Tomás Sánchez (1550–1610) became influential through his revision and elaboration on laws regarding marriage and sex, and particularly on the subject of rape. The Roman view on rape (or *raptus*) as "theft" had been carried over into early modern Christian culture. *Raptus* (or abduction), according to Sánchez, was a crime of larceny against a woman's parents, or against her husband, and a crime against chastity if extramarital sex was involved. Sánchez was slightly radical when he iterated that *raptus* "was not exclusively a male crime, for it could also be perpetrated by a woman either against a man or another woman." Also significant is the fact that Sánchez added abduction to the list of violent acts, as a kind of psychological coercion by the perpetrator toward his victim: "[Any] passionate and importunate pleading by the perpetrator who implored his victim to run away with him or begged tearfully for her sexual favors, constituted the force necessary to qualify the act as *raptus*."[18]

Catholics and Protestants both continued to follow the lead of St. Augustine and other Church Fathers in officially condemning prostitution, while still condoning the existence of the prostitute as a "necessary evil" and a regulator of sexual lust. During the late thirteenth and fourteenth centuries, prostitutes in various Italian cities were outlawed and expelled in 1259, 1266, 1314, and 1327. Although men were still allowed to have concubines in the earlier medieval period, stricter laws against concubinage were being enforced by the late 1300s, and this practice transferred over into the early modern period. Ecclesiastical law, for the most part, maintained its aversion to the prostitute, but legal writers and theologians left the door open for toleration of prostitution and possible salvation in the case of true repentance, in light of the various reasons that led a woman into such a lifestyle: poverty, rape, or being sold into harlotry by her parents. Courts were also known to flex the rules and allow prostitutes as "credible witnesses in impotence cases."[19] There was an uneasy feeling about prostitution, which had become a "public utility," with governments and religious leaders like the English Bishop of Winchester even owning or receiving rents from brothels. By the end of the sixteenth century, however, brothels in certain municipalities were being shut down, and prostitutes who operated privately were heavily penalized.

Male and female homosexual acts, as well as acts of bestiality, came under the umbrella of sin and sodomy. These acts were considered crimes against nature, and were severely punished by both Catholic and Protestant law in the sixteenth and seventeenth centuries. Whereas writers and judges in earlier centuries had placed less emphasis on "lesbian" acts and transvestite activity, early modern authorities stressed their concern by making punishments more severe for such transgressive and societally destabilizing acts. During this period, masturbation also came under the banner of "the unnatural" alongside sodomy, although the death penalty was not required for masturbation. The chief reason for this aversion to masturbation was the fact that its main objective was to experience the pleasure of orgasm. The Jesuit priest Tomás Sánchez was convinced that "even spontaneous orgasm . . . was wrong and should be fended off, if at all possible. A person who felt a sexual climax coming on, save during marital intercourse, should lie still . . . avoid touching the genitals . . . make the sign of the cross, accompanied by fervent prayers beseeching God not to allow him to slip into orgasmic pleasure."[20]

INTRODUCTION

British writers like John Fisher (1459–1539) believed that sex and the experience of orgasm and semen emission came under the rubric of lechery, as something that "attacked both body and soul," with orgasm being the result of "the filthy lust of the flesshe," which "robbed men of vital energy and exposed them to dangers both moral and physical."[21] Fisher's view suggests a trace of Aristotelian philosophy, but also mirrors a part of the belief system of some Eastern (e.g., China, Japan, Korea) and Southeast Asian (e.g., Thailand, Vietnam) religions, such as Daoism and Buddhism. Here Buddhism and Daoism have some common ground with Christianity, in its ambivalence toward the physical, and in its division of higher from lower self, soul from body.

Religious attitudes toward sex in Judaic thought during this period reflected the belief that all human behavior was supposed to reflect a sense of God's holiness. Sex between a husband and wife was seen as positive, and the pleasure of both a right. Spiritual purity in the sexual act was illustrated through bodily purification rituals. One example of this was expressed in the *niddah*, or family purity ritual during a woman's menstrual period. *Niddah* is described in the Torah as a ritual impurity, and sexual relations are prohibited while a woman is menstruating. A woman who is *tum'ah*, or impure, is classed among women who have just given birth, or among individuals who have come into contact with a dead body (*Tum'at met*). A woman continues to be in a state of *niddah* until she experiences *taharah* (purification) through a *mikvah*, or ritual bath. The *taharah* process involves a minimum of eleven days (twelve for Ashkenazi Jews). Sexual intercourse with a woman who is *niddah* required self-sacrifice or *Yehareg ve'al ya'avor*, which literally means "One should be killed and not transgress." Thus, the punishment for sex during menstruation was the same as murder, adultery, idolatry, and various types of homosexual acts and incest. Judaism's strict observance of bodily rituals constructed sexual relations as symbolic of the couple's spiritual purity in the presence of a holy God.

Despite being free of the concept of original sin, Eastern religions too had a sometimes ambivalent attitude toward sexuality. While sex was more usually seen as something of the body that distracted the soul from higher pursuits, there were schools of thought which privileged human sexuality and made it part of the path to higher spiritual attainments. Practitioners of the Tantric school in both Hinduism and Tibetan Buddhism maintained that human experience is the manifestation of a universal energy that comes from the gods. They used physical ecstasy, both metaphorically and in practice, for the godly purposes of procreation, as a metaphor for ultimate spiritual unity, and to achieve a higher form of pleasure. In the early modern period, some Daoist communities (in the sexual practices among the laity) believed that the loss of semen was equated with a loss of balance in energy between mind and body, and practiced sexual yoga and retention practices to enhance longevity. Buddhism, of which Daoism is a derivative, shared with Hindus the belief in *nirvana*, a state of highest happiness, where the practitioner is said to experience perfect peace and freedom from the suffering that is caused by desire (lust, anger, craving). However, Tantra provided a way of achieving *nirvana* through the harnessing of desire to achieve oneness through the combining of yin (female) and yang (male) energies.

In Islamic areas, which included the peoples from northern and eastern Africa as far as India, procreation was regarded as the major purpose for marriage, according to the Qur'an. The Qur'an also stated that Allah gives companionship and love as marital gifts, yet the text is not specific on the details that characterize the significance of such companionship or love. Thus, Muslim jurists depended on the *hadiths* for clarity, and wrote manuals on how to treat wives and the role of sex in marriage, including the right of women to sexual satisfaction. The Qur'an also presented an ambiguous position for contraceptive practices, and jurists debating the practice of *coitus interruptus*, and the conditions under which it was acceptable. Early modern Islamic views on contraception reflected the medieval writings of the Shafi'i jurist al-Ghazali (1058–1111), who declared that as far as procreation was concerned, there was no basis for prohibiting *coitus interruptus*, since the causes of pregnancy relied first on marriage, then on intercourse, ejaculation, and the settling of semen in the womb, respectively, and inseparably—since there was no basis for prohibiting marriage, there could be no basis for making pregnancy mandatory. Extramarital intercourse, one of the few acts that the Qur'an describes specific punishments for, was regarded as *zinä*, or unlawful intercourse. Stoning or lashing was given to the offenders, dependent upon the marital status of the individuals involved.

In Africa, south of the Muslim lands in the west and northeast, the sheer number and variety of religions and attitudes toward sexuality make it difficult to make sweeping generalizations on African religious views on sexuality. There were hundreds of different tribes and cultures across the continent, ranging in size from a few hundred people to the size of city states on the eastern coast and large empires in the north. Culturally, tribes and cultures ranged from the very matriarchal to the very patriarchal, while some placed great emphasis on virginity and others placed little importance upon it. Fertility rituals sometimes had religious meaning attached, and many tribes and cultures produced spectacular examples of sexually themed art and fetishes.

In surveying religious traditions and their laws and customs surrounding sexual practice, the diversity and points of similarity are intriguing. This volume, and indeed this entire series, offers an in-depth look at these and other themes in cultural studies. Suggestions for further reading are provided at the end of each entry for those seeking a deeper understanding of the topics.

NOTES

1. Helmut Puff, *Sodomy in Reformation Germany and Switzerland, 1400–1600* (Chicago: University of Chicago Press, 2003), 7.
2. David M. Halperin, "Forgetting Foucault: Acts, Identities, and the History of Sexuality," in *Sexualities in History: A Reader*, ed. Kim M. Phillips and Barry Reay (New York: Routledge, 2002), 45.
3. Valerie Traub, "The (In)Significance of 'Lesbian' Desire," in *Queering the Renaissance*, ed. Jonathan Goldberg (Durham, NC: Duke University Press, 1994), 65.
4. Mary Fissell, "Gender and Generations: Representing Reproduction in Early Modern England," in Phillips and Reay, *Sexualities in History*, 105.
5. Jennifer L. Morgan, "Male Travelers, Female Bodies, and the Gendering of Racial Ideology," in *Bodies in Contact: Rethinking Colonial Encounters in World History*, ed. Tony Ballantyne and Antoinette Burton (Durham, NC: Duke University Press, 2005), 54.
6. Ibid.
7. As quoted in Morton M. Hunt, *The Natural History of Love* (New York: Alfred A. Knopf, 1959), 176.
8. As quoted in ibid., 202.
9. Guido Ruggiero, *Binding Passions: Tales of Magic, Marriage, and Power at the End of the Renaissance* (New York: Oxford University Press, 1993), 128–29.
10. Karen Vieira Powers, *Women in the Crucible of Conquest: The Gendered Genesis of Spanish American Society* (Albuquerque: University of New Mexico Press, 2005), 11.
11. Tony Ballantyne and Antoinette Burton, ed. *Bodies in Contact: Rethinking Colonial Encounters in World History* (Durham, NC: Duke University Press, 2005), 3.

12. Caroline Walker Bynum, *Fragmentation and Redemption: Essays on Gender and the Human Body* (New York: Zone Books, 1991), 175.

13. Elaine Pagels, *Adam, Eve, and the Serpent* (New York: Vintage Books, 1989).

14. James A. Brundage, *Law, Sex, and Christian Society in Medieval Europe* (Chicago: University of Chicago Press, 1987), 557.

15. Rosemary Ruether, *Christianity and the Making of the Modern Family* (Boston: Beacon Press, 2000), 77.

16. Ibid., 79

17. Bucer's views on divorce appear in his treatise "Marriage, Divorce and Celibacy." This treatise was included in his commentary on Matthew, Mark, and Luke. John Milton's "The Doctrine and Discipline of Divorce" clearly explains his stance.

18. Brundage, *Law, Sex, and Christian Society*, 570.

19. Ibid., 512.

20. Ibid., 571.

21. As quoted in Brundage, *Law, Sex, and Christian Society*, 490.

FURTHER READING

Brundage, James A. *Sex, Law and Marriage in the Middle Ages*. Burlington, VT: Variorum, 1993; Bullough, Vern L., and James Brundage. *Sexual Practices and the Medieval Church*. Buffalo: Prometheus Books, 1982; Coletti, Theresa. *Mary Magdelene and the Drama of the Saints*. Philadelphia: University of Pennsylvania Press, 2004; Sachedina, Zulie. "Islam, Procreation and Law." *International Family Planning Perspectives* 16, no. 3 (September 1990): 107–11; Thapar, Romila. *Asoka and the Decline of the Mauryas*. Oxford: Oxford University Press, 1997.

Guide to Related Topics

AFRICA AND ASIA
Africa
Asia
Buddhism
Caste
Castration
Chinese Treasure Fleets
Confucianism
Daoism
Eunuchs
Exploration and Colonization, European
Footbinding
Harem/Seraglio
Hinduism
'Ishq
Islam
Kama Sutra
Middle East
Polygamy/Polyandry
Sati
Sikandar Lodhi
"The Story of Layla and Majnun" (Ganjavi)
Sufi Romances
Zinä

CHILDREN AND BIRTH
Abortion and Contraception
Adolescents
Bastardy
Childbirth
Childhood
Churching
Fatherhood
Foundlings and Orphans
Infanticide
Midwives
Motherhood
Obstetrical Manuals
Pregnancy
Premarital Sex

EUROPE AND AMERICA
Americas (North and South)
Architecture, European
Aretino, Pietro
Art, European
Berdache
Borgia, Lucrezia
Calvin, John
Celibacy
Christianity
Churching
D'Aragona, Tullia
Diane de Poitiers
Diaz del Castillo, Bernal
Elizabeth I, Queen of England
Europe
Exploration and Colonization, European
Fonte, Moderata
Forteguerri, Laudomia
Gilles de Rais
Henry III, King of France
Henry VIII, King of England
Joan of Arc
Julian of Norwich
La Malinche
Literature, European
Luther, Martin
Marguerite de Navarre
Marlowe, Christopher
Raleigh, Sir Walter
Reformation
Savonarola, Michele
Shakespeare, William
Witches

GEOGRAPHICAL REGIONS AND PRACTICES
Africa
Americas (North and South)
Architecture, European
Art, European
Asia
Berdache
Caste
Castration
Celibacy
Chinese Treasure Fleets
Eunuchs
Europe
Exploration and Colonization, European
Footbinding
Harem/Seraglio
Literature, European
Middle East
Sati
Slavery
Zinä

INDIVIDUALS
Aretino, Pietro
Borgia, Lucrezia
Calvin, John
D'Aragona, Tullia
Diane de Poitiers
Diaz del Castillo, Bernal
Elizabeth I, Queen of England

Fonte, Moderata
Forteguerri, Laudomia
Gilles de Rais
Henry III, King of France
Henry VIII, King of England
Joan of Arc
Julian of Norwich
La Malinche
Luther, Martin
Marguerite de Navarre
Marlowe, Christopher
Raleigh, Sir Walter
Savonarola, Michele
Shakespeare, William
Sikandar Lodhi
Villon, François

Legal Issues
Annulment
Bastardy
Bestiality
Brothels
Divorce
Domestic Violence
Dowry
Homosexuality
Incest
Infanticide
Marriage
Premarital Sex
Rape
Slavery
Witches

Literary Works, Themes, and Authors
Aretino, Pietro
The Book of the Courtier (Castiglione, 1528)
Calvin, John
Diaz del Castillo, Bernal
Eros
The First Blast of the Trumpet Against the Monstrous Regiment of Women (Knox, 1558)
Fonte, Moderata
Forteguerri, Laudomia
Ganymede
Index of Prohibited Books
Julian of Norwich
Kama Sutra
Literacy
Literature, European

Love
Love Songs
Luther, Martin
Malleus Maleficarum (Kramer, 1486)
Marguerite de Navarre
Marlowe, Christopher
Obstetrical Manuals
The Perfumed Garden for the Soul's Delectation (al-Nafzawi, 15th Century)
Platonic Love
Pornography
Printing
Raleigh, Sir Walter
Shakespeare, William
"The Story of Layla and Majnun" (Ganjavi)
Sufi Romances
Theatre
The Travels of Sir John Mandeville (c. 1366)
Villon, François

Marriage
Adultery
Annulment
Betrothal
Chastity
Concubines
Divorce
Domestic Violence
Dowry
Harem/Seraglio
Love
Marriage
Mistresses
Polygamy/Polyandry
Premarital Sex
Remarriage/Widows
Sati
Virginity
Zinä

Religion, Religious Issues, and Reformers
Adultery
Annulment
Bastardy
Betrothal
Brothels
Buddhism
Calvin, John

Celibacy
Chastity
Christianity
Churching
Confucianism
Daoism
Divorce
Hinduism
Homosexuality
Incest
Incubi/Succubi
Index of Prohibited Books
Infanticide
Islam
Judaism
Lesbianism
Luther, Martin
Magic, Love, and Sex
Malleus Maleficarum (Kramer, 1486)
Marriage
Masturbation
Mikveh
Mystics
Pederasty
Penitential Practices
Polygamy/Polyandry
Premarital Sex
Prostitution
Reformation
Remarriage/Widows
Trent, Council of
Virginity
Witches
Zinä

Reproduction and the Body
Abortion and Contraception
Castration
Childbirth
Childhood
Eunuchs
Footbinding
Hermaphrodites
Impotence
Marriage
Masculinity
Masturbation
Medicine
Menstruation
Midwives
Pregnancy

Savonarola, Michele
Science
Venereal Disease

SEXUALITY AND SEX PRACTICES
Adultery
Anal Sex
Bestiality
Brothels
Courtesans
Cross-Dressing
Homoeroticism
Homosexuality
Lesbianism
Magic, Love, and Sex
Masturbation
Mistresses
Oral Sex
Pederasty
Premarital Sex
Prostitution
Rape
Virginity
Zinä

SOCIAL AND CULTURAL ISSUES
Abortion and Contraception
Actors
Adultery
Architecture, European
Art, European
Bastardy
Berdache
Betrothal
Brothels
Caste
Castration
Chastity
Churching
Concubines
Cross-Dressing

Divorce
Domestic Violence
Dowry
Eunuchs
Footbinding
Foundlings and Orphans
Homosexuality
Incest
Infanticide
Lesbianism
Literacy
Love
Love Sickness
Love Songs
Magic, Love, and Sex
Marriage
Masculinity
Masturbation
Medicine
Midwives
Mistresses
Pederasty
Platonic Love
Pornography
Premarital Sex
Printing
Prostitution
Rape
Remarriage/Widows
Sati
Science
Slavery
Theatre
Venereal Disease
Virginity
Witches
Zinä

WOMEN AND WOMEN'S ISSUES
Abortion and Contraception
Adultery

Bastardy
Borgia, Lucretia
Chastity
Childbirth
Churching
Concubines
Courtesans
D'Aragona, Tullia
Diane de Poitiers
Divorce
Domestic Violence
Dowry
Elizabeth I, Queen of England
The First Blast of the Trumpet Against the Monstrous Regiment of Women (Knox, 1558)
Fonte, Moderata
Footbinding
Forteguerri, Laudomia
Joan of Arc
Julian of Norwich
La Malinche
Lesbianism
Marguerite de Navarre
Marriage
Menstruation
Midwives
Mikveh
Mistresses
Motherhood
Obstetrical Manuals
Pregnancy
Prostitution
Rape
Remarriage/Widows
Sati
Virginity
Witches
Zinä

Chronology of Selected Events

1401 Mongol ruler Tamurlane (Timur the Lame) conquers and destroys Baghdad.

1405 A Chinese fleet under the command of Zheng He transports 28,000 Chinese across the Indian Ocean as far as India, Africa, and the Middle East in search of trade and influence.

1407 Beginning of construction of the Forbidden City in Beijing, which is completed in 1420.

1415 Public brothels are legalized in Florence, Italy; Henry V of England defeats the French at Agincourt, one of the most important battles of the Hundred Years War.

1428 The Mexica and their allies establish the Aztec Empire in Mesoamerica.

1431 The English burn Joan of Arc (Jeanne d'Arc) for heresy and witchcraft in the marketplace of Rouen, France; the last of the Chinese treasure fleets sails to the eastern coast of Africa.

1434 An expedition sponsored by Prince Henry of Portugal ("The Navigator") goes south of Cape Bojador (on the western coast of Africa, south of the Canary Islands), ushering in the age of European exploration.

1438 Inca Yupanki comes to power and begins the building of the Inca Empire in Peru.

1440 Upon coming to the throne of Benin in western Africa, Oba Ewuare Ogidigan bans sexual intercourse in his kingdom after two concubines poison each other—a mass emigration from Benin ensues; execution of French nobleman Gilles de Rais, who was found guilty of the rape and murder of hundreds of children, mostly male.

1441 First shipment of African slaves arrives in Portugal.

1450 Johannes Gutenberg, a German goldsmith, invents the first European printing press with moveable type.

1451 Founding of the Vatican Library; the Iroquois Five Nations Confederacy is founded around this time in North America.

1452 Birth of Leonardo da Vinci near Vinci, Italy.

1453 Constantinople falls to the Ottoman Turks, who rename the city Istanbul.

1454 Publication of the Gutenberg Bible.

1460 Construction begins on Machu Picchu, the great mountaintop city of the Incas.

1461 Ottoman emperor Mehmed II conquers Trebizond, the last outpost of the Christian Byzantine Empire.

1468 Lorenzo the Magnificent, along with his brother Guiliano, becomes ruler of the Italian city-state of Florence.

1469 Birth of Nanak, founder of Sikhism, in Lahore, India.

1475 Coffee is served in a public place for the first time at Kiva Han in Istanbul; a law is enacted allowing a Turkish woman to divorce her husband if he does not supply her with her daily quota of coffee.

1480 Founding of the Spanish Inquisition; death of Matope leads to end of kingdom of Great Zimbabwe; rise of the city-states of Mombasa, Maline, and Kilwa along the east coast of Africa.

CHRONOLOGY OF SELECTED EVENTS

1485 Richard III of England is killed at the Battle of Bosworth Field; Richard's supplanter, Henry VII, founds the Tudor dynasty in England.

1486 Publication of the *Malleus Malleficarum* (*The Hammer of the Witches*), a handbook for witch hunters.

1490s Foundation of the Songhai Empire in West Africa.

1491 The Inca Empire of Peru is the largest empire on earth, with the longest road system on planet (25,000 miles); Prince Henry, the second son of Henry VII and future king of England as Henry VIII, is born at Greenwich Palace.

1492 King Ferdinand and Queen Isabella exile the Jews from Spain after conquering the last Muslim kingdom on the Iberian Peninsula; sailing for Spain, the Italian explorer Christopher Columbus arrives in the West Indies.

c. 1493 Arrival of syphilis in Europe.

1497 Incited by the preacher Girolamo Savonarola, citizens of Florence burn their luxuries on Shrove Tuesday—this event comes to be called "the bonfire of the vanities"; Savonarola is later excommunicated and executed.

1500 Start of the Atlantic slave trade.

1501 Shah Esma'il of Iran starts his reign by converting the country from Sunni to Shi'ia Islam.

1502 In Mexico, Montezuma II becomes ruler of the Aztec Empire; the first African slaves appear in the New World—they are brought to the Caribbean after the near extermination of the native Arawak Indians forces the Spanish to find a new source of labor to work the plantations of the New World.

1503 Prince Henry of England is betrothed to his elder brother's widow, Catherine of Aragon, daughter of Ferdinand and Isabella of Spain.

1505 Pope Julius II issues a papal bull dispensing any impediments to the marriage of Prince Henry of England and Catherine of Aragon, including Catherine's prior marriage to Henry's late brother, Prince Arthur.

1506 Syphilis appears in China.

1509 Henry VIII accedes to the throne of England and marriages his late brother's widow, Catherine of Aragon.

1513 Publication of Eucharius Rösslin's *Rosengarten für swangere Frauen und Hebammen* (*Rosegarden for Midwives and Pregnant Women*), a guide for midwives.

1516 Sir Thomas More publishes *Utopia*; birth of Princess Mary, later Mary I of England and the only child of Henry VIII and Catherine of Aragon to survive to adulthood.

1517 Martin Luther nails his 95 Theses to a church door in Wittenberg, Germany, marking the start of the Protestant Reformation.

1519 The Spanish adventurer Hernan Cortés lands in Mexico at Vera Cruz; birth of Henry Fitzroy, future duke of Richmond, Henry VIII's illegitimate son by Elizabeth Blount.

1520 Accession in Constantinople of the Ottoman sultan Suleiman I (The Great).

1521 Ferdinand Magellan, a Portuguese explorer in the service of Spain, arrives in Polynesia; chocolate is imported to Spain from Mexico; the Spanish, led by Hernan Cortés, conquer Tenochtitlan, the capital of the Aztec Empire, thus destroying the Aztec state.

1522 The first mixed-race (*mestizo*) child is born in the New World to La Malinche and Hernan Cortés—the child is named Martin; birth of Sen no Rikyuu, who had the greatest influence on the development of the *chado*, or Japanese tea ceremony.

1525 Henry VIII begins a brief sexual liaison with Mary Boleyn, the sister of Anne Boleyn, and a former mistress of Francis I of France.

1526 King Afonso of the Kongo Empire sends two letters to the Portuguese king strongly protesting the capture of free individuals for slavery by the Portuguese; the Muslim emperor Babur defeats Ibrahim Lohdi at the first battle of Panipat thereby beginning the establishment of the Mughal Empire in India.

1527 Lacking sons and having fallen in love with a woman of his court, Anne Boleyn, Henry VIII applies to Pope Clement VII for an annulment of his marriage to Catherine of Aragon on the grounds that the marriage is invalid due to Catherine's prior marriage to Henry's late brother; Rome is sacked by the armies of the Holy Roman Emperor Charles V, the nephew of Catherine of Aragon.

1528 Publication of Baldassare Castiglione's *The Courtier*, which becomes the manual for how ideal Renaissance courtiers should behave.

1529 The troops of Sultan Suleiman end their siege of Vienna and return to Belgrade, thereby halting the westward expansion of the Ottoman Empire; the failure of a legatine court to grant an annulment of his marriage leads Henry VIII to seek other means to free himself from Catherine of Aragon.

1531 Europeans begin cultivating tobacco in Santo Domingo.

1532 Abortion becomes a capital offense in the Holy Roman Empire.

1533 Henry VIII secretly marries a pregnant Anne Boleyn; birth of Amina of Zazzau, a capable and fearless Hausa warrior queen in the savannah region of western Africa; Henry VIII breaks with Rome and declares himself head of the English Church, which is thereby empowered to annul his marriage to Catherine of Aragon; birth of Princess Elizabeth, the future Elizabeth I of England, the daughter of Henry VIII and Anne Boleyn; the pope excommunicates Henry VIII.

1534 Arrival of the French explorer Jacques Cartier in what would later become Canada; St. Ignatius Loyola founds the Jesuit order; the pope declares valid the marriage of Henry VIII and Catherine of Aragon.

1535 Executions of Sir Thomas More and Bishop John Fisher for their opposition to Henry VIII's break with Rome.

1536 Execution of Anne Boleyn for treason and adultery.

1537 Pope Paul III declares that "Indians themselves indeed are true men" and must be treated well; birth of Prince Edward, the future Edward VI, Henry VIII's long-awaited son, by his third wife, Jane Seymour.

1539 The first printing press is set up in the New World in Mexico City.

1540s Cities in Italy start enforcement of laws dictating dress and curtailing movement of courtesans.

1541 Spanish arrive in Peru under Francisco Pizarro, who overthrows the Inca Empire.

1542 Founding of New France in Canada; Katherine Howard, the fifth wife of Henry VIII, is executed for treason and adultery; Joao Cabrilho of Spain arrives in California; Antonio de Mota becomes first European in Japan.

1545 Opening of the Nineteenth Ecumenical Council of the Catholic Church, known as the Council of Trent.

1547 Ivan IV (the Terrible), Grand Prince of Moscow, becomes Tsar of Russia; death of Henry VIII of England and of Francis I of France, the later possibly of syphilis; Edward VI, a nine-year-old boy, becomes king of England.

1549 St. Francis Xavier reaches Japan.

1553 Mary I, the first English queen regnant, restores the English Church to Catholicism.

1555 Tobacco arrives in Spain.

1558 John Knox publishes *The First Blast of the Trumpet Against the Monstrous Regiment of Women* criticizing the regime of Mary I in England; accession of Elizabeth I (The Virgin Queen) to the throne of England; death of Roxelana Sultan, wife of Suleiman I (The Magnificent)—a former slave from the Ukraine, Roxelana rose in the harem and convinced Suleiman to marry her, an almost unheard-of thing.

1560 Jesuit Jasper de Cruz becomes the first European to personally encounter tea and write about it.

1561 Establishment of the Luba Empire in southern Zaire.

1562 John Hawkins initiates the English Atlantic slave trade with slaves from what is now Sierra Leone in West Africa.

1563 Catholic doctrine on marriage as a sacrament is established at the nineteenth session of the Council of Trent.

CHRONOLOGY OF SELECTED EVENTS

1564 The Tridentine Index or *Index of Prohibited Books*, a list of books censored by the Roman Catholic Church as being dangerous to faith, is established by Pope Pius IV; William Shakespeare is born in Stratford, England.

1565 Spain lays claim to the Philippine Islands.

1567 The Portuguese establish colonies near what is now Rio in Brazil.

1570 The Japanese open the port of Nagasaki to outside trade; Hiawatha and Dekanawidah form the Iroquois League in North America; Pope Pius V issues the bull *Regnans in Excelsis*, which declares Elizabeth I of England excommunicated and deposed.

1571 The naval Battle of Lepanto, in which a European coalition that included Spain, the pope, and Venice defeated a Turkish fleet, is fought off western Greece.

1572 The St. Bartholomew's Day Massacre, a royally sanctioned slaughter of French Protestants, occurs in Paris and throughout the kingdom.

1573 End of the Ashikaga shogunate in Japan.

1574 Henri, duke of Anjou, who is suspected of homosexuality, succeeds his brother, Charles IX, as Henri III of France.

1577 The English explorer Sir Francis Drake launches his voyage of circumnavigation.

1580 Sir Francis Drake returns to England, thus completing his three-year voyage of circumnavigation.

1582 Devised by Pope Gregory XIII, the Gregorian calendar replaces the old Julian calendar in Catholic countries—it will not be introduced into England until 1752.

1584 The Dutch Protestant leader, William of Orange, is assassinated by a Catholic fanatic.

1585 Sir Walter Raleigh sends a colonizing expedition to Virginia, a portion of the east coast of North America that is named for Elizabeth I of England, the "Virgin Queen."

1586 Due to hardship and the hostility of the local native, Raleigh evacuates his colonists from Virginia.

1587 Elizabeth I of England consents to the execution of her Catholic cousin, Mary, Queen of Scots; Sir Walter Raleigh sends out a second English colonizing expedition to Virginia.

1588 The English defeat the Spanish Armada, which was launched against England by Philip II of Spain in part as a response to the execution of Mary of Scots.

1589 Murder of Henri III of France.

1590 Toyotomi Hideyoshi unifies Japan; upon returning to Virginia after a three-year absence occasioned by the Armada invasion, John White finds the English colonists vanished; Edmund Spenser publishes the first three books of *The Faerie Queen*.

1591 At the Battle of Tondibi, the Songhai Empire falls to the army of the Sultan of Morocco, which is armed with guns; Gao and Timbuktu come under Moroccan control.

1592 Sir Walter Raleigh is imprisoned in the Tower of London for seducing and impregnating one of Queen Elizabeth's maids of honor.

1593 English playwright, spy, and homosexual Christopher Marlowe is murdered at an inn in Deptford.

1598 The first opera—*Dafne* by Jacopo Peri—is performed in Florence.

1600 The British East India Company is founded and begins to conduct trade with East Asia.

1603 Death of Elizabeth I of England; Tokugawa Ieyasu establishes a military dictatorship, the Tokugawa shogunate, over Japan and moves the residence of the emperor and thus the capital of Japan to Edo (modern-day Tokyo).

1616 Death of William Shakespeare.

The Encyclopedia

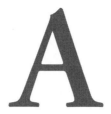

ABORTION AND CONTRACEPTION. The ability to control fertility—either through contraception or abortion—has been important throughout history and in all cultures. In **Europe**, the knowledge of how to do so has existed at least since the time of the ancient civilizations of Greece, Egypt, and Rome (McLaren 1990, 6; Riddle 1992, viii, 2–7). Above and beyond the need to conceal evidence of illicit sexual relationships, fertility control was important within **marriage** for the control of family size at times of economic hardship and because constant childbearing was perceived as detrimental to women's health and to the health of their existing children (McLaren 1990, 142–46). Works by Hippocrates and Galen contain many recipes for agents that can be used as abortifacients or contraceptives. Islamic medical texts from the ninth century CE were based on this Hellenistic learning and subsequently translated from Arabic into Latin so that, by the thirteenth century, western European physicians had assimilated and likely were using this ancient medical knowledge (Riddle 1992, 76–81, 129–30). Renaissance humanists retranslated original Greek and Roman medical texts in the fifteenth and sixteenth centuries, but it is clear that, in Europe, attitudes towards the control of fertility from the Middle Ages onward were shifting toward a more restrictive and prohibitive outlook (Riddle 1992, 144–46; Riddle 1997, 89–92). Instead of viewing such measures positively, ecclesiastical and secular authorities sought to make them sinful if not downright criminal. Both Catholic and Protestant religious authorities condemned the use of contraceptives and abortifacients but legal attitudes toward birth control differed from region to region. In 1532, when the Holy Roman Emperor Charles V codified German law for the first time in his *Constitituo Criminalis Carolina* contraception and abortion were equated with murder, while English Common Law of the same time did not define the killing of a child still in the womb as felonious (Riddle 1997, 126–29).

ABORTION. For many women in early modern Europe, inducing an abortion was the first line of defense against unwanted pregnancy and so it was regarded as a form of contraception. Attitudes toward any deliberate effort to end a pregnancy varied according to a woman's circumstances. If it was used to conceal an illicit sexual relationship (usually so by unmarried women), then the practice was condemned or even used as evidence to support accusations of further sexual criminality or **infanticide** (Gowing 2003, 142). However, if a married woman sought an abortion to protect her own health or that of her family, then her action could be considered justified (McLaren 1984, 107). The timing of any attempt at abortion was crucial to establishing its effectiveness or criminality and depended on the understanding of when a fetus was thought to possess a soul. In the early modern period, "ensoulment" was thought to occur on "quickening," around the fourth month of pregnancy (McLaren 1984, 108; Riddle 1992, 127; Wiesner 1993, 48, 94). Consequently, taking measures to end an unwanted pregnancy before quickening was not thought of as abortion but as "restoring the menses," although any attempt to end a pregnancy after quickening was considered murder (McLaren 1990, 160–61). Contemporary opinion of the time considered that hardening secular, religious, and legal measures against contraception and infanticide drove women toward abortion (McLaren 1990, 159).

Methods used to induce abortion included beatings, tight lacing of the clothing (McLaren 1984, 101), letting blood from the feet or thighs (Gowing 2003, 47; McLaren 1984, 101), and herbal abortifacients, either taken orally or as pessaries. The most commonly recommended herbs were ergot of rye, pennyroyal (a member of the mint family), and savin (juniper) (McLaren 1984, 104; Riddle 1997, 54).

An increase in the levels of legal and moral condemnation of contraception and abortion led to an association in the public mind between the knowledge of such agents and criminality. Inevitably, women suffered most from this association. Beginning in the Middle Ages and continuing throughout the sixteenth and seventeenth centuries, it is possible to trace the transfer of the expert knowledge of fertility control from male, university-educated physicians to female midwives who inhabited the more popular world of printed herbals and the oral transmission of knowledge (Myrsiades 2002, 4; Riddle 1992, 157; Riddle 1997, 89–91). The fifteenth-century witch-hunters' handbook, **The Malleus Maleficarum,** or *The Hammer of the Witches* (1486), defined a witch as someone who practiced any means of limiting the size of a family, either through contraception, abortion, **castration**, or sterilization (cited Myrsiades 2002, 4–6; Riddle 1997, 111). In England, the oath taken by midwives bound them not to use witchcraft, sorcery, or herbs and potions that would cause an abortion (Gowing 2003, 159). Consequently, in early modern Europe, ancient knowledge of fertility control was increasingly associated with magic, superstition, criminality, and unruly female behavior.

CONTRACEPTION. In early modern Europe, the simplest method of contraception was abstinence or continence, but Catholic and Protestant teachings from the **Reformation** onward (influenced by the writings of St. Augustine) emphasized that procreation was the only reason for marriage, thus making sexual intercourse a marital duty. Indeed, it was thought that contraception used by married couples was a worse sin than if it was used by the unmarried (McLaren 1990, 149–50). It seems that one of the most widely used and effective contraceptive methods (and the most widely condemned) was onanism, or *coitus interruptus*. The method was condemned because it was non-procreative intercourse and so, like abstinence, had no place in marriage. Outside marriage, *coitus interruptus* was associated with other non-procreative sexual acts such as sodomy (McLaren 1984, 58–61, 75–81).

The knowledge of contraceptives most obviously inherited from ancient medicine was that of herbal potions made from plants such as rue, mint, savin (juniper), willow, pennyroyal, and agnus castus (also called chaste tree) and taken by women (McLaren 1984, 72–75; Riddle 1997, 54). The same herbs were used in pessaries, tampons, and douches (McLaren 1990, 154, 157). Other herbal remedies, such as hemlock, were taken or worn by men as anaphrodisiacs (McLaren 1984, 72). Recipes for these potions and lotions were printed in herbals and were also passed on orally, either within families (mother to daughter) or by **midwives**. These remedies increasingly were rejected by trained physicians and, by the eighteenth century, there was a decline in general belief about their efficacy. Their longevity of use in medical and herbal texts and in oral traditions, however, suggests that there was some level of effectiveness (McLaren 1990, 154; Riddle 1997, 144).

The only new contraceptive produced during the early modern period was the condom. First described in 1564, it was designed not to prevent pregnancy but to protect men from syphilis, and was consequently associated with prostitution (McLaren 1984, 82–86; McLaren 1990, 157). There is no evidence of condoms being described as contraceptive devices in the sixteenth and seventeenth centuries. *See also* Anal Sex; Witches.

Further Reading: Bicks, Caroline. *Midwiving Subjects in Shakespeare's England*. Aldershot: Ashgate, 2003; Gowing, Laura. *Common Bodies: Women, Touch and Power in Seventeenth-Century England*. New Haven, CT: Yale University Press, 2003; McLaren, Angus. *Reproductive Rituals: The Perception of Fertility in England from the Sixteenth Century to the Nineteenth Century*. London: Methuen, 1984; McLaren, Angus. *A History of Contraception from Antiquity to the Present Day*. Oxford: Blackwell, 1990; Myrsiades, Linda. *Splitting the Baby: The Culture of Abortion in Literature and Law, Rhetoric and Cartoons*. New York: Peter Lang, 2002; Riddle, John M. *Contraception and Abortion from the Ancient World to the Renaissance*. Cambridge MA: Harvard University Press, 1992; Riddle, John M. *Eve's Herbs: A History of Contraception and Abortion in the West*. Cambridge, MA: Harvard University Press, 1997; Wiesner, Merry E. "The Midwives of South Germany and the Public/Private Dichotomy." In *The Art of Midwifery: Early Modern Midwives in Europe*, edited by Hilary Marland, 77–94. London: Routledge, 1993.

Lynn Robson

ACTORS. The advent of acting as a profession, rather than an amateur pasttime, came during the latter half of the sixteenth century in western Europe. Previously, acting had been the province of amateurs with other main employment, and who participated only occasionally in the production of mystery and miracle plays. As drama became more secularized, acting troupes were formed, although very little is known about them before 1545. However, these early actors cannot have been well-regarded by society at large since they were often considered little better than vagabonds, and could be prosecuted at law for vagrancy. Moral objections to the new secular theater included the questionable nature of the acting profession itself, predicated as it was on pretense, subterfuge, and the assumption of characters and positions other than one's own. One consequence of the resulting stigma was the adoption of stage names by French public-theater actors for the purpose of disguise. Despite such objections, in England, Italy, and Spain, theatrical popularity resulted in the formation of licensed, and for the first time, fully legal companies of players and playhouses.

At the height of the English Renaissance, an actor's month could involve fifteen different plays in repertory, and the addition of a new play in rehearsal every two weeks, with profits limited to company-sharers. The first such English company, the Earl of Leicester's Men, was headed in 1574 by an actor named James Burbage (creator of the first playhouse erected in London, known simply as the Theatre, in 1576). His son, Richard Burbage, originated some of William Shakespeare's most renowned tragic roles, such as Othello, Hamlet, Richard III, and King Lear. Other actors of this time included tragedian Edward Alleyn, famous for the Marlovian roles of Doctor Faustus, Edward II, and Tamberlaine, and comedians such as Richard Tarleton, Will Kempe, and Robert Armin, who played the famous fools of Shakespearean drama. The style of these actors is hard to determine; some scholars believe it to be realistic, while others believe it to be formalist and conventionalized, due in part to female parts being played by boys. While strictly enforced in England, the barring of women from the stage was far from universal. In Spain, women were legally allowed to act from 1587 through 1596, while in Italy and France, *commedia dell'arte* troupes typically consisted of seven men and three women. The preeminent actor of the Gelosi Company, the most famous of these troupes, was Isabella Andreini (1562–1604).

Customs regarding women on the stage varied in Asia as well. In Japan, the highly stylized *Noh* drama, originated by the actors Kan'ami and his son Zeami, of the Kanze troupe, was the dominant theatrical form from the fourteenth to the seventeenth centuries. As codified by Zeami, Noh theater was an austere, strictly conventionalized, and entirely male-dominated affair, featuring a main actor (*shite*), his companions (*tsure*), and secondary characters (*waki*), as well as parts played by boy actors (*kokata*). Conversely, in Ming dynasty China, the critic Pan Zhiheng (1556–1622) cited an actress, Yang Chaochao, as the supreme actor of her time, and noted for her psychologically realistic performances.

Indian and Persian theater of this period was relatively undistinguished, due to Islamic distaste for human representation in art. In India, regional folk theater forms (i.e., Bengali *jatra*, Keralite *kathakali*) did flourish in rural areas as family troupes made acting a hereditary profession. However, because of the lack of records associated with folk arts, the absence of a stage-play tradition, and the ephemeral nature of theatrical performances, little can be said about professional actors in India, Africa, and the New World. *See also* Shakespeare, William; Theater.

Further Reading: Brown, John Russell, ed. *The Oxford Illustrated History of Theatre*. Oxford: Oxford University Press, 1995; Chambers, E.K. *The Elizabethan Stage*. Oxford: Clarendon Press, 1922; Fei, Faye Chunfang, ed. *Chinese Theories of Theater and Performance from Confucius to the Present*. Ann Arbor: The University of Michigan Press, 1999; Gurr, Andrew. *The Shakespearean Stage: 1574–1642*. 3rd ed. Cambridge: Cambridge University Press, 1992; Richards, Kenneth, and Laura Richards. *The Commedia Dell'Arte: A Documentary History*. Oxford: Basil Blackwell Ltd, 1990; Yoshinobu, Inoura. *A History of Japanese Theater I: Up to Noh and Kyogen*. Yokohama, Japan: Kokusai Bunka Shinkokai (Japan Cultural Society), 1971.

Balaka Basu

ADOLESCENTS. Early modern European society had an ambivalent attitude toward both adolescents and adolescence, ranging from idolization to disparagement, but it was not ambivalent about the existence of such a stage in life nor about its definition. Following Isidore of Seville's six-part subdivision of the course of human life, adolescence (*adulescentia*) was the fourth period in human development, coming immediately after childhood (*puerizia*) and just before youth (*iuventus*). It spanned ages fourteen to twenty-eight and coincided with a period of intense sexual development and growing maturity (*Etymologies*, XI.ii). Because of this sudden spurt in sexual development, adolescents were seen as particularly prone to concupiscence and very much in need of education. Good teaching and firm direction would allow them to grow into upright and responsible adults. Not surprisingly, then, adolescence was seen as a particularly crucial period in a person's development, for it marked the point when an individual moved from the "innocence" of childhood into the "responsibility" of adulthood. For males, the classical image of Hercules at the crossroads came to represent adolescence as a time of choice between one or the other path in life, between proper or improper behavior, virtue or vice, and, ultimately, between salvation and damnation. When describing the ages of life in his treatise *Della vita civile*, the Florentine historian Matteo Palmieri clearly drew on this myth when using the letter Y to represent the course of life. Palmieri explained that infancy (birth to age seven) and childhood (seven to fourteen years of age) constituted the stem of the letter Y, while adolescence was the point of bifurcation, the moment of choice between the two paths that lay ahead, the path of virtue and that of vice. For women the case was somewhat different, for early marriage catapulted them immediately into motherhood and, by extension, adulthood. There was no need to educate women on proper career and lifestyle choices, for this had already been done for them by their male relatives when they chose their husband or their convent for them.

Education and discipline were, therefore, the key to the successful rearing of an adolescent male. Aside from the personal contribution of parents and tutors, who provided direction in the family and at school, there were other venues that contributed to the education of an adolescent, such as apprenticeships in a shop (for males) or service in a household (for females). In Florence, in particular, lay religious confraternities provided adolescents (in this case, males aged thirteen to twenty-four) with yet another venue for personal growth, this time by educating the youths in basic skills (reading, writing, singing) and in the faith (rituals, beliefs, traditions) and also by giving them valuable experience in management, organization, finances, and other skills necessary in running an organization with, at times, hundreds of members and sizeable property. Adolescents thus became emblematic not only of the innocence and purity of their society (a role they shared with children), but also, and especially, of that society's vitality and potential. For this reason, they were often prominently featured in royal entries or in official civic ceremonies, both in life and in paintings.

That is not to say, however, that adolescents were model members of their society or that they were always seen in a positive light. The violent behavior of male adolescents at festivities such as Carnival, or even in the routines of daily life, is well documented in chronicles and legal documents. In the case of female adolescents, their innate weakness (as understood by current medical and moral concepts based on Aristotelian philosophy) left them prone to sexual misbehavior and excess. Contemporary moralists and reformers such as St. Bernardine of Siena railed against the manners and mannerisms of adolescents, whom he found to be too obsessed with sex, while reformers such as Girolamo Savonarola tried to redirect their secular entertainments to more religious and spiritual ends. Recently, Ottavia Niccoli has argued that the violence of male adolescents was an endemic element of early modern society, that it was long accepted as a "voice" from God speaking through these "innocents," but that in the wake of the religious reforms of the sixteenth century such adolescent violence was seen as unacceptable and actively discouraged.

Court records throughout Europe clearly indicate that working-class adolescent women, as young as thirteen or fourteen years of age, were often the object of unwanted sexual attention, both in the workplace and on the street. In the wealthy and in the noble classes, they were used, instead, as pawns in the family's marriage strategies. Adolescent males were also sexually active, but generally they did not marry until after their adolescence. In Florence, for example, a man usually contracted his first marriage sometime in his mid-thirties, while a woman did so sometime in her late teens. This generational discrepancy between husbands and wives led to a variety of actual and imagined problems that contemporary society acknowledged, but was unable to solve—the high number of young widows to be cared for, and the constant concern with cuckoldry are just two of the most obvious.

The late age of marriage for males also meant that adolescent males (that is, men in their teens and twenties), who more often than not were still celibate, had to seek other venues for sexual gratification, be that in the company of prostitutes or of each other. As Michael Rocke has shown, adolescent **homosexuality** was so widespread in Florence that it could be seen as the norm; not surprisingly, in various parts of Europe **sodomy** itself came to be known as "the Florentine vice." The pattern was clear and simple: a young man in his early teens would serve as the passive partner to an older adolescent's active sexual gratification; at about age eighteen, the "passive" male would, in turn, find himself a younger friend and become the "active" partner in a new sexual relationship. Such a practice was seen as a phase in an adolescent male's sexual maturation and, generally, was not viewed as problematic unless it extended into adulthood; that is, past the age of marriage.

Further Reading: Ariès, Philippe. *Centuries of Childhood: A Social History of Family Life*. New York: Vintage Books, 1965; Eisenbichler, Konrad. *The Boys of the Archangel Raphael: A Youth Confraternity in Florence, 1411–1785*. Toronto: University of Toronto Press, 1998; Eisenbichler, Konrad, ed. *The Premodern Teenager: Youth in Society, 1150–1650*. Toronto: Centre for Reformation and Renaissance Studies, 2002; Isidore of Seville. *The Etymologies*. Cambridge: Cambridge University Press, 2006; Niccoli, Ottavia. *Il seme della violenza. Putti, fanciulli, mammoli nell'Italia tra Cinque e Seicento*. Bari and Rome: Laterza, 1995; Polizzotto, Lorenzo. *Children of the Promise: The Confraternity of the Purification and the Socialization of Youths in Florence, 1427–1785*. Oxford: Oxford University Press, 2004; Taddei, Ilaria. *Fête, jeunesse et pouvoirs. L'Abbaye des Nobles Enfants de Lausanne*. Lausanne: Université de Lausanne, 1991; Taddei, Ilaria. *Fanciulli e giovani. Crescere a Firenze nel Rinascimento*. Florence: Leo S. Olschki, 2001; Trexler, Richard C. "Ritual in Florence. Adolescence and Salvation in the Renaissance." In *The Pursuit of Holiness in Late Medieval and Renaissance Religion*, edited by Charles Trinkaus and Heiko A. Oberman, 200–64. Leiden: E.J. Brill, 1974.

Konrad Eisenbichler

ADULTERY. In early modern Europe, and in many non-Western societies of the time, adultery was defined as voluntary sexual intercourse between a married individual and a person who was not his or her spouse. Attitudes toward adultery varied widely, from those of the Toda people of southern India, who attached no social stigma to extramarital sex, and the Nuer people of the Sudan, who willingly accepted any children born of adultery, to Tudor England, where adulterous women were whipped through the streets, and various Muslim societies, where adulterers could be executed.

In western Europe, adultery was viewed as a serious moral offense. One seventeenth-century moralist declared "corrupting a man's wife" to be "the worst sort of theft, infinitely beyond that of goods" (Macfarlane, 242), and, in the mid-sixteenth century, the Catholic Council of Trent condemned adultery as a "defilement of the marriage bed" (Catechism of Trent [www.cin.org]). Adultery also drew widespread social disapproval, as evidenced by the early modern English practice of hanging horns on the house of a man who was known in the community to have been cuckolded by his wife. However, despite frequent calls, especially by clerics and secular social commentators, for more severe penalties, punishments for adultery in early modern Europe were often relatively light. In England, adulterers were tried in ecclesiastical courts, where the usual punishments were fines or public confession and humiliation. In court records, adultery was often not distinguished from sexual relations between unmarried persons, with both acts simply being described by some general term, such as "fornication."

In Europe, a clear double standard pervaded the whole issue of adultery. Because of the importance of property rights and legitimate inheritance, the laws and society as a whole considered adultery committed by married women to be worse than adultery committed by married men. As Samuel Johnson wrote in the eighteenth century, adultery "introduced confusion of progeny," and for this reason a woman who broke her marriage vows was "so much more criminal" than a man who did the same (Macfarlane, 243). Henry Home, Lord Kames, a prominent Scottish jurist of the same era, condemned the adultery of wives as "an alienation of affection from the husband, which unqualifies [the wife] to be his friend and companion; and . . . tends to bring a spurious issue into the family, betraying the husband to maintain and educate children who are not his own (Macfarlane, 242–43). Marital infidelity by kings, noblemen, and other men of property was frequent and condoned; wives were expected to accept it and keep silent, even when illegitimate children resulted from their husbands' liaisons. Marital infidelity by queens and upper class wives was altogether more serious. The alleged adultery of **Anne Boleyn**, the second wife of **Henry VIII**, led to her execution in part because her actions threw doubt on the legitimacy of Princess Elizabeth (*see* **Elizabeth I**) and thus clouded the royal succession.

European women of all classes were treated more harshly than men by the courts and the law when they committed adultery. In England and western Europe, an unmarried woman who bore the child of a married man was usually stripped half naked and whipped in public before suffering a year-long confinement in a house of correction. Her offense was largely economic; unless her lover voluntarily took responsibility for the child or could be obliged by the court to provide support, her child became an extra charge upon the local parish, whose members thus suffered in their purses for her adultery. The double standard also applied when it came to ending an adulterous **marriage**. Although true **divorce** was unavailable in early modern England, the ecclesiastical courts granted **annulments** (such as the English Church granted Henry VIII in 1533) and allowed separations. Men who could prove adultery in their wives could obtain a separation, but wives of adulterous husbands could have a separation only if they proved adultery and some other marital offense, such as cruelty or desertion. By the end of the seventeenth century, actual divorce became possible for well-connected Englishmen who had the money and patience to see a private bill through Parliament, but for most men, and all women, desertion or adultery were the only remedies for a bad marriage.

Despite the legal and social penalties that were technically attached to it, adultery in early modern Europe was, in practice, widely tolerated and thus frequently committed. Although the records of English church courts are full of cases of suspected adultery—one tiny Essex village had ten such cases in a three-year period between 1587 and 1589—most historians believe that the vast majority of adulterous unions never made it to the courts. Many contemporary observers, such as the famous diarist Samuel Pepys, commented on the frequency of adultery, and the tolerance commonly accorded to it. By the seventeenth century, adultery was more frequently a matter of jest than a matter for the courts, as indicated by the joke about the woman, who, upon hearing from her husband that Parliament was considering a law calling for all cuckolds to be cast into a river, asked him, "Husband, can you swim?" (Mcfarlane, 241).

In early modern Muslim communities, Islamic law (*shari'a*) condemned adultery as a great sin in both men and women, and anyone convicted of ***zinä*** (which included adultery) could be stoned or whipped to death. However, punishments were usually harsher and more swiftly applied for women, who could be beaten or killed by a father or brother (although an aggrieved husband might also kill his wife's lover). However, such drastic punishments gradually became less frequent and Islamic tradition, rather than seeking the dissolution of marriages disrupted by adultery, came to encourage a reconciliation of the spouses mediated by the two families. In Jewish communities, as among Christians, adultery was forbidden by the seventh commandment. By the early modern period, the ancient punishment of stoning anyone found guilty of adultery had largely given way to the practice of dissolving adulterous marriages. Jewish law forbade a man to continue living with a wife who had committed adultery; he was obliged to give her a "get," or bill of divorce, and she was prohibited from thereafter marrying her lover. *See also* Bastardy; Christianity; Islam; Judaism.

Further Reading: Bouhdiba, Abdelwahab. *Sexuality in Islam.* London: Routledge and Kegan Paul, 1985; Epstein, Lewis M. *Sex Laws and Customs in Judaism.* New York: Ktav Publishing House, 1967; Macfarlane, Alan. *Marriage and Love in England 1300–1840.* Oxford: Blackwell, 1987; Philips, Roderick. *Putting Asunder: A History of Divorce in Western Society.* Cambridge: Cambridge University Press, 1988; Stone, Lawrence. *The Family, Sex and Marriage in England 1500–1800.* New York: Harper and Row, 1977.

John A. Wagner

AFRICA. Africa is a vast continent populated by thousands of different cultures and ethnic groups of varying size. The early modern period was one of great upheaval in Africa, as empires within the continent rose and fell, and large areas began to be colonized by external European powers. From the eighth through the eleventh centuries, the Maghreb (North Africa and the Sahara Desert area) became predominantly Muslim, and **Islam** was also a major force down along the Swahili Coast (the east coast of Africa from Somalia to Mozambique), where African and Arab traditions and cultures met and blended together. The Christian kingdoms of Nubia and Ethiopia were often troubled during this process, and early intrusions along the western and eastern coasts by the Portuguese, who began to trade, colonize, and enslave natives with and without the permission of local governments, began to destabilize the continent. This article will focus on precolonial sub-Saharan Africa (for northern Africa, please *see* **Middle East**). Sub-Saharan Africa can generally be divided into three different regions: West Africa, East Africa, and then Central and South Africa. These regions were populated by thousands of different cultures ranging in size from small tribes of twenty to thirty to large empires encompassing millions of people. Central and South Africa were primarily home to the Bantu, who composed approximately a third of Africa's population.

Most African societies were patrilineal but throughout Africa there were no single fixed models or gender roles. Sexual norms varied between the societies and between class, age, religion, and ethnic backgrounds. Initiation rites in many societies were important, as were taboos. In some areas of West Africa, it was taboo to show obvious pleasure in intercourse, although a libation to the ancestors could make things right again. Ceremonies marked a number of life transitions such as birth, coming of age, and **marriage**. All of these societies possessed their own traditions. For example, among the Gusii in modern day Kenya, a child was considered an adult at eight years of age. Among the Bemba, the coming-of-age ceremony could last up to a month. In East Africa, among Muslim populations, female circumcision was widely practiced. Among the Ganda in Uganda, sex was only allowed to take place in the dark. Status and rank within these societies was often distinguished through a variety of scarification, tattoos, hairstyles, and dress.

Sexual relations among many societies were very casual and revolved around reproduction. This casualness in some cultures made prostitution an acceptable profession that was considered a legitimate business, and widows and divorced women often supported themselves through prostitution. **Homosexuality** and same-sex relationships were tolerated in many cultures and in some cultures they were part of a life cycle phase or initiation ritual. Among the Hausa in northern Nigera, homosexuality was practiced privately between older and younger men. In Yoruban tribes, physical contact such as handholding between men was not considered sexual. In present day Cameroon, female-female marriages are allowed. However, these unions are social in nature and not sexual.

The majority of African societies, like the Igbo, Yoruba, and the Vai of West Africa, were patrilineal, patrilocal, and polygamous; however, countless exceptions existed. The Ashanti of Ghana, eastern Nigeria, and Benin were matrilinear, and strong kinship systems predominated throughout the continent. Living arrangements varied. For example, among the Asante, spouses continued to live in the houses where they were born. In other cultures and marriage systems, women circulated instead of wealth. Families would exchange women or men would marry many women. Younger children would follow their mothers to her new husband's house but when they grew older they joined a male family member's family.

In patrilineal societies, descent and inheritance was anchored around the father and patriarch. These societies tended to be stricter than matrilineal ones. Often pre-pubescent marriages, either infant or child marriages, were arranged. These forged family and tribal alliances but they also effectively eliminated premarital sex. In matrilineal societies, all children belonged to the mother. There were few controls on female sexuality. Women controlled their bodies and kept their children. Often one of the mother's brothers became the social father of the children. In Lozi society (northern Zambia), there was little if no punishment for sexual activity, **adultery** was pervasive, **divorce** common, and fosterage was the common practice, but the biological father of the child was recognized.

In many cultures, **premarital sex** was forbidden but the meaning of the term was also interpreted differently. For example, among the Kikuyu in East Africa, mothers regularly checked the genitalia of their daughters to ensure that they had not had intercourse. If they had, they were punished severely. In the case of premarital **pregnancy** among the Tswana, the family put the child to death, at birth.

In East and South Africa, the taboo of premarital sex applied only to penetration that resulted in the breaking of the hymen. As long as this line was not crossed, a large assortment of sexually erotic activities were practiced, most notably *coitus inter crura*, or penetration between the thighs. This permissiveness has been attributed to societies such as the Zulus, who had to maintain a large unmarried warrior class.

Marriage was almost universally a very important act, as it joined kinship groups, established social bonds, and produced children, and there were a wide variety of marriage types. Many marriages could be characterized as relationships of affinity. Some were temporary while others were permanent. Marriages were often based on establishing social linkages and family and or tribal alliances, rather than affection. Almost always, a **dowry** or bride wealth was paid for a wife. This was considered as compensation for the loss of a daughter and her contribution to the family, and gave the husband the rights to the sexual and economic services of his wife. Polygamous marriages were common but practiced primarily among those in senior or leadership positions and the rich.

A variety of marriage systems were maintained. In many cultures it was preferable and expected to marry a close relative. The choice could be a niece, a cousin, a half sister or even a granddaughter. Marriages between cousins were favored in Central and

South Africa. In some societies, "in-law marriages" were expected. In these marriages, for example a husband would marry his wife's brother's daughter, his niece-in-law. Levirate marriages were also common, where a man would marry the widow of his older brother. Similarly, there were sororate marriages, where a man would marry his wife's sister if his wife died or even if she was still alive.

At least forty precolonial cultures practiced "woman marriage," primarily in West Africa. This arrangement allowed a woman to legally marry one or more women. These were not sexual unions but marriages, which allowed for the augmentation of kinship and family structure. In some cases, as among the Igbo, a female child was designated as a "male" daughter to fill an empty gender position. A female husband often married inside the family, often a brother's daughter. She would choose the male genitor, who fathered her wife's children. A separate hut was built for the genitor's visits but the female husband's wife/wives were required to live in the household.

While sex was casual in many cultures, adultery in many others was forbidden or punished harshly. However, adultery was interpreted differently within different groupings. Women who were married into a family as the wives of older brothers or of the father sometimes discretely copulated with male family members. This was not considered adultery. Among the Bantu, a brother occasionally had sex with his brother's wife before she had her first child. Husbands, when they became old, sometimes permitted their brother or even a son to have sex with his younger wives.

Customs differed greatly among cultures regarding when not to engage in sexual intercourse. Female sexual abstinence was practiced primarily during pregnancy, sometimes for three years after the birth of a child or for a year after the death of a child. Women over forty frequently abstained from sex because it was thought to be unseemly for a grandmother to have sexual intercourse. Additionally, they also thought that they had enough children. *See also* Christianity; Divorce; Polygamy/Polyandry.

Further Reading: Bock, Phillip K. "Love Magic, Menstrual Taboos, and the Facts of Geography." *American Anthropologists*. New Series. 69, no. 2 (April 1967): 213–17; Caldwell, John C., Pat Caldwell, and I.O. Orubuloye. "The Family and Sexual Networking in Sub-Saharan Africa: Historical Regional Differences and Present Day Implication." *Population Studies* 46, no. 3 (November 1992): 385–410; "Marriage Systems." In *Africa: An Encyclopedia for Students*. Vol. 3, edited by John Middleton. New York: Charles Scribner, 2002; Shillington, Kevin G., ed. *Encyclopaedia of African History*. Vol. 1. New York: Fitzroy Dearborn, 2005.

Mark David Luce

AMERICAS (North and South). Romantic relationships and sexuality in the Americas in the early modern age were necessarily impacted by the process of colonization. The native lifestyles in the North were affected by the French and British newcomers, while in the rest of the Americas the influence of the Spanish and Portuguese colonizers was dominant. The main consequence of this situation was a particular articulation of social views and practices based predominantly on the concept of race, as represented by the geopolitical composition of the emerging population of American Indians, Europeans, Africans, and African-Americans.

The Spanish conquest was a highly gendered warfare process, but so had been the conflicts between the native populations, as the early Spanish and Italian chroniclers attested. According to a 1494 letter written by Christopher Columbus's doctor, Diego Alvarez Chanca, when the Columbus expedition first arrived in the Caribbean its members discovered that the Caribs (the native population whose name is the etymological source of the word "cannibal") were in the habit of castrating children taken prisoner, after which they used them sexually throughout their adolescence and then killed and ate them (*see* **Castration**). Later on, in Mexico, it would be found that the Nahuatl word for a powerful warrior (*tecuilónti*) meant "I make someone into a passive." Similar attitudes existed throughout the Andes also. However, the **rape** of young war prisoners was common practice in Europe too, and the Spaniards were no exception. The main source on the atrocities committed by the Spanish conquistadors, particularly in South America, is Father Bartolomé de las Casas's *Brevísima relación de la destrucción de las Indias* (*A Brief Account of the Destruction of the Indies*), published in 1552, which also indicates, as other contemporary sources do, that **cross-dressing** and cross-gender behavior were quite widespread among the natives.

The main historical source on social practices in the New Spain (modern Mexico) is the *Historia General de las cosas de la Nueva España* (*General History of the Things of New Spain/Florentine Codex*) compiled by Fray Bernardino de Sahagún between 1540 and 1585. While Mexican machismo has pre-Columbian roots in Aztec culture, the Spanish colonization enhanced it with the classical elements of dominant Mediterranean, particularly Iberian (with strong Muslim/Arab influences) **masculinity**, whereby women were regarded as inferior to men and were used mainly for procreation. This view was applied to the native female population as well, a famous case being that of **La Malinche** (c. 1502–c. 1529 or 1551–1552), an indigenous woman of Aztec descent who became the mistress of Spanish conqueror Hernán Cortés (1485–1547), to whom she bore a son. Illustrative of the problematic racial mix of Mexico is the multiplicity of La Malinche's cultural image, which alternates between victimized mother of the emerging Mexican people and a frequent association with the image of Virgin Mary, and the evil whore whose sexuality caused her to betray Aztec men to the Spanish conqueror (an Aztec Eve, as Sigmund Freud would later put it). A popular nickname for La Malinche in Mexico is the pejorative La Chingada ("the fucked one"); nevertheless, this name has been nostalgically and assertively incorporated into the

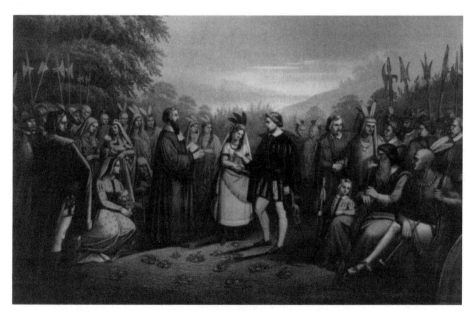

A nineteenth-century print showing a large gathering of Native Americans and Englishmen for the wedding ceremony between Pocahontas and John Rolfe. Courtesy of the Library of Congress.

battle cry "*¡Viva México, hijos de La Chingada!*" ("Long live Mexico, children of the Great Whore!"), which is currently used in Mexico to celebrate Independence Day on September 16. At the same time, Cortés's image served as the prototype for the traditional model of the Mexican strong man, popularly described as *el chingón* ("the fucker"), the carrier of *huevos de oro* ("golden balls"). Sahagún also mentions the parental practice common among natives of deciding the gender–identity inclinations of sons, seen as innate, and then raising them accordingly, along the masculine or the feminine behavioral models.

A somewhat different development took place in North America following the settlement of Jamestown in 1607. The early English and Dutch settlers, whose beliefs about sexuality were shaped by the Protestant **Reformation**, viewed the family as a "little commonwealth" ruled by the husband and condemned sexual activity outside **marriage**, but also added marital love to procreation as a justification for sexual intercourse. Nevertheless, courtship and marriage continued to be determined by wealth, love serving as a rationale mainly for the lower classes. The Puritan settlers and their goals of maintaining a stable family life and implementing a marital reproductive sexuality were challenged not only by the local conditions, initially less than favorable beyond the New England area, but also by the sexual practices of the native populations, which they found fascinating and disturbing at the same time.

One main aspect of this challenge is the fact that the native peoples did not associate sexuality, nudity, or cross-dressing with sin, shame, or guilt, but, quite to the contrary, with spiritual and visionary qualities. **Homosexuality** was not treated differently than heterosexuality, and cross-dressing, more common among the male population, did not affect one's social standing (*see* **Berdache**). In contrast to European practice, sexuality was not regarded as marital property and conflicts of an erotic nature were resolved through the formation of a new union. Also, **prostitution** did not exist prior to the arrival of the Europeans and rape was rare, yet forbidden, and native men were known not to have raped English women fallen captive during the colonial wars. In contrast, European settlers, particularly the Spaniards, would rape native women on a regular basis as a right of conquest.

There also took place a lifestyle differentiation between the early colonial areas due to the social composition of the migrant groups. In New England, there existed a relative middle-class (farmers and craftsmen) homogeneity, while the population of the Chesapeake colonies (Maryland and Virginia) ran across the social spectrum, from gentry to servants. This difference translated into cohesive family life and higher birth rates in the Puritan New England, and more common promiscuity in the southern colonies, where the high men-to-women ratio gave women a certain marriage security, regardless of their sexual past. The first recorded interracial marriage in North America occurred in Virginia in 1614—between John Rolfe, the first successful tobacco exporter, and Pocahontas, later known as the London socialite Lady Rebecca Rolfe, daughter of the eastern Algonquian chief Powhatan and one of his many wives. In all colonies, with the exception of North Carolina, interracial marriages with Native Americans were tolerated in the beginning. However, they would become rarities in the aftermath of Pocahontas's death in 1617, at the age of twenty-two. John Rolfe later returned to Virginia with their son and remarried in 1620. In 1622, he was killed, along with one-third of the Virginia tobacco planters, in a native assault led by Opechancanough, the half-brother of Pocahontas's father.

Nevertheless, the Puritan norm had its own internal challenges, exercised by fellow Englishmen of a more adventurous inclination. Such was the case with

Thomas Morton (c. 1576–1647), a lawyer and social reformer who in 1625 established the Merry Mount plantation in Plymouth, an experiment where English and Indian men and women would engage in casual, extramarital sexual activities. Homosexuality might have also been practiced. The profusely hedonistic May Day celebrations that he organized—particularly the erection of a suggestive eighty-foot maypole—finally led to his banishing back to England for licentiousness. There was also the case of Samuel Terry, the constable of Springfield, Massachusetts, who had a long court record. In 1650, he was sentenced to whipping for masturbating in public at the Sabbath sermon. In 1661, he was fined five pounds for presumed **premarital sex** because his wife gave birth five months after their wedding. In 1673, he was fined again, along with eight other men, for indecent performance in a play.

Both the Chesapeake and the New England colonies legally enforced morality, with drastic consequences for fornication, **adultery**, out-of-wedlock **pregnancy**, rape, and sodomy (see **Anal Sex**), but the laws were more drastic and more extensively enforced in New England. Although rarely enacted, even capital punishment was prescribed in the Massachusetts Bay colony for adultery, rape, and sodomy. One such case was that of Mary Latham, who was hanged in 1645, at the age of eighteen, for having committed adultery with twelve men. In 1636, male homosexuality was first assigned the death penalty in Plymouth, where it seems to have been more of a problem, or at least more prosecuted. However, leniency was extensively exercised, whipping being the more common punishment, and it appears that only the very obvious cases were prosecuted. Occasionally, trumped up charges were brought against troublesome individuals who might not have engaged in homosexual acts. Plymouth is also the location of the first recorded homosexual incident, involving five young men who had committed the act of buggery on the high seas in 1629, aboard the ship *Talbot*, as they were sailing into Massachusetts Bay from England, where they were sent right back. The only execution for homosexuality in New England took place in 1646, in New Haven, where William Plaine, a married man who reportedly had engaged in sodomy back in England, was convicted for repeatedly engaging in **masturbation** with numerous other men. In 1711, buggery would cease to be prosecuted in New England.

Lesbianism was inscribed as a capital offense only in New Haven in 1655, but it was removed only ten years later when the colony was incorporated by Connecticut. It was not otherwise prosecuted, except for one 1649 New England case involving Mary Hammon and Sarah Norman. Inexplicably, Sarah, a married woman, was sentenced to make a public statement of "unchast behavior" while Mary was absolved. This might be connected to the fact that the same year Sarah's name appeared in the accusations of homosexuality brought against Teage Jones by Richard Berry and which included claims of "unclean" practices between Jones and Mrs. Norman. Interestingly enough, Berry changed his mind and admitted that he had lied, for which he was whipped. It appears to have been a case of homosexual jealousy since three years later both men, and more of their friends, were ordered by the court to "part theire uncivell liveing together." Berry himself also had a wife, a thief convicted for milking somebody else's cow and for stealing a scarf, some bacon, and some eggs.

In cases of zoophilia, the punishment included having to witness the execution of one's "partner" (see **Bestiality**). The year 1642 seems to have been a busy year in this area for the courts. Also in Massachusetts, William Hacketts, prior to his own hanging, had to watch the execution of the cow he had committed buggery with. Thomas Grazer (or Granger) of Plymouth, by the age of sixteen, had had intercourse with "a mare, a cow, two goats, five sheep, two calves and a turkey." He was court ordered to identify the five sheep out of a lineup and witness their execution before his own. George Spencer of New Haven was executed for having had intercourse with a sow, based on the fact that the animal had given birth to a deformed fetus that was claimed to resemble Spencer. A similar case took place in 1647, again in New Haven, where another sow gave birth to a deformed fetus and a certain Thomas Hogg was proven to have been involved with the sow when he was ordered to fondle her and instant signs of manifest lust between them were recorded. The records also show as further proof, that the next sow Hogg was ordered to fondle did not react in any way to his advances. However, he was sentenced to jail time only and the following year he was already released.

In the southern colonies, there was more laxity. Such was the case with Captain William Mitchell, member of the Maryland governor's council, who not only "fornicated" with his live-in girlfriend, but also got a married woman pregnant and helped her to have an **abortion**. However, he was only charged with being an atheist and mocking religion, rather than for his other crimes, for which the punishment was a fine of five thousand pounds of tobacco. Tolerance with regard to sexual transgression eventually started to increase everywhere toward the end of the seventeenth century. The surge in the number of Africans brought over as slaves after 1670, particularly in the vaster, more agricultural south, also affected sexual practices. Due to the shortage of white women, some white men married black women, a legally tolerated act until late in the seventeenth century.

In the French areas of Canada (known as New France and settled in 1534) and Louisiana (settled in 1682), interracial marriages between French men and native women were actually adopted as a policy for alliance, a way to avoid warfare. In fact, the vast majority of the North American fur traders, whether English, French, or Spanish, were married to native women, business facilitation being many times a factor. Nevertheless, in the Spanish areas, like New Mexico, the strong sense of class and honor caused the local aristocracy, consisting in a limited number of families, to maintain their dominance by intermarriage. *See also* Africa; Christianity; Exploration; Slavery.

Further Reading: D'Emilio, John, and Estelle B. Freedman. *Intimate Matters: A History of Sexuality in America*. 2nd ed. Chicago: University of Chicago Press, 1997; Godbeer, Richard. *Sexual Revolution in Early America*. Baltimore: Johns Hopkins University Press, 2002; Hodes, Martha, ed. *Sex, Love, Race: Crossing Boundaries in North American History*. New York: New York University Press, 1999; Jackson, Charles O. *The Other Americans: Sexual Variance in the National Past*. Westport, CT: Praeger, 1996; Smith, Merril D., ed. *Sex and Sexuality in Early America*. New York: New York University Press, 1998; Trexler, Richard C. *Sex and Conquest: Gendered Violence, Political Order, and the European Conquest of the Americas*. Ithaca, NY: Cornell University Press, 1995.

Georgia Tres

ANAL SEX. Anal sex has a long history; its practice both among heterosexuals and homosexuals dates back to classical times. Reactions against anal sex have been both cultural and religious over the centuries. In Europe during the Middle Ages, anal sex was dubbed "buggery" and was sometimes punishable by death. Churches condemned the practice as unnatural because the sex act could not result in **pregnancy**, which was considered the ultimate and, for some religions, the only goal of sexual activity. St. Peter Damian later created another term for the practice—sodomy. Use of this term has continued into modern times and the term has at various times been employed to cover a multitude of offenses, including **bestiality** and treason, but essentially the term "sodomy" refers to anal sex between male partners.

In Renaissance England, where boys were sent off to boarding school at an early age and isolated from contact with women, sodomy quite naturally grew as a way to vent adolescent male sexual energy. There is no indication that punishments for boys engaging in anal sex were particularly cruel; Renaissance societies were generally tolerant of their children. Sodomy among adult men was, on the other hand, the subject of state laws beginning in England with **Henry VIII**'s Buggery Act in 1533 and continuing into the mid-seventeenth century with statutes enacted by the Puritan Commonwealth. Originally, accusations of buggery were a matter for ecclesiastical courts, but when the **Reformation** brought new power to the state, practices considered moral abominations came under state jurisdiction. There is scant evidence, however, that executions were frequent. In fact, no more than a handful of executions for sodomy are recorded over the entire English Renaissance, and those were cases in which anal sex was just one of many accusations brought against the man accused.

In Renaissance literature, references to anal sex were usually playful. In lyric poetry, there are sodomitical references in the poems of Richard Barnfield, who begins his "Affectionate Shepherd" poem with the line, parodying Caesar, "I came, I saw, I viewed, I slipped in." In comedies by Ben Jonson, like *Epicoene*, for example, there are suggestions of male-male anal penetration. There are, however, occasional references to sodomy in serious plays. In William **Shakespeare**'s *The Two Noble Kinsmen*, Arcite tells Palamon that they should leave the city of Thebes where "crimes of nature" apparently abound. The most notorious anal sex scene in Renaissance drama is the execution of the king in Christopher **Marlowe**'s play *Edward II*. After crushing Edward under a table, the jailor takes a red-hot poker and inserts it into the king's anus, a kind of reflective execution for Edward's sexual dalliance with his male lover Piers Gaveston. *See also* Homosexuality.

Further Reading: Bredbeck, Gregory. *Sodomy and Interpretation: Marlowe to Milton*. Ithaca, NY: Cornell University Press, 1991; Crompton, Louis. *Homosexuality and Civilization*. Cambridge, MA: Belknap Press, 2003; Dynes, Wayne R., ed. *The Encyclopedia of Homosexuality*. New York: Garland Publishing, 1990; Morin, Jack. *Anal Pleasure and Health: A Guide for Men and Women*. San Francisco: Down There Press, 1998.

George Klawitter

ANNULMENT.   Annulment declares a **marriage** void, null, or non-binding due to a problem of impediment, form, or consent. An annulled marriage is invalidated and the parties retain the legal and/or spiritual status they possessed prior to the marriage. While an annulment effectively ends a marriage, it differs from a **divorce** in that it is as if an annulled marriage never occurred, thus leaving the participants free to marry a different partner as if for the first time without impediment. Several conditions may present such impediments, including the following:

- consanguinity (marriage to a close blood relation)
- affinity (marriage to a deceased partner's parent or child)
- non-consummation (impotence, excessive youth or age)
- previous religious vows

An annulment based on a problem of form might be issued if the marriage ceremony was not performed by a licensed, authorized official (either ecclesiastical or civic), or if the marriage was not performed under the current law of the country in which it took place. Finally, a marriage might be annulled due to a provable lack of consent, such as force, constraint, insanity, or duress, at the time of marriage.

Virtually all cultures, governments, and religions provide guidelines or precedents for the termination of marriage. Traditional Jewish law, for example, provides an option for divorce, the "get," Islamic divorce, or *talaq*, can be obtained for a variety of reasons similar to those listed above, and for Shi'ite Muslims the early and disputed practice of *mut'a*, or "fixed-time marriage," allows a couple to separate after a prespecified time without obtaining the *talaq*, or legal divorce. Finally, all sects of **Christianity** provide options for divorce as well as for annulment. All modern state governments that allow civil marriages have established guidelines and procedures for the dissolution of civil marriage, and individual countries usually attempt to include provisions in legislation that consider the requirements of the major religion(s) present within their country, which often depends on the degree to which the state government incorporates or espouses an official, state-approved religion. Today, annulment can be sought within both state and church governments in most countries because marriage can be contracted both legally and ecclesiastically. In the early modern period, the issue of whether the state or the church should have authority to grant annulments was a contentious and widely debated issue involving issues of sovereignty and national and papal jurisdiction.

Historically, marriage laws and regulations fell under familial, tribal, or ecclesiastical purview, and annulments were not a legal concern. In pre-Reformation Europe and in the Catholic states after the **Reformation**, the papacy regulated all marital issues because the church viewed marriage itself as a sacrament and thus a spiritual contract separate from secular governmental jurisdiction. In addition, most medieval governments recognized the spiritual authority of the papacy and were connected to the church, and papal decrees provided universally applicable canon law in Europe. For medieval kingdoms, whose secular authority fluctuated over time, the Church's ecclesiastical authority was often more durable and established than the authority of the state government. However, as independent nation-states increasingly distinguished between national sovereignty and papal authority, especially after the Reformation, secular challenges to ecclesiastical law became more common. The result was increased government legislation in areas previously considered solely ecclesiastical, as well as monarchs and governments who considered their own authority equal or superior to that of Rome—and as able to resolve disputes such as annulment, which had previously been considered purely religious issues.

These tensions were exemplified in the unique case of **Henry VIII** of England (r. 1509–1547). Henry annulled or attempted to annul four of his six marriages, including his unions with his first wife, Catherine of Aragon; his second wife, Anne Boleyn; his fourth wife, Anne of Cleves; and his fifth wife, Katherine Howard. Each annulment rested on different grounds. Catherine of Aragon was the widow of Henry's elder brother Prince Arthur, who died in 1502. Henry married Catherine on his accession in 1509 under a dispensation from Pope Julius II. When, by the late 1520s, the marriage had only produced one daughter and no male heir, Henry sought annulment on grounds of consanguinity. In 1533, after Henry had broken with Rome, Archbishop Thomas Cranmer declared Henry's marriage invalid, and a week later Henry married Anne Boleyn; unfortunately, Anne's inability to produce a male heir, as well as her alleged adultery, resulted in an annulment and her execution for treason in 1536. Henry annulled his marriage to his fourth wife, Anne of Cleves, in 1540 after only six months on the grounds that the marriage had never been consummated.

His marriage to his fifth wife, Katherine Howard, ended in an annulment-execution on grounds of adultery and treason in 1542. The annulment of Henry's first marriage ultimately resulted in Henry's excommunication by the pope, England's break with Rome, the establishment of the Church of England, and the introduction of the Oath of Supremacy, whereby English subjects swore to accept Henry as head of the English Church. There were many other important cases of annulment in the early modern period, but Henry's marital troubles had the deepest and most lasting impact in early modern Europe. *See also* Elizabeth I, Queen of England; Islam; Judaism.

Further Reading: Bowker, John, ed. *The Oxford Dictionary of World Religion.* New York: Oxford University Press, 1997; Jenks, Richard. *Divorce, Annulments, and the Catholic Church: Helpful or Hurtful?* New York: Haworth Press, 2002; Martos, Joseph. "Marital Dissolution in Medieval and Modern Times." In *Catholic Divorce: The Deception of Annulments,* edited by Pierre Hegy and Joseph Martos. New York: Continuum Press, 2000; Robinson, Geoffrey. *Marriage, Divorce and Nullity: A Guide to the Annulment Process in the Catholic Church.* London: Geoffrey Chapman, 1984; Scarisbrick, J. J. *Henry VIII.* Berkeley: University of California Press, 1968; Smith, Jonathan, ed. *The Harper Collins Dictionary of Religion.* San Francisco: HarperCollins, 1995; Valbuena, Olga. *Subjects to the King's Divorce: Equivocation, Infidelity, and Resistance in Early Modern England.* Bloomington: Indiana University Press, 2003.

Barbara Zimbalist

ARCHITECTURE, EUROPEAN. Architecture in the Renaissance was considered one of the fine arts, or as was said then, "the noble arts," together with painting and sculpture, her sisters, and governed like them by their father, design. Architecture was considered to have two parts: its beauty and its ornaments. If beauty came from the ideas of order and proportion embodied in the basic forms of the design, it was through the patterns of the ornaments, controlled as they were by rule and decorum, that the order of architecture could be more openly expressed, as it had been in all the models of classical architecture still standing in Italy and, especially, in Rome.

Such ideas about the nature and principles of design served at the highest level to suggest architecture might represent the unity and beauty in God's universe. Yet at a more practical level, these details reviving the form of classical art, served to reconnect this architecture, both formally and politically, to the great traditions of antiquity, long destroyed by the Goths when Constantine moved to the East and Rome was ravaged by wave after wave of foreign invaders. According to Renaissance scholars, the first moment this new architecture appeared was in the Cathedral of Pisa, built in 1016, where the front was decorated by numbers of antique columns, suggesting once again what good design might be.

But it was not for another two centuries, in the work of Brunelleschi in Florence, that a more fully ordered and self-conscious style of classicizing architecture was established in such designs as those for the Ospedale degli Innocenti (begun 1419), the great dome on the Cathedral (begun 1420) and the two churches of San Lorenzo (begun 1421) and Santo Spirito (begun 1436). It was then at the Palazzo Medici-Riccardi by Michelozzo di Bartolommeo (begun 1446) and at the Palazzo Pitti (begun 1458) that a new form of domestic architecture was also established.

The next stage in the development of the new architecture came in the 1450s with the work of Leon Battista Alberti, who designed a number of important buildings in Florence such as the façade of the church of Santa Maria Novella (1455–1460) and the Palazzo Rucellai (1455–1460), but also worked further afield, in Rimini at the Tempio Malatestiano (begun 1450) and in Mantua on the Cathedral of S. Andrea (begun 1470). He also wrote a treatise, dealing with all the practical and theoretical matters of architecture, modeled very clearly on the example of the Roman writer Vitruvius. With his work done, all was set for the next generation of architects, Bramante and Michelangelo above all, to expand the language of classical design even further and often on a scale not imagined before. The most important examples of the work of the new generation were the library at San Lorenzo, Florence, begun in 1525 by Michelangelo, the so-called Tempietto at San Pietro in Montorio, Rome (1502) by Bramante, and the great complex of the Vatican and St. Peter's, literally built from the materials of ancient Rome, that was begun under the patronage of Pope Julius II in the first decade of the sixteenth century and completed later that century by Michelangelo and Giacomo della Porta.

And, if in the fifteenth century there had been some other cities like Pienza, Urbino, and Ferrara where such principles of design were picked up by patrons for their own purposes, in places like Genoa and Venice and Milan the influence of this new architectural style did not emerge until the next century in combination with local traditions of building and decoration. The great public buildings in Venice designed in the 1540s by the Florentine Jacopo Sansovino or the buildings in Milan designed by Galeazzo Alessi, such as the church of S. Maria di Carignano in Genoa (1549) and the Palazzo Marini (1558) reflect these influences. The last great figure of this period was Andrea di Pietro (known historically as Palladio), for not only did he write a treatise on architecture that in the age of printing was now widely distributed, but in and around Venice and Vicenza he designed a range of buildings. Both secular and religious, more modest in their language than those of Bramante and Michelanglo, they were usable by all those in Europe, gentlemen and princes alike, who now modeled their lives and their culture on the examples of Italy. The great example of Polladio's work is the so-called Villa Rotonda (1566–1567) in Vicenza, which came to be copied often in later years.

By now the first Italianate buildings had also begun to appear in France at Fontainbleau (begun 1528) and at the Louvre in Paris (begun 1546), a trend continued into the seventeenth century with the extensions to the east front of the Louvre (begun 1667) and the vast palace of Versailles (begun 1669). By now there were Italianate buildings in Spain, as with the palace of Charles V in Granada (begun 1526) and the Escorial, near Madrid (begun 1563). Also by now, if far further away and later, the first classically influenced buildings began to appear in England during the reign of Queen **Elizabeth I**, in houses built by private patrons, like Longleat (begun 1572) and Hardwick Hall (begun 1590). In the seventeenth century, there were various buildings designed for James I and Charles I by Inigo Jones on the clear model of Palladio, such as the Banqueting House at Whitehall, London (1619–1622) and the Queen's House at Greenwich (1616–1635), which were followed later by Christopher Wren in his buildings at Oxford and Cambridge and, after the Great Fire of London in 1666, with St. Paul's Cathedral (begun 1670) and the great complex of the Royal Hospital, Greenwich (begun 1695). By this time, both in Europe and beyond in the Americas, the architecture of Italy, whatever the local variations, had becames the dominant style of design and it stayed so until in the nineteenth century, when industrialization and the political claims of new nations called for new types of building and new forms of design that could no longer be accommodated in this language.

Further Reading: Heydenreich, L., and W. Lotz. *Architecture in Italy: 1400 to 1600.* Translated by M. Hottinger. Harmondsworth: Penguin, 1974.

David Cast

ARETINO, PIETRO (1492–1556). The Italian poet, playwright, and satirist Pietro Aretino was described as the "scourge of princes" for his merciless literary attacks lampooning the rich and powerful in Italian Renaissance society. He was born in Arezzo, a city in the Republic of Florence, on April 20, 1492, the son of a shoemaker. His real name is not known because he was ashamed of his father's modest roots and claimed instead to be the bastard son of a nobleman, adopting the name "Aretino" after his birthplace. He spent his youth in Perugia, where he painted and wrote poetry and although he claimed to have little formal education, he developed a lifelong interest in art and vernacular literature. In 1517, he moved to the Roman household of the wealthy and influential banker and patron of the arts, Agostino Chigi, where he developed a taste for the high life.

His early claim to notoriety and fame began when he wrote a series of outrageous pasquinades, a type of witty political and personal verse, attacking the rivals for the papacy of his patron and the favored candidate, Cardinal Giulio de'Medici. When the austere Adrian VI was elected Pope instead of Medici in 1522, Aretino found it prudent to leave Rome. He entered the court of Federigo Gonzaga, marquis of Mantua, where he formed a deep and lasting friendship with Giovanni de'Medici, the dashing condottiere known as Giovanni delle Bande Nere. When Adrian VI died in 1523, Giulio de'Medici was finally elected pope as Clement VII, and Aretino returned to Rome. Despite the protection of the Medici pope, Aretino was forced to leave Rome again in 1524 when, inspired by paintings of Giulio Romano engraved by Marcantio Raimondo, he wrote a series of matching pornographic verses. The illustrations showed various prominent Roman citizens and churchmen in compromising sexual positions with well-known courtesans. When the book, known as *The Sixteen Positions* (*I Sedici Mode*), was published complete with Aretino's verses, it was promptly banned and most copies were rounded up and destroyed. No complete original copy remains extant, but various other artists have since contributed to it. Aretino and Romano managed to escape capture and prosecution, but the engraver Raimondo was thrown into prison. Due to the influence of his papal patron, Aretino was able to return to Rome only to leave again after narrowly escaping an assassination attempt orchestrated by the chief victim of his vicious penmanship, Bishop Giovanni Giberti.

In 1527, after the death in battle of his friend Giovanni de'Medici, the loss of whom left him devastated, Aretino settled in the Republic of Venice, where he found the political climate more favorable than in Rome. Living in style in a house on the Grand Canal, often with a full household of guests, he prospered and continued to wield his influence over well-known figures, who preferred no mention of their names by Aretino in his writings to a critical mention. While writing and publishing his vast collection of letters, he also turned his hand to other genres and wrote some highly esteemed devotional works. Aretino commented on the political and social world around him as he saw it, while criticizing what he saw as the hypocritical attitudes of his day. He wrote several plays on this theme, among them *The Cortegiana,* published in 1525. The first part of *The Dialogues* (*I Ragionamenti*) published in 1534, describes the hypocrisy and pretensions of Roman society in the form of a dialogue between prostitutes. In the dialogue, Nanna, the mother courtesan, is advising her daughter Pippa on her career choices—she may choose among becoming a wife, a nun, or a courtesan. Pippa reaches the conclusion that the career of courtesan is the most honest and honorable choice.

The establishment of the Venetian tribunal of the Holy Office of the Inquisition in 1542 led to a more severe climate of moral policing in Venice. Many of Aretino's works were declared lewd and put on the ***Index of Prohibited Books***, although a brisk black market still flourished, and printers published his books under a pseudonym. Aretino's friend, the Venetian painter Titian, immortalized him in a famous portrait, in which the artist captures Aretino's love of life and laughter. Aretino died on October 21, 1556, from a fit of apoplexy whilst laughing too loudly at his own joke. Today, Aretino stands as a political and social realist, a free thinker who opposed and exposed many of the repressive moralistic trends of his time. *See also* Pornography.

Further Reading: Cleugh, James. *The Divine Aretino (Pietro of Arezzo, 1492–1556, A Biography)*. London: Anthony Blond, 1965; Chubb, Thomas Caldecott, ed. *The Letters of Pietro Aretino*. Hamden, CT: Archon, 1967; Hutton, Edward. *Pietro Aretino: The Scourge of Princes*. Boston: Houghton-Mifflin Company, 1922; Putnam, Samuel, ed. and trans. *The Works of Aretino*. 2 vols. New York: Covici-Friede, 1933.

Mary Hewlett

ART, EUROPEAN. In its revival of the traditions of Greece and Rome, the Renaissance brought back the forms of art and the parts of a literature taken up so often with sexual and erotic material. Sexual imagery can occasionally be seen in medieval art, as with images of Bathsheba or the Golden Age, and in the many more direct images of sexual activities found in the margins of manuscripts or on the minor parts of church architecture and furnishings, such as corbels or the woodcarvings of choir stalls. But, in its focus on the representation of the body, the Renaissance had access to a far richer vein of sexual imagery with the rediscovery of pagan mythology and its stories of human and divine love.

On a neo-Platonic level, the explanation and excuse for all such representation came from the idea that the human body, in all its external beauty, might stand also as the token of a more inward spiritual beauty. At another, more practical level, it is clear the ever increasing number of sexual images of love and romance on birth salvers and cassoni, or marriage chests, reflected a thriving private market for such objects, decorated often, as in examples by Apollonio di Giovanni, with scenes of Mars and Venus or allegories of the Triumph of Chastity or Love. Moreover, especially in the sixteenth century, there were the patrons of the courts, ready always for representations of sexual adventure, as in the famous series of the loves of the Gods, produced in the 1530s by Correggio for Mantua or the several pictures done in the 1550s by Titian for the court of Philip II in Spain. There were occasional stories of love and sexual desire in the Bible or the Apocrypha that also were subjects of art in the Renaissance, as of David and Bathsheba, in paintings by Raphael and Paris Bordone. With the story of Susanna and the Elders, in paintings by Jacopo Tintoretto, the spying of the old men, looking surreptitiously at the naked body of Susanna, could mirror the more open gaze of the spectator. Something of the same moral ambiguity was implied with classical mythology, whatever the particular moral meaning, by such subjects as that of Tarquinius and Lucretia or the rape of the Sabines, as in the examples by Titian and Domenico Beccafumi, where the attraction for the male viewer depended both on the brutality of the theme and the evident beauty of the female figures.

It was only rarely, as with depictions of Diana, the chaste virgin huntress, that the moral tables were turned, as in the story of Actaeon, who when having stumbled on Diana and her companions bathing, as in the pictures by Parmigianino and Domenichino, was turned into a stag and torn apart by her hounds. Yet, in the story of Endymion, sent to sleep forever in return for his perpetual youth, it was seen in the paintings by Taddeo Zuccaro and Luca Giordano that even Diana could fall in love,

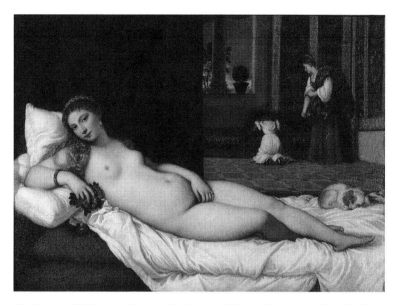

The Venus of Urbino, by Tiziano Vecellio, c. 1538. © The Art Archive/Galleria degli Uffizi Florence/Dagli Orti (A).

visiting him chastely at night. For artists there were always also the stories of Venus herself, sometimes seen in her twofold nature as a symbol of both sacred and profane love, as in the painting by Titian, sleeping, as in the painting by Giorgione, unaware of those looking at her, or at her toilet, as again in paintings by Titian, where she lay reclining on a couch while Cupid held up a mirror in which she, and we, then see her reflection.

Frequent also were the stories of her many loves, as with the subject of Mars, where often less, as in the painting by Botticelli, was said of her infidelity than of the exemplary devotion the lovers shared. The story of her passion of Adonis was depicted by Giorgio Vasari and Paolo Veronese, and many more general pictures of Venus and Cupid or of the Judgment of Paris were painted by Raphael and Ippolito Scarsellino, allowing the female body to be seen in all its glory not once but three times. To which might be added the story of Atalanta and Hippomenes, as in a painting by Guido Reni, where Atalanta, if a strong huntress like Diana, was defeated in a foot race when she stopped to pick up the golden apples purposefully given to Hippomenes by Venus.

To what extent these pictures are to be seen as intentionally erotic is difficult to determine. Yet it is clear that all such imagery, whatever its final purpose, was couched in a language both culturally and stylistically elevated that could serve as a defence against the strictures of the Church and still preserve it for the limited elite that had access to it. It was also this elite audience, especially with the advent of printing, that consumed more pornographic images, even if such a category of art had not yet been defined, as in the famous instance of *The Sixteen Positions*, prints of sexual intercourse, designed by Giulio Romano and published by Marcantonio Raimondi in 1524, and accompanied by poems by **Pietro Aretino**. Needless to say, all such pornographic imagery, whether in print or in pictures, was designed for the male viewer, women perhaps having neither the desire nor the access to commission anything of this nature for themselves. It might be noted that there are several subjects—**Ganymede**, David, and Atys-Amorino, for example—that seem to contain strains of homoerotic (*see* **homoeroticism**) imagery. These strains become more apparent when the subject is treated by an artist like Donatello, whose sexual personality was spoken of by contemporaries in these terms. It is difficult to know how to read what we see, however, especially since art was not then concerned with the self-expression that modern artists are used to and even the definition of homosexuality itself was so distinct from how we define it now. All we can say, as elsewhere, is that these images also were produced for an elite, private audience. *See also* Eros.

Further Reading: Lucie-Smith, E. *Sexuality in Western Art*. Revised ed. London: Thames and Hudson, 1991; Talvacchia, B. *Taking Positions: On the Erotic in Renaissance Culture*. Princeton, NJ: Princeton University Press, 1991.

David Cast

ASIA. The impact and influence of the Indian and Chinese civilizations on Asia and the world, both culturally and religiously, has been immeasurable. The early modern period (1500–1800) in Asia, primarily in India and China, was a pivotal historical point, as it was an era during which a multitude of changes, initiated by nascent Western imperialism and the increase of world trade, had a profound effect on the area. Foreign intrusions and the subsequent establishment of Western colonies began to alter traditions and introduced new customs, sensibilities, and prohibitions throughout the Asian world.

By 1500, the Indian subcontinent had become an astoundingly diverse mixture of peoples, cultures, religions, and sects. The Muslim rulers of India, the Mughals, were ethnically Turkish but culturally Persian, while the majority of their subjects were Hindus, Buddhists, or Jains. The structure of society revolved around the major beliefs, laws, and customs of **Hinduism**, **Buddhism**, and **Islam**. Rather than stay static and apart, however, the ideas and beliefs of each system and culture were synthesized in a multitude of permutations.

This interaction of cultures was notably marked by the success of the expansion of Islam on the subcontinent, which spread to Bengal in the form of Sufism, a form of Islamic mysticism. Islam allowed for social mobility in a land and culture that was rigidly regulated by a complex system of class and caste, resulting in an eclecticism of beliefs and practices. It created a new Muslim population, which adopted Muslim law and social practices, ultimately allowing for an even more diverse society to emerge. Social class and education contributed to and regulated customs.

Hindu society was stratified by class and caste but it had always been open to sexuality. Among the educated, sex and love manuals, of which the **Kama Sutra** is the best known today, were available. They included illustrations of a multitude of coital positions and instructed the reader on the importance of foreplay and female orgasm. Biting, scratching, cooing, slapping, and other acts were added to augment and to extend pleasure.

In Hinduism, the vulva (*yoni*) was considered a sacred place of pleasure and the phallus (*linga*) was an object of veneration. Sexual union was considered a way of communing psycho-spiritually. Certain Hindu shrines and sects had temples that were centers for such veneration. At some temples barren women came to copulate with priests to become fertile, and many of these types of temples also gained revenue to support their employees through the activities of a cadre and class of devoted temple prostitutes. Diverse sects existed that included a range of ascetics, celibates, and even necrophiliacs.

Hindu society condemned **bestiality, rape, incest, adultery**, and sex outside of the proper **caste**. Laws regulating these crimes were laid down with the first-century CE *Law Code of Manu*, and both adopted and adapted to various degrees, at differing times, by the populations of Burma, Thailand, Cambodia, and Indonesia, where cultural and doctrinal beliefs varied. Hindu and Indian beliefs extended into Southeast Asia and, as a result, the region was heavily influenced by Indian culture, music, art and architecture, as well as law.

Buddhism had also emerged from India and pervaded all of Asia, bringing with it a new set of cultural practices as missionaries were sent abroad and India itself became a destination for pilgrimage and study. Large numbers of Buddhist monks and nuns established monasteries throughout eastern Asia and practiced celibacy. Buddhism, like Hinduism, had different paths within it, which included the Tantric school, where followers practiced a type of sexual yoga. Tantric Buddhism became predominant in Tibet, Nepal, and Bhutan.

China in the early modern era was an agrarian civilization. Vast distances, rugged mountains, harsh terrain, and deserts had largely separated and isolated it from outside influences. The Chinese (Han) considered themselves racially superior to all, and thought of China as the one country which stood directly beneath Heaven—the priviledged "Middle Kingdom." Chinese society was stratified and feudal, and both Confucianism and Daoism were strong stabilizing influences on Chinese society that were also complimented by Buddhism.

The Confucian and Daoist traditions recognized the different sexual natures of males and females. These differences were elaborated within the concepts of the *yin* and *yang*. The *yin* was negative, passive, weak, female, and destructive, while the *yang* was positive, active, strong, male, and constructive. Based on the principles of *yin/yang*, numerous works on sexology were written. The subject matter of these manuals covered everything from the selection of partners and flirting to all aspects of sexual intercourse.

A large corpus of Daoist classics included works on sexual practices, medicine, household manuals, and special practices for women. A form of sexual yoga similar to Tantrism was practiced, in which the overwhelming principles concerned the uniting of the *yin* and the *yang*. The strengthening of life force (*ch'i*) was believed to be essential for long life and health. In Daoist belief, male ejaculation depleted the *ch'i*, and males could increase their *ch'i* and add to it by gaining *ch'i* through the orgasms of their female partners while not ejaculating themselves. Masters could copulate with many different partners for hours to promote health and also gain more pleasure than through simple ejaculatory sex. Most of the literature of Daoist sexual practices is concerned with "paired practices," but many works were also written to promote female "solo practices."

All people married within their class and at all levels **concubines** were purchased for their beauty. The wives of the Emperors had no special status and were chosen for rulers by magistrates. During the Ming Dynasty (1368–1644), chastity became almost a cult. The remarrying of widows was discouraged and rates of **divorce** by mutual consent declined because of the stigma attached to it. However, husbands could still divorce their wives for seven main reasons: sterility, lewdness, insubordination to in-laws, talkativeness, stealing, jealousy, and lastly, a loathsome disease. Also during this period, young Daoist couples often engaged in free sensual and sexual behavior directed and commanded by a master teacher, who shouted orders to them. Hundreds of fictional erotic works of varying degrees were written during this period, which afford a picture of courtly love and romance among the elite. Prior to this period, there had been official efforts to censor and suppress erotic literature.

Chinese civilization had a tremendous influence on the cultures of eastern Asia, from Mongolia to Korea, Japan, and Indochina, leading to similar social structures and attitudes throughout the region.

After a century and a half of civil war, Japan began to unify and stabilize under Tokugawa Ieyasu, and to isolate itself from the Asian mainland and the rest of the world. The dominant Japanese philosophy of the time was Neo-Confucianism, which stressed the importance of morals, education, and a hierarchical order in government and society, although Buddhism and Shintoism were also important. A strict, four-class system existed, with the *samurai* at the top of the social hierarchy, followed by peasants, artisans, and merchants. These four classes, or **castes**, were rigid and did not allow for social advancement. People with professions that were considered impure, such as tanners, formed a fifth class, the *eta*, and were considered social outcasts.

In Kyoto, Japan, in 1589, the first walled-in "pleasure quarter" was constructed based on those of the Ming dynasty in China and in 1617, after petitioning the government, brothel owners in Edo (present-day Tokyo) were allowed to create a courtesan quarter. This established the practice of restricting all prostitutes and **brothels** to a quarter of a city, where a set of standard rules was applied to all.

In accordance with Japanese social classes, there were corresponding classes of courtesans and prostitutes. At the beginning of the Tokugawa period many high-ranking *samurai* were killed in power struggles during a reformation of the political order. This displaced many daughters and young wives, who became destitute and turned to **prostitution** to support themselves. As a result, these earlier **courtesans** formed a very cultured and elegant class. There were many different classes of courtesans within these pleasure quarters, and over time, more classes were created. The lowest class, the *sancha-joro*, were illegal bathhouse women, and they were rounded up and placed within the pleasure quarters during this period. In 1751, the institution of the *geisha* was created but the skills and education of these courtesans were far below the level of those first top courtesans of the first "pleasure quarters."

The early modern period was a time of great social change throughout Asia. A rising merchant class and changes in trade and economy had enormous impact on all classes, along with increased urbanization and Western imperialism. The proliferation of Islam in Southeast Asia and the advent of **Christianity** and its proponents throughout the continent changed, pressured, and influenced traditional values and practices in profound ways. *See also* Confucianism; Daoism; Remarriage/Widows.

Further Reading: Orr, Leslie C. *Donors, Devotees and Daughters of God: Temple Women in Medieval Tamilnadu*. New York: Oxford University Press, 2000; Ruan, F. F. *Sex in China: Studies in Sexology in Chinese Culture*. New York: Plenum Press, 1991; Van Gulik, R. H. *Sexual Life in Ancient China, a Preliminary Survey of Chinese Sex and Society ca. 1500 B.C. till 1644 A.D.* Leiden: Brill, 2003; Wile, Douglas, ed. *Art of the Bedchamber: The Chinese Sexual Yoga Classics Including Women's Solo Meditation Texts*. Albany: State University of New York Press, 1992.

Mark David Luce

B

BASTARDY. Bastardy was a legal term for illegitimacy and referred to the act of bearing or fathering a child out of wedlock, as well as to the condition of a child born in such circumstances. In societies that practiced **polygamy** or concubinage, particularly in **Asia** and **Africa**, children born outside of marriage usually carried no social stigma and were not barred from inheriting property. In Europe, the spread of **Christianity**, with its insistence on monogamy, and the rise of an increasingly individualistic society, in which rights of property and inheritance were highly important, led to the development of the concept of bastardy and the legal and social rules that defined and maintained it.

In much of early modern Europe, the parents of illegitimate children were liable for criminal prosecution, while the children were denied inheritance rights and, in some cases, certain civil rights. Bastardy had a strong economic component and usually only became a criminal matter if the local community was obliged to support the child because the parents either could not or would not do so. If the father had the means to support the child and undertook to do so, or if the mother's family was willing and able to do so, prosecution of either parent for bastardy rarely occurred. As a result, most bastardy prosecutions, especially in England and western Europe, were of unmarried lower-class young women, often working as servants, who, abandoned by their lovers, could not support a child on their own. Such women were brought before the ecclesiastical courts in both Catholic and Protestant countries, where they would be sentenced to make public confession and to serve a year in the local house of correction. Because of social attitudes toward sex and women and the difficulty of proving paternity—the legal dictum was *mater certa est* ("the mother is certain"), the same double standard that differentiated consequences for men and women in regards to **adultery**, applied to bastardy. If the putative father could be found and brought before the court, the usual result was only an order to provide support.

In cases where a servant or peasant girl was seduced, usually with false promises of **marriage**, by a man of similar social class, the local authorities would seize the father, if he had not fled, and compel him to marry his pregnant lover, thus legitimizing the child and, hopefully, creating an economic unit that could support it. If the man had fled, the young woman usually faced prosecution. If the young woman had been impregnated by someone of a higher social class, such as the master of the house in which she was employed or one of his brothers or sons, marriage was out of the question even if it had been offered to accomplish the seduction. In such cases, the woman was often married off to a man of her own class who was willing to have her and her child. Young women who had acquired a reputation for promiscuity were, once pregnant, in the worst predicament, since they would be scorned by the community as fornicators and often unable to identify with certainty the fathers of their children.

Among the nobility and propertied classes, illegitimacy was not the social stigma it was among the lower classes, although illegitimate children were barred from inheriting the family estate. **Henry VIII**, although he had an acknowledged illegitimate son, Henry, duke of Richmond, broke with the pope and the Roman Catholic Church in his efforts to contract a new marriage and have a legitimate son to succeed him on the English throne. Nonetheless, kings and noblemen frequently had many illegitimate children. In the fifteenth century, Edward IV of England had numerous **mistresses** and probably numerous bastards, although only two are known for certain since the king did not openly acknowledge them and made quiet provision for their support. Edward's seventeenth-century successor, Charles II, was known to have had at least a dozen bastards by seven different women, all of them affectionately acknowledged and provided for by the king. However, both monarchs were easily outdone by Augustus the Strong, king of Poland and elector of Saxony, who by his death in 1733 had over 350 acknowledged bastards. Once again, the double standard prevailed. Despite the inheritance bar, the illegitimate sons of the upper classes were usually well educated and suffered little in terms of careers and marriages. As Lord Mulgrave remarked in the eighteenth century, "bastardy is of little comparative consequence to the male children" (Stone, 534). Illegitimate daughters faced far more uncertain futures; the only career open to women of the upper classes was marriage and illegitimate girls had bleak prospects since they could expect little in the way of a **dowry** to attract a suitable husband. *See also* Concubines; Pregnancy.

Further Reading: Hambleton, Else L. *Daughters of Eve: Pregnant Brides and Unwed Mothers in Seventeenth-Century Essex County, Massachusetts*. New York: Routledge, 2004; Ingram, Martin. *Church Courts, Sex and Marriage in England, 1570–1640*. New York: Cambridge University Press, 1987; Macfarlane, Alan. *Marriage and Love in England 1300–1840*. Oxford: Blackwell, 1987; Stone, Lawrence. *The Family, Sex and Marriage: In England 1500–1800*. New York: Harper and Row, 1977; Wrightson, Keith. *English Society 1580–1680*. New Brunswick, NJ: Rutgers University Press, 1982.

John A. Wagner

BERDACHE. Berdache is a term used by seventeenth-century French explorers to describe Native American men who dressed like women, adopted the social roles and mannerisms of women, and often engaged in sex with other men. Believing that men who dressed and behaved as women were demeaning themselves, Europeans who encountered berdaches in the sixteenth and seventeenth centuries were both puzzled and offended by the phenomenon. For early modern Europeans, all sex that was not for procreation was considered the crime of sodomy, and was severely punished. A 1533 English statute, for instance, prescribed death for men convicted of engaging in **anal sex** with one another.

Because most of what we know about berdaches in the early modern period comes from accounts written by Europeans, it is difficult to determine just how such individuals were viewed and treated by their own people. Historians and social commentators of sixteenth and seventeenth-century America have long debated the role of the berdache in Native American societies. Some argue that being a berdache was a spiritual matter, and that assuming a different gender identity was an accepted and even respected calling, completely divorced from sexual behavior; others, however, simply define berdaches as homosexuals. Today, some Native Americans reject the term "berdache" as offensive and too laden with inaccurate European conceptions of sex and gender, and prefer instead such terms as "two-spirit person" or "woman-man."

The first descriptions of berdaches come from the early and mid-sixteenth century and depict individuals encountered among many different peoples, including the Native peoples of Canada, the Great Lakes region, the American Southwest, Louisiana, and Florida. Although allowance must be made for the confused or disapproving perceptions of European missionaries and explorers, to whom the notion of a "two-spirited" individual was beyond comprehension, it does appear that the status and role of a berdache varied somewhat from group to group. In the 1530s, the Spanish explorer Cabeza de Vaca described as "effeminates" men among the tribes of Florida who dressed as women and did the work of women, but who also hunted with the men and carried heavy burdens. In 1564, a French explorer in Florida, René Goulaine de Laudonniére, mistakenly called the berdaches he encountered "hermaphrodites," and said that they had a special role caring for the sick and infirm, being strong enough to carry the ill about until they recovered (Williams, 67). In the 1670s, Father Jacques Marquette, writing of berdaches among the Illinois and neighboring peoples, reported that their advice was sought and followed in council and that they passed "for Manitous—that is to say, for spirits—or persons of consequence" (Williams, 17).

Europeans were particularly horrified by berdaches who had sexual relations with other men—relations between two berdaches were rare—or who completely adopted the mannerisms of women. Cabeza de Vaca, who "saw one man married to another" among the Florida Indians, denounced the practice as "a devilish thing" (Williams, 110). Writing in the 1680s, the Spanish cleric Fernandez de Piedrahita declared that "the abomination of sodomy was freely permitted" among the Lache Indians of Colombia, whose headmen often preferred a berdache over a woman (Williams, 87). Pierre Liette, who lived with Mississippi Valley Indians in the 1690s, scornfully described the appearance and manner of berdaches he encountered as follows:

> [They] are girt with a piece of leather or cloth which envelops them from the belt to the knees, a thing all the women wear. Their hair is allowed to grow and is fastened behind the head. They are tattooed on their cheeks like the women and also on the breast and arms, and they imitate their [the women's] accent, which is different from that of the men. They omit nothing that can make them like women. (Williams, 73)

However, while all berdaches took on the gender roles of women as defined within their group, not all had sexual relations with men, and some moved back and forth between male and female attire and male and female activities. A Crow berdache named Osh-Tisch ("Finds Them and Kills Them"), earned his name by donning male clothes and heroically leading a war party against the Lakota. In a more extreme example, an Osage war leader became a berdache in response to a vision, but still frequently went to war dressed as a man.

Although less noted by European observers, female berdaches—women who dressed and acted as men—existed among some Native American groups. They were often allowed to participate in male activities and sometimes to take other women as wives. *See also* Homosexuality.

Further Reading: Lang, Sabine. *Men as Women, Women as Men: Changing Gender in Native American Cultures.* Austin: University of Texas Press, 1998; Roscoe, Will. *Changing Ones: Third and Fourth Genders in Native North America.* New York: St. Martin's Press, 1998; Sayre,

Gordon. "Native American Sexuality in the Eyes of the Beholders 1535–1710." In *Sex and Sexuality in Early America*, edited by Merril D. Smith. New York: New York University Press, 1998; Williams, Walter L. *The Spirit and the Flesh: Sexual Diversity in American Indian Culture.* Boston: Beacon Press, 1986.

John A. Wagner

BESTIALITY. Sex between humans and animals existed in both legend and reality in Renaissance Europe. The amours of the classical Greek and Roman gods in animal form were well-known to humanists, particularly through the ancient Roman poet Ovid's frequently translated and commented-upon text, *Metamorphoses*. The story of Queen Pasiphae, who fell in love with a bull and conceived the Minotaur by him, was particularly prominent in literature. Traditional European legends also incorporated bestiality. Olaus Magnus (1490–1558), a Scandinavian humanist historian, recounted the legend that the royal line of Denmark was descended from a woman and a bear. Bestiality was often linked with witchcraft, as demons would allegedly take on animal or monstrous form to have intercourse with **witches**. Common animal forms used in witchcraft accounts included toads, goats, and cats. Goats were particularly suited for this role, as they were strongly associated with lust.

Although intercourse between women and animals is relatively common in mythology, legend, and literature, anti-bestiality legislation was aimed almost entirely at men, who comprised the vast majority of those charged and convicted of it. The condemnation of bestiality by **Christianity** and **Judaism** originated in the laws recorded in the Book of Leviticus, which forbade any man or woman from "lying with any beast," something that was considered an abomination. Unlike many Levitical bans, this prohibition was not only taken by Christianity from Judaism, but strengthened and intensified. Bestiality was also forbidden in Islamic *shari'a* law. During the Middle Ages, bestiality had become a matter for criminal enforcement rather than just religious penance, and by the fifteenth century it was a capital offense in some parts of Europe. Catholicism and Orthodox Christianity both put bestiality with other sexual offenses, such as anal intercourse and sex between men, in the category of sodomy.

Enforcement of laws against bestiality was aimed principally at rural populations, and particularly at herdsmen, and played little role in urban society. Despite the presence of often harsh anti-bestiality laws, however, enforcement was erratic, and bestiality was often treated casually, as a matter of little consequence, in day-to-day life. In the sixteenth century, bestiality laws were more strongly enforced in the Catholic lands around the Mediterranean, where the Inquisition held sway over sexual offenses, than it was in France or northern Europe. The Aragonese Inquisition saw a peak of the enforcement of bestiality laws, along with a campaign against male sodomy, from 1570 to 1630, when bestiality convictions were even more likely to result in execution than sodomy convictions. Immigrant farm workers from France were particularly likely to be targeted.

The belief that intercourse between man and animal could lead to monstrous offspring was widespread, adding to the horror with which bestiality was presented by preachers and moralists. The Franciscan Observant preacher Giacomo della Marca (1391–1476) recounted stories of pig-human, cow-human, and dog-human monsters to warn his listeners away from the horrible sin. *See also* Anal Sex; Homosexuality.

Further Reading: Salisbury, Joyce E. *The Beast Within: Animals in the Middle Ages.* New York and London: Routledge, 1994; Wiesner-Hanks, Merry E. *Christianity and Sexuality in the Early Modern World: Regulating Desire, Reforming Practice.* London and New York: Routledge, 2000.

William E. Burns

BETROTHAL. Betrothal is a ceremony in which the future **marriage** of a man and a woman is agreed upon. In some early modern societies, individuals as young as infants could be betrothed, years before any actual wedding took place. Betrothal rituals could, alternatively, be performed close to or in connection with the nuptials, depending on the local mores. While matrimony was a communal and public event in many early modern cultures, betrothals were usually celebrated more privately, with close friends and relatives as witnesses. However, because of the social importance of marital institutions and the need to maintain order and paternal authority, clandestine betrothal or wedlock was discouraged and even punished in many regions. For instance, Islamic communities deemed it inappropriate to wish to marry a woman already betrothed to another man, and betrothals were to be open and honorable, not clandestine.

Sometimes the good offices of go-betweens were used in presenting a suit for marriage, and mediators—even matchmakers—could accompany suitors or present the suit instead for them. Whether the consent of the fathers and guardians, or even the agreement of the principal parties themselves, was necessary in making the match varied over cultures. Once the consent of the guardian and/or the prospective bride and groom were obtained, the couple was considered betrothed, either immediately or after special rites.

In many cultures, the betrothal involved social and religious rituals and unilateral or mutual exchanges of gifts involving both families or kin-groups, especially when the couple was high on the social scale. In these cases, a more formal marriage process tended to accompany high status and large property interests. The role of betrothals also reflected the local honor code In some regions stressing **virginity**, the bride's **chastity** was closely guarded until the wedding, although elsewhere more contact between the couple after a formal betrothal could be allowed. In some regions, all children born to betrothed couples were considered legitimate.

Certain societies judged the betrothal the most important ceremony of the marriage process precisely because it included contractual elements, unilateral or mutual gifts, and the participation and consent of parents and kin. The wedding was considered only the implementation of the agreement. Similarly, various societies considered betrothals binding though dissoluble, although the unilateral breach of a contract could cause legal, financial, or social repercussions, such as paying compensation, formal prosecution, or even open enmity. In China, betrothal gifts from the groom's family to the bride's were an important part of the engagement ceremony. After the receipt of the betrothal gift, the bride's family could not break off the union with impunity (prosecution was possible). Among Orthodox Christians living in eastern Europe and Russia, betrothals (*obručenie*) were obligatory and public ceremonies were performed in church. Once ecclesiastical betrothal had taken place, it was nearly as binding as marriage, and marriage to another was considered adultery. A betrothal could also be combined with the wedding, with each ritual performed successively.

In some areas of western Europe, betrothal and marriage were partially amalgamated under the influence of the medieval Catholic ecclesiastical doctrine. The church distinguished between mutual vows in the present tense (constituting indissoluble marriage) and in the future tense (a breakable engagement, transformed into matrimony by subsequent intercourse). By using the wrong phrase, the couple might accidentally get married instead of becoming engaged, or vice versa. The canon Tametsi, introduced at the **Council of Trent** (1563) separated informal unions based on betrothal or marriage promises from sacramental matrimony by insisting on clerical solemnization, two witnesses, and previously announced banns. The Latin term *sponsalis* ("of a betrothal") came from *sponsa* ("spouse"), which confused and blurred the terminology of engagement and wedlock in European languages with Latin roots or influences. Even today, "betrothal" is occasionally used synonymously with irrevocable marriage vows instead of an engagement.

Many Jewish communities also tended to fuse the betrothal (*kiddushin*), linked to the payment of a bride-price and signing the marriage contract, and the nuptials into a single ceremony. Even when a longer period elapsed between the *kiddushin* and the wedding, betrothals were considered binding, fidelity was required, and dissolution was only possible by formal divorce. In early modern Italy, match-making (*tenaim*) came to closely resemble the *kiddushin* as the rituals were largely parallel: exchanging gifts, setting the conditions of the union in legal and written form, and publicizing the decision to marry. *See also* Adultery; Bastardy; Christianity; Islam; Judaism.

Further Reading: Harrington, Joel. *Reordering Marriage and Society in Reformation Germany.* Cambridge: Cambridge University Press, 1997; Korpiola, Mia. *Between Betrothal and Bedding: Marriage Formation in Sweden, 1200–1600.* Leiden: Brill, 2007; Levin, Eve. *Sex and Society in the World of the Orthodox Slavs, 900–1700.* Ithaca, NY: Cornell University Press, 1989; Weinstein, Roni. *Marriage Rituals Italian Style. A Historical Anthropological Perspective on Early Modern Italian Jews.* Leiden: Brill, 2004.

Mia Korpiola

BOLEYN, ANNE. See Henry VIII

THE BOOK OF THE COURTIER (Baldassare Castiglione, 1528). Written by Baldassare Castiglione (1478–1529), an accomplished Italian writer and diplomat, *Il cortegiano* (*The Courtier*, or, as usually rendered in English, *The Book of the Courtier*) was one of the most popular and important literary works of the European Renaissance, influencing such later writers as Edmund Spenser and William **Shakespeare**. A treatise in dialogue form, *The Courtier* is divided into four books that describe in detail the attributes of the ideal courtier, including his appearance, manner, attainments, and political service, as well as the qualities of his perfect female companion. Full of wit and wisdom, and written in a lively, dramatic style, *The Courtier* served for centuries as the chief European guide to social and sexual interaction, defining proper behavior and correct manners.

The son of a professional soldier in the service of the marquis of Mantua, Castiglione undertook humanistic studies in Milan before returning, upon his father's death in 1499, to Mantua to serve the marquis as soldier and diplomat. In 1504, he entered the service of the duke of Urbino, who sent Castiglione to represent him at the royal courts of England and France, the ducal court of Milan, and the papal court at Rome. He returned to the service of the duke of Mantua in 1516, the same year he married Ippolita Torelli, the daughter of Bolognese nobility. In 1524, Pope Clement VII named him papal nuncio to Spain, where Castiglione resided until his death of plague on February 8, 1529.

Castiglione began writing *The Courtier* sometime around 1513, and had largely completed it by 1518, although he spent the next decade revising the work. Having sent the manuscript to his friends for comments and corrections, Castiglione finally submitted it for publication in 1528, when he began to fear that the various circulating copies of the text would lead to a pirated edition. The work was an immediate success in Italy and soon gained great popularity throughout western Europe, being translated into Spanish in 1534, French in 1537, English (by Sir Thomas Hoby) in 1561, and even into Latin in 1571.

The Courtier is set at the court of Urbino in 1506, during a visit by Pope Julius II and his entourage and during a time when the author was himself absent from court. This device allowed Castiglione, whose characters in the book were real people, to include among his interlocutors individuals who were not otherwise part of the court at Urbino, and to exclude himself from the dialogue, which he claims to record as it was reported to him. Written in vernacular Italian, rather than in the literary Tuscan used by Petrarch (1304–1374) and other noted authors of the Italian Renaissance, *The Courtier* is dedicated to Alfonso Ariosto, the cousin of a close friend, who, at the urging of Francis I of France, encouraged Castiglione to write about the perfect courtier. Each of the characters in *The Courtier* is a recognized authority on the subject of his discourse: Pietro Bembo (1470–1547), for instance, speaks on Neoplatonic love, the topic of his 1505 work, *Asolani*. Although female characters appear in *The Courtier*, especially in the dialogue on the ideal court lady in Book 3, they are never active participants and serve only to ask questions and moderate discussions.

Book 1 opens as the courtiers and ladies gather to play a game designed to "portray in words a perfect courtier." The subsequent discussions define the ideal courtier as a nobleman proficient in the use of arms and delighting in physical activity, but also skilled in arts and letters and able to perform in each of these areas with grace and style, and without apparent effort. Proper outward appearance is also vital for a courtier, who must always avoid affectation. Book 2 discusses the proper display of courtly qualities, especially through the use of finally honed conversational skills that illustrate the courtier's charm, wit, humor, learning, and discretion. Book 3 defines the court lady, who exhibits most of the qualities of her male counterpart, although with a greater emphasis on physical beauty and the exercise of discretion to preserve reputation. Book 4 describes how the ideal courtier should serve his prince, a discussion that eventually becomes a debate on the relative merits of monarchies and republics. Resuming a theme brought up in Book 3, the discussion finally turns to the topic of love and how the courtier should progress from physical love to a pure idealized love. Although many later works on "courtesy" and social relations attempted to imitate *The Courtier*, none was as successful or brilliant a portrait of sixteenth-century Renaissance courts as Castiglione's masterpiece.

Further Reading: Burke, Peter. *The Fortunes of the Courtier: The European Reception of Castiglione's Cortegiano*. University Park: Pennsylvania State University Press, 1996; Castiglione, Baldassare. *The Book of the Courtier*, edited by Daniel Javitch. Translated by Charles S. Singleton. New York: W.W. Norton and Company, 2002; Castigilione, Baldassare. *The Courtier*. Translated by Sir Thomas Hoby. London, 1561 (available on Renascence Editions Website at http://darkwing.uoregon.edu/rbear/courtier/courtier.html; Hanning, Robert W., and David Rosand, eds. *Castiglione: The Ideal and the Real in Renaissance Culture*. New Haven, CT: Yale University Press, 1983; Woodhouse, J. R. *Baldesar Castiglione: A Reassessment of "The Courtier."* Edinburgh: Edinburgh University Press, 1978.

John A. Wagner

BORGIA, LUCREZIA (1480–1519). Thanks to later stories, novels, and films, the name Lucrezia Borgia today evokes images of a femme fatale embroiled in Machiavellian intrigue. In actuality, the real Lucrezia did not actively participate in crimes perpetrated by her father, Pope Alexander VI, or her brother, Cesare Borgia, and seems to have been more their pawn than their accomplice.

Born in Subiaco, Lucrezia was the third child of Rodrigo Borgia, a Spanish cardinal serving in Rome, and his Italian mistress, Vanozza Catanei. From the age of three, she was raised by Rodrigo's cousin, Adriana de Mila. Before she reached eleven, her father initiated and ended for her engagements to two Spanish nobles. In 1492, when Rodrigo became Pope Alexander VI, he negotiated her engagement to Giovanni Sforza, who was twice her age, and Lucrezia was married at the age of thirteen, as was not uncommon for elite women of the early modern period. When the Sforza connection gave little advantage, Alexander declared Giovanni impotent, a cause for an **annulment**, and ended the marriage in March 1497. In anger, Giovanni accused Alexander of wanting Lucrezia himself. Rumors that Lucrezia had incestuous relations with her brothers Cesare and Juan also abounded. After Lucrezia fled to the convent of San Sisto in that year, another rumor developed that claimed she had become pregnant by her father's messenger, Pedro Calderon, who was later found murdered. In 1498, Lucretzia gave birth in secret to a child of mysterious paternity who was named Giovanni, but became known as the *infans Romanus* (child of Rome); Pope Alexander declared that Giovanni was Cesare's son but privately acknowledged him as his own, although it is now uncertain whether Giovanni was born of an incestuous relationship Lucretia may have had with her brother or father or of her relationship with Calderon.

In the same year, 1498, Lucrezia was wed to Alfonso D'Aragona, nephew of the King of Naples. Both seventeen, they unexpectedly fell in love. When this **marriage** too lost its utility for the Borgias, Alfonso fled, fearing Cesare, whom popular opinion suspected of being responsible for the murder of his own brother, Juan. Upon his return, Alfonso was attacked by unknown assailants; Lucrezia nursed Alfonso in the Borgias' Vatican quarters. A month later, Cesare's henchman, Micheletto, tricked Lucrezia into leaving the room and Alfonso was murdered by suffocation, catapulting Lucrezia into mourning.

Losing little time, Alexander pursued a match for Lucrezia with Alfonso d'Este, aged twenty-four, who was the eldest son of the Duke of Ferrara. The Duke did not welcome an alliance with the bloody Borgias, but through the efforts of Cesare's emissary, pressure from King Louis XII of France, and a 200,000-ducat **dowry**, he capitulated. When the wedding finally took place, Borgia enemies circulated rumors of wedding party debauchery.

Ferrara, known for the arts and the intellectual attainments of women such as Alfonso's sister, Isabella d'Este Gonzaga, attracted Lucrezia. Furthermore, she was eager to leave Rome. Forced to leave behind Rodrigo, her son from her brief second marriage, and to send back the huge retinue with which she entered Ferrara, the young matron had the added challenge of meeting and charming her new relatives, tasks that she successfully accomplished. Two years later, in 1503, Lucrezia's father, Pope Alexander, died suddenly; without his father's protection, Cesare's fortunes fell. The d'Estes, though encouraged to send Lucrezia away, chose to let her remain.

In 1505, the Duke of Ferrara died. With her husband Alfonso the new ruler, and encouraged by Lucrezia, the Ferrarese court attracted artists, poets, and intellectuals, with poet Pietro Bembo as a major admirer of the duchess. Lucrezia continually exerted political influence on behalf of Cesare until he died in 1507. She then turned to her brother-in-law Francesco Gonzaga for protection. When Alfonso traveled, Lucrezia administered affairs of state and deployed soldiers. She made charitable donations and frequently retreated to San Bernardino, a convent she established. By all accounts, she was a devoted mother. Before her end, Lucrezia had at least nine known pregnancies, but only four children survived to adulthood. At thirty-nine, she died after giving birth yet again and was deeply mourned by all who knew her.

Lucrezia's legacy took on mythic proportions as she came to be depicted by many literary figures. She appears in novels written by Alexandre Dumas, Victor Hugo, Mario Puzo, John Faunce, Roberta Gellis, and Gregory Maguire. Gaetano Donizetti created an opera about her; a 1949 film, *Bridge of Vengeance* (*Mask for Lucretia*), starred Paulette Goddard. These fictional portrayals focus on the steamier stories about Lucrezia despite the more balanced views of contemporary historians. *See also* Annulment.

Further Reading: Bellonci, Maria. *Lucrezia Borgia*. Translated by Bernard and Barbara Wall. London: Phoenix Press, 2000; Bradford, Sarah. *Lucrezia Borgia*. New York: Viking, 2004; Corvo, Frederick Baron. *A History of the Borgias*. New York: Modern Library, 1931; Erlanger, Rachel. *Lucrezia Borgia: A Biography*. New York: Hawthorn Books, 1978; Gregorovius, Ferdinand. *Lucrezia Borgia: A Chapter from the Morals of the Italian Renaissance*. New York: Phaidon Publishers, 1948; Shankland, Hugh, ed. and trans. *The Prettiest Love Letters in the World: Letters Between Lucrezia Borgia and Pietro Bembo*. Boston: David R. Godine, 1987.

Sally Ann Drucker

BROTHELS. Until the middle of the sixteenth century, municipal and licensed brothels flourished in a number of European towns, including Strasbourg, Basel, Augsburg, Frankfurt, Nuremburg, Munich, Seville, Avignon, Toulouse, Dijon, Paris, Sandwich, Southampton, and Southwark, across the Thames from London. Authorized red-light districts existed in Venice and Florence. In Japan, the establishment of the three state-run pleasure districts in Kyoto, Edo, and Osaka, surrounded by broad moats and gated entries, began in 1589. In fifteenth-century Europe, civic and religious authorities continued to view male sexual desire as a potential threat to public order when left unsatisfied. **Prostitution** was seen as a necessary evil that protected honest women and men, and that needed to be carefully regulated to protect virtuous women and prevent crime. Historians have viewed a range of demographic issues—higher ages at the time of marriage, declining populations, and a possible disproportion in sex ratio—as concomitant factors producing a climate of tolerance.

In some areas, the town itself took on the responsibility and profit of running a brothel. Elsewhere, brothels were "farmed" to individual investors, often respected public figures, who bought authorization from a municipality or clergymen land-holders to run and receive a portion of the revenue from a brothel; the bishops of Winchester, for example, were the landlords of the stews of Southwark. Authorized brothels were largely run by men, although in England and France women, known as bawds, were responsible for supervising prostitutes. Supervision included checks for venereal disease and pregnancy, limitation of a sex worker's social and sexual relationships, enforcement of bans against fancy clothing and of requirements for wearing identifying marks, and, in some cases, the illegal use of beatings and intimidation, for which bawds were fined if they were caught.

Towns throughout Europe began to close authorized brothels in the mid-sixteenth century. Historians have sometimes linked this to the public health crisis posed by the most severe syphilis epidemics of the 1490s (*see* **Venereal Disease**). More recent studies have emphasized the shift in sexual morality and attitudes toward individual responsibility for sexual transgression produced by the **Reformation** and Counter-Reformation. In addition, the proliferation of clandestine prostitution resulted in a high degree of competition for the market.

Illegal brothels in this period were a far cry from the high-end fantasy brothels of the nineteenth century; indeed, the line between lodgings and brothel was not always evident. Taverns and inns had rooms where prostitutes could take their clients.

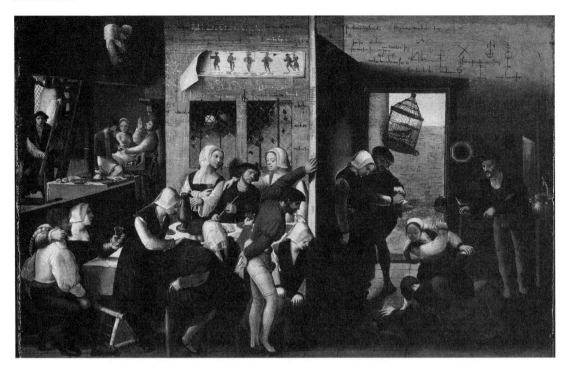

Lockere Gesellschaft or *Scene in a Tavern*, by Jan Sanders van Hemessen, c. 1540. © The Art Archive.

A lodging house might rent to several prostitutes. Bath houses offered beds to prostitutes and their customers and, by the fourteenth century, yielded their name, "stews," to places where prostitution occurred. A woman or man might house several prostitutes and secure clients for them or serve as a procurer for clergymen, sailors, foreigners, and army encampments. The eventual growth of illegal "bordels," as brothels were called until the seventeenth century, probably occurred in relation to the criminalization of prostitution. Sex workers who had been able to work independently or in legal institutions increasingly needed houses to pay off authorities, madams and procurers to negotiate for them, and the physical protection of pimps to avoid being fleeced, blackmailed or harassed. *See also* Concubines; Courtesans.

Further Reading: Karras, Ruth Mazo. *Common Women: Prostitution and Sexuality in Medieval England*. Oxford: Oxford University Press, 1996; Norberg, Kathryn. "Prostitutes." In *A History of Women in the West. Volume 3: Renaissance and Enlightenment Paradoxes*, edited by Natalie Zemon Davis and Arlette Farge, 458–74. Cambridge, MA: Harvard University Press, 1993; Otis, Leah Lydia. *Prostitution in Medieval Society: The History of an Urban Institution in Languedoc*. Chicago: University of Chicago Press, 1985; Powers, Karen Vieira. *Women in the Crucible of Conquest: The Gendered Genesis of Spanish American Society, 1500–1600*. Albuquerque: University of New Mexico Press, 2005; Sone, Hiromi. "Prostitution and Public Authority in Early Modern Japan." In *Women and Class in Japanese History*, edited by Hitomi Tonomura, Anne Walthall, and Wakita Haruko. Translated by Akiko Terashima and Anne Walthall, 169–85. Michigan Monograph Series in Japanese Studies, 25. Ann Arbor: University of Michigan, Center for Japanese Studies Publication Program, 1999.

Pamela Cheek

BUDDHISM. By the early modern period, Buddhism had been almost completely eradicated in India, its country of origin, by Muslim invaders. However, two great branches of Buddhism flourished in Ceylon, Tibet, Indo-China, China, Korea, and Japan: one was Mahayana, and the other Theravada, or Tantric Buddhism.

At the heart of Buddhism are the teachings of its fifth-century BCE spiritual founder the Buddha ("Enlightened One"), who taught that following the Eight-Fold Noble Path would lead to *nirvana*, the end of suffering. Becoming a Buddhist monk or nun in a monastery or nunnery, even for a season, became a common practice amongst followers as a step toward liberation from *karma*, the cycle of cause and effect set in motion by personal actions.

Buddhist ethics teach a hypothetical imperative in which actions are or are not performed to achieve enlightenment. There are no moral absolutes in the Buddhist perspective, therefore an action's integrity is decided in the context of the situation. One of the steps on the Eight-Fold Noble Path includes the elimination of sexual misconduct from one's life; the definition of misconduct is defined contextually. Ultimately, impulses motivating sexual roles and actions are governed by the ultimate goal of attaining enlightenment.

Buddhist monks were expected to be celibate and generally were in the school of Mahayana Buddhism. However, in some Vajrayāna Buddhist schools, **marriage** by monks was permissible. Monastic practices and ordinary life among Buddhists was usually tolerant of sexual practices that satisfied its ethic. Prior to significant Western contact, Buddhism did not describe **homosexuality** as sexual misconduct.

In Japan, the general Buddhist attitude toward sex was that it is natural, like eating, and is acceptable in its appropriate place. The same attitude existed toward homosexuality. It was somewhat common for Mahayana Buddhist monks to take younger monks as lovers. Ihara Saikaku (1643–1693) prior to becoming a Buddhist monk, wrote racy stories of the merchant class, and as a monk he celebrated male homosexuality in his book, *The Great Mirror of Male Love* (1687). Some Japanese Buddhists did come to oppose homosexuality, however, and some masters of Zen, an austere Japanese variant on Buddhism, warned monks that homosexuality would cause them to go straight to hell and to acquire very bad karmic results. Opposition to immorality by some Buddhist leaders led to the suppression of Kabuki theater in Japan. By 1625, the unbridled licentiousness of the theater was officially viewed as a social threat, so women and boys were forbidden to participate in the performances.

Tantric Buddhism developed in India and spread throughout Asia, most famously in Tibet. Practice focused on achieving enlightenment through spontaneous action, using mandalas, mantras, and sexual imagery. Tantric Buddhists rejected the original Buddhist attitude of detachment from the world, and, instead, emphasized the importance of the body as a vehicle for achieving *nirvana*, which was defined as the achievement of ultimate oneness. Sexual union was considered a powerful symbol of oneness, as it took the prime duality of the world, male and female energy, and made it one. Both sexual images and, on occasion, physical sexual union were used to describe and experience a transcendent understanding of oneness.

Buddhism opposed **abortion** as the taking of a life and as an action that brings *karma*. During the Edo period in Japan, which began in 1603, families were allowed to practice **infanticide** or abortion during times of famine. *See also* Asia; Celibacy; Islam.

Further Reading: Cabezon, Jose Ignacio. *Buddhism, Sexuality and Gender.* New York: State University of New York Press, 1992; Stevens, John. *Lust for Enlightenment: Buddhism and Sex.* Boston: Shambhala Publications, 1990.

Andrew J. Waskey

C

CALVIN, JOHN (1509–1564). One of the most important leaders of the Protestant **Reformation**, John Calvin combined an emphasis on strict morality and decorum with a generally more positive view of sexuality than that more commonly prevalent in the Catholic Church. Calvin treated sexuality as God-given and natural, even rebuking St. Paul for saying that it is better to marry than to burn, since **marriage** was good in itself rather than a lesser evil. Like other Christians, he viewed marriage as the only state in which sex was legitimate although, as a Protestant, he did not accept the Catholic definition of marriage as a sacrament. To his mind, the Catholic Church's promotion of **celibacy** went against nature, and in many cases resulted in sexual abominations practiced by clergy and monks. Calvin approved of sexual pleasure within marriage and denounced the common practice of marrying young women to old men as going against human sexual nature. When Calvin himself married in 1540, at the urging of the Strasbourg pastor Martin Bucer, he sought a woman known for modesty and care for her household rather than for beauty. Calvin's marriage to the widow Idelette de Bure seems to have been happy. He spoke of the bitter pain caused by her death in 1549, but despite the urgings of some of his associates, did not remarry.

As the spiritual leader of the city of Geneva, Calvin was deeply involved with legal issues relating to sexuality. The institution that oversaw many of these issues, the Consistory of Ministers and Elders, had been created at Calvin's instigation, and Calvin exerted a dominant influence within it as permanent head of the Company of Pastors. The precedent set by Geneva was important as Calvinism—the beliefs and practices that developed from Calvin's writings and teachings—spread throughout Europe, and similar institutions were set up in Calvinist states. Calvin himself was fully trained in Roman law, and helped draw up a new code of marriage law for Geneva. This code, unlike the Catholic canon law it replaced, allowed for **divorce** in the case of **adultery**. Calvin's own brother, Antoine, sought a divorce from his wife Anne Le Fert, a move which Calvin himself fully supported and worked to advance. This was an early example of a divorce in which both parties remarried. *See also* Christianity.

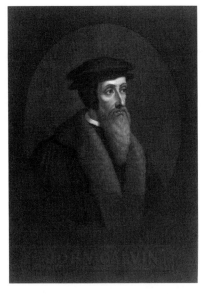

An undated portrait of John Calvin. Courtesy of the Library of Congress.

Further Reading: Bouwsma, William. *John Calvin: A Sixteenth Century Portrait.* New York and Oxford: Oxford University Press, 1988; Kingdon, Robert M. *Adultery and Divorce in Calvin's Geneva.* Cambridge, MA: Harvard University Press, 1995.

William E. Burns

CASTE. Caste (*varna*) is one of two major intertwined principles in **Hinduism**, the other being allegiance to the Vedas, a set of four ancient Indian texts. While the origins of India's caste system are obscure, they probably originated with the subjugation of the original Dravidic population by invading Aryan tribes about 3,500 years ago. There are four castes in India, which stratify the population into four groups based on social function. The Aryans formed the top caste, the Brahmins, who served as priests and scholars; Kshatriyas served as the rulers and warriors; Vaishyas worked as craftsmen, merchants, traders, and farmers; and Sudras became the servants of the higher castes.

Caste was justified in the *Rig Veda* (one of the four Vedas), which stated that the Brahmin, Kshatriya, and Vaishya castes were *dvijas*, or "twice-born." Members could undergo a "rebirth" ceremony at about the age of twelve to become "twice-born." The members of the Sudhra caste were not considered twice-born and could not become students of the Vedas. Learning even a part of the Vedas could cause a Sudra to be severely punished.

The mythic story of the origin of the castes tells how people were created from parts of the body of the god Purusha. From Purusha's mouth came the Brahmins; from his two arms came the warrior Kshatriyas; from his two thighs came the merchant Vaishyas; and from his two feet came the Sudras. Around 1500 BCE, the *Laws of Manu* codified the *varna* system and added the Chandalas (or Kandalas, i.e., the "untouchables") as people recognized as social outcastes. Chandalas were so lowly they were considered to be outside the caste system. A person could be born a Chandala in several ways. One way was to be born the child of a Sudra father and a Brahmin caste mother. Opposition to such unions was based on the belief that caste miscegenation caused confusion between the castes. If confusion occurred, then the system of *samsara* and reincarnation would not be fulfilled. To rebel against birth in a particular caste is to incur *karma* (lit., action or deed) that will bring one to birth in a lower caste or level in the next reincarnation. The *Laws of Manu* describe in detail the possible combinations of children from **marriage**s between the castes and their polluted mixed offspring. Brahmin men could marry women of their own castes and of three lower castes. The children produced by their unions are given different caste names. The *Laws* then assigned to them different occupations, suggesting this is how occupational castes arose. Intermarriages and other occupational assignments led to the creation of several thousand sub-castes called *jati*, which means "births," and thus refers to lineage or race.

The "untouchables" at the casteless bottom of Indian society lacked *varna* and were therefore held as vile and utterly lacking in merit. To them was left the meanest of labors. As social outcasts they did the sanitation work of washing clothes (*dhobi*) and scavenging garbage (*bhangi* or *chura*) and further polluted themselves by working with leather (*chamar*).

The *varna* system created a complex system of purity and impurity. Purity regulations occur in a number of areas of life, especially in the areas of touch and marriage. Touch is a very sensitive area. If a Shudra should accidentally touch someone of a higher caste, such as a Brahmin, then the Brahmin would be contaminated and extensive rites of purification would be necessary to remove the stain. Marriage is permitted only between members of the *jati* of a *varna*. This endogamous practice has led to complicated family kinship relations.

In the early modern period, the caste system withstood a number of attacks. After destroying **Buddhism** in India, early modern Muslim invaders substituted their own Islamic anti-caste teachings for the anti-caste teachings of Buddhism. The Bhakti movement, which gained strength in India between 1200 and 1700, also challenged the caste system by promoting cults of devotion to a particular Hindu deity or form of a god. Doing so minimized the role caste in religion by elevating the role of devotion: practitioners believed that singing and dancing with loving care before Krishna or Shiva, for example, mattered more to the god than the caste of the devotee. The Lingayats, another devotee movement, also opposed to the caste system. Wearing a lingam as a sign of devotion to Shiva, they rejected the Vedas and the caste system. *See also* Islam.

Further Reading: Hutton, J. H. *Caste in India: Its Nature, Function and Origins*. Cambridge: Cambridge University Press, 1952; Kulke, Herman, and Dietmar Rothermund. *A History of India*. New York: Barnes & Noble, 1986; Omvedt, Gail. *Buddhism in India: Challenging Brahmanism and Caste*. Thousand Oaks, CA: Sage Publications, 2003; Sharma, Ursula. *Caste*. New York: Open University Press, 1998; Smith, Brian K. *Classifying the Universe: The Ancient Indian Varna System and the Origins of Caste*. New York: Oxford University Press, 1994; Warshaw, Steven. *India Emerges: A Concise History of India from Its Origin to the Present*. Berkeley, CA: Diablo Press, 1992.

Andrew J. Waskey

CASTIGLIONE, BALDASSARE. *See The Book of the Courtier*

CASTILLO, BERNAL DÍAZ DEL. *See* Díaz del Castillo, Bernal

CASTRATION. The social ramifications of the word "castration" have made it a complex concept throughout history. Originally a technique used to control animals (particularly cattle) and to manage their populations, castration soon came to be used in and on human populations, where it could refer to the physical or metaphysical removal of the testicles and/or penis. The *Oxford English Dictionary* (*OED*) cites its earliest use in the English language as 1420, when it was simply defined as the "removal of the testicles; gelding." The *OED* gives the earliest definition of the verb *castrate*; "To deprive of vigour, force, or vitality"; without any reference to the testicles, citing the earliest example in Thomas Martin's *Marriage of Priestes* in 1554: "Ye *castrate* the desires of the flesh" (emphasis added).

For centuries the biggest debate in the West regarding castration revolved around its spiritual necessity. Physically, castration deprived a man of what was considered to make him a man: the ability to reproduce. Spiritually, the issue rested with Matthew 19:12, where Jesus refers to those who make themselves **eunuchs** (men usually castrated after puberty) for the kingdom of heaven. Whether John Wycliffe's "geldingis" (in his fourteenth-century English translation of the Bible), the King James Version's "eunuch," or the Vulgate's *eunuchi*, designated by *ipsos castraverunt* or those who "castrate themselves," some interpreted the injunction literally, and others, like St. Augustine, did so figuratively. This figurative command helped separate most early Christians from pagans, but also from other early Christians like Origen, who literally castrated themselves to be closer to God. Medieval Catholic Church leaders condemned the practice, though their own choirs employed castrati, men castrated before puberty to create a uniquely high singing voice. Interestingly, **Reformation** leaders such as Martin **Luther** later condemned the celibate clergy as nothing more than self-castration, which itself leads to fornication without restraint because a castrated man lacks the power to impregnate.

Many cultures of the time, and still today, believe that reproductive power constitutes manliness. Within his testicles, a man carries multitudes, and without those testicles, unable to spread his seed, that same man is powerless. Despite the removal of their reproductive organs, however, in the classical through the early modern period (and beyond in many parts of the world) some man were able to gain *more* power after castration. In Byzantium and the Persian kingdoms, kings and sultans employed eunuchs to guard their bedchambers and wives. Rulers trusted eunuchs because they did not have power to procreate. This not only ensured that the eunuchs could not impregnate the rulers' wives, but it ensured that by the eunuchs' protection, other men could not do the same. In addition, these same rulers often placed eunuchs in charge of their armies. In China, eunuchs held enormous political power under the Ming Emperors, who employed them for their personal loyalty to the crown.

Most Europeans had little or no contact with authentic eunuchs, but they were familiar with castration as a punishment. Modern researcher Jacqueline Murray has theorized that this knowledge spurred a castration anxiety throughout medieval Europe. Courts (formal and informal) punished rapists, sodomites, adulterers, and sometimes fornicators by castration, which was often far more brutal than a simple gelding. These public spectacles sometimes included the devouring of the complete genitals by an animal or burning them in front of the condemned man. And, because a medieval understanding of anatomy suggested that the male and female reproductive organs were the same (the female's inverted and therefore inferior), a woman could also face castration—and often symbolically did so when she lost her **virginity** to fornication. *See also* Adultery; Celibacy; Christianity.

Further Reading: Finucci, Valeria. *The Manly Masquerade: Masculinty, Paternity, and Castration in the Italian Renaissance*. Durham, NC: Duke University Press, 2003; Murray, Jacqluine. "Sexual Mutilation and Castration Anxiety: A Medieval Perspective." In *The Boswell Thesis: Essays on Christianity, Social Tolerance, and Homosexuality*, edited by Matthew Kuefler, 254–72. Chicago: Chicago University Press, 2006; Taylor, Gary. *Castration: An Abbreviated History of Western Manhood*. New York: Routledge, 2000.

William John Silverman, Jr.

CELIBACY. Celibacy can be understood as deliberate abstention from sexual activity, whether for a short period or a lifetime. Many religious and philosophical traditions advocate temporary abstention to promote health, hygiene, or spiritual purity; lifelong celibacy is rarer and more controversial. Lifelong celibacy is not the same thing as deciding to remain unmarried for a stipulated time, nor is it the same thing as simply happening to remain single through lack of finding a suitable spouse. Rather, celibates deliberately renounce the opportunity to create new family ties. Such renunciations typically occur as part of a commitment leading to a particular kind of religious life, as a priest, shaman, oracle, monk, or nun. This sacrificed opportunity sets the celibate apart from "normal" life. It frees the celibate from the inevitable distractions of **marriage** and children, ideally allowing him or her to approach each individual they meet with equal interest and compassion. Celibates may also choose abstinence and singleness to store up and channel spiritual strength. The celibates in Asia, Europe, and Mesoamerica during the early modern era avoided not just marriage but also sexual contact, while those of non-Christians in sub-Saharan **Africa** may have included some expectation that women oracles might have some sexual contact.

The traditions that most encourage celibacy have been **Buddhism** (the Buddha invented monastic life, and during his lifetime gave permission for not just men but also women to become monks) and **Christianity**. At the start of this period both traditions had places for male and female celibates. Buddhist religious leaders of both sexes are typically celibate; at the start of the early modern era, Catholic priests were celibate, while Orthodox and Oriental Orthodox Christians, although they ordained married men, accorded their highest esteem to celibate priests. Both traditions marked celibates with distinctive dress and required them to give up personal ownership of most possessions. Christian celibates were usually esteemed, and in Tibet and Japan we know this was also true of Buddhist celibates.

To the Chinese, who practiced very nearly universal marriage, celibacy was somewhat suspicious, despite the centuries-old presence of Buddhist and Daoist monks and nuns. Monks, in particular, were thought to be sexually unnatural, and likely to have chosen celibacy as a means of gaining sexual access to boys and innocent women. Women celibates were less subject to the suspicion that they were sexual predators, but it could be difficult for unmarried women to become celibates. Chinese families did not permit girls to become nuns or recluses; rather, girls who refused marriage usually had to do so over strong family opposition, often running away.

Women's obedience to and reverence for their husbands had strongly sacred connotations in early modern China. Therefore, widows were strongly encouraged not to remarry; indeed, widow suicides were highly revered. If a woman's fiancé died before the marriage was consummated, she could gain great esteem by refusing further marriage. Thus, many occupants of Chinese monasteries were widows.

In Japan, Buddhism had received intermittent state support since the Nara period, and there were state-sponsored monasteries and convents for men and women. Some members of Buddhist convents and monasteries entered as children, but monasticism was more often the choice of adults—women and men who had already married once. Buddhist monks and nuns also acted as mendicant religious teachers and fundraisers. During this period it was still common for women's convents to be founded for the purpose of providing widows with a safe haven, and these houses did not typically last past the lifetimes of their first inhabitants.

Neither **Islam** nor **Judaism** had traditions of monasticism or celibacy, and both religions expected their adherents to marry. At the start of the early modern era there were probably more celibate people per capita in western Europe than anywhere else. These numbers dwindled significantly toward the end of the era. Before the Protestant **Reformation**, most families in western and central Europe hoped that at least one son or daughter would enter the church. Boys could become priests, friars, or monks, and girls could become nuns or, later in the era, sisters.

Some people chose celibacy over family opposition or as older adults. However, more typically, parents chose religious careers for their children before the children reached puberty, just as parents chose their children's spouses. Girls in particular often went to convents that had held many generations of their family members, joining a community where they already had an elder aunt or cousin. It was not uncommon for widows to take shelter in convents and to remain there in seclusion their whole lives, especially before decisions made at the Council of **Trent** (convened three times between 1545 and 1563) led the Roman Catholic Church to restrict nuns' freedom to interact with visitors or to leave the convent. In the fourteenth, fifteenth, and early sixteenth centuries many pious women, called *beguines* or *beatas*, banded together less formally, living or worshipping communally as celibate adults—whether as widows or virgins—without taking official vows. The spread of Protestantism created whole countries where religious celibacy was considered deviant and, in Great Britain, was actually forbidden. In England, Scotland, and parts of Germany, monasteries and convents were seized and some of the inhabitants turned out, with nuns clinging to their convents longer than monks. Protestant pastors were strongly encouraged to marry. Yet, in Catholic and Orthodox regions, celibates continued to be widely admired. The sixteenth and seventeenth centuries saw the founding of numerous new religious orders dedicated to service in the community, teaching, and evangelism.

Celibacy does not seem to have been widely practiced among pre-Columbian men and women of the **Americas**, nor to have been a central feature of most African religious practices. In Mesoamerica, Aztec priestesses had to be virgins and celibate. If they married, they had to leave the priesthood. The early modern era brought Roman Catholic Christianity as well as conquest to the New World, introducing the concepts of a celibate priesthood and of celibate monasticism. Native American and African-descended men became priests, tertiaries (associates of a religious order) and monks, and some Native American women became tertiaries and nuns. *See also* Annulment; Betrothal; Chastity; Daoism; Hinduism; Virginity.

Further Reading: Carrasco, Davíd, with Scott Sessions. *Daily Life of the Aztecs: People of the Sun and Earth.* Westport, CT: Greenwood Press, 1998; McNamara, Jo Ann. *Sisters in Arms: Catholic Nuns Through Two Millennia.* Cambridge, MA: Harvard University Press, 1996; Ruch, Barbara, ed. *Engendering Faith: Women and Buddhism in Premodern Japan.* Ann Arbor: Center for Japanese Studies, The University of Michigan Press, 2002; Wijayasundara, Senarat. "Restoring the Order of Nuns to the Theravadin Tradition." In *Buddhist Women Across Cultures: Realizations*, edited by Karma Lekshe Tsomo, 79–90. Albany: State University of New York Press, 1999.

Pamela McVay

CHASTITY. From the Latin word *castus* ("pure"), "chaste" is sometimes used synonymously with "virginal" or "celibate," but more strictly refers to the abstention from unlawful sexual relations whether inside or outside of **marriage**. Thus chastity, unlike **virginity**, is a condition that applies to the married as well as the unmarried. For example, one frequently treated figure in various works of art and literature throughout the early modern period is the Roman matron Lucretia, whose portrayal as the epitome of a chaste married woman bestowed upon her a status equivalent to that of a virgin.

From Edmund Spenser, who described chastity in Book Three of the *Faerie Queene* as "the fairest virtue, far above all the rest," to John Milton, whose *Comus* was written in honor of chastity, the moral implications of chastity led toward an idealization, particularly of female chastity, which reflects the Neo-Platonism of Renaissance thinking. Seen as a physical condition that reflected a spiritual state, chastity was viewed as a connection between the material world of the body and the spiritual world of the soul. This relationship between physical chastity and spiritual status is paralleled by the position assigned to the Virgin Mary by the Catholic Church as mediatrix between humans and God, and between earth and heaven, a position that gained heightened attention during the early modern period.

In the church, chastity fell within the larger classification of the moral virtue of temperance, a virtue that enabled one to moderate one's passions, appetites, and desires in accordance with the dictates of reason. Notably, St. Augustine defined chastity not according to the act but according to the desires, calling chastity "a virtue of the mind," thereby exempting victims of **rape** from charges of unchastity. Yet, despite this consideration of the will, the locus of chastity was the body. With the emphasis on chastity's connection to inner virtue and bodily restraint, vows of chastity taken by men and women within the church were less subject to the double standard of chastity found outside the church.

While chastity was rooted in and treated as an issue of morality both inside and outside the church, the social and political import of a woman's chastity led to a gendered view of chastity in larger society. It was upon women's chastity alone that the proper transmission of wealth and property within a patrilinear system of inheritance depended, so while the moral import of chastity might be equal for men and women, its social and political import depended almost entirely on the chastity of women. The sexual transgression of a woman, whether that of a married woman against her husband or that of an unmarried woman against her father, was cause of no less than the disordering of an entire household as well as future households, and thus the disordering of society as a whole. Beyond this, a legal status that positioned women as essentially the property of men gave **adultery** by women more farther-reaching consequences than male adultery. For a man to be made a cuckold by his wife was to undermine not only his entire household but also his very manhood. Such anxieties are addressed directly by the ever-present cuckolding plots in literature throughout the early modern age, from Geoffrey Chaucer's *Canterbury Tales* in the late fourteenth century to many of the dramas of the English Restoration period in the late seventeenth century.

Such a gendered view of chastity was reinforced by the medical ideas of the age. Humoral theories held that the physiological constitution of a woman, whose internal organs were subject to greater heat, predisposed her to inordinate sexual desires and disorders such as "hysteria." Women's chastity thus became the subject of scrutiny and advice in both medical literature and conduct literature, creating a two-pronged approach to ensuring chastity, one external and the other internal. So while medical experts recommended such treatments as cooling baths for the treatment of an overheated uterus, moralists and social critics urged the internalization of honor and virtue as a means of maintaining chastity from within.

This location of chastity in the realm of desire thus expanded the definition and signs of chastity well beyond mere sexual behavior. Behavior considered to be unchaste, in women particularly, was broadly defined and included immodest speech, dress, and behavior; impure thoughts; and wandering eyes. Such behavior was routinely proscribed in conduct manuals that were widely circulated throughout the early modern period. This same literature praised chastity as both an external adornment of a woman as well as an internal delicacy of feeling and repulsion toward lewdness of any kind. Ironically, while the categories of chaste and unchaste behavior included a wide spectrum of sexual offenses, women themselves were categorized as either "chaste" or "unchaste" based on their engagement in any of these wide-ranging behaviors. *See also* Celibacy; Medicine.

Further Reading: Ariès, Philippe, and Andre Bejin. *Western Sexuality: Practice and Precept in Past and Present Times.* Oxford: Basil Blackwell, 1985; Baines, Barbara J. *Representing Rape in the English Early Modern Period.* Lewiston, NY: The Edwin Mellen Press, 2003; Chedgzoy, Kate, Melanie Hansen, and Suzanne Trill, eds. *Voicing Women: Gender and Sexuality in Early Modern Writing.* Keele, UK: Keele University Press, 1996; Dixon, Laurinda S. *Perilous Chastity: Women and Illness in Pre-Enlightenment Art and Medicine.* Ithaca, NY: Cornell University Press, 1995; Fletcher, Anthony. *Gender, Sex, and Subordination in England, 1500–1800.* New Haven,

CT: Yale University Press, 1995; Turner, David M. *Gender, Sex, and Civility in England, 1660–1740*. Cambridge: Cambridge University Press, 2002.

Karen Swallow Prior

CHILDBIRTH. During the early modern period, childbirth was a natural process invested with great meaning by society and individuals. Dominated by women, the mysteries of the childbed drew on religious and customary practices seeking safe deliverance for the mother and child. In Europe, some childbirth practices faced increasing scrutiny under the influence of the **Reformation**, new scientific thought, and the anxiety of the witch-craze, but little change resulted.

After the quickening in the second trimester of **pregnancy**, expectant women began to ready themselves for giving birth. First-time mothers relied upon the advice of older female relatives; in Europe, that meant mothers, and in China, often aunts and grandmothers. Virgins were usually excluded from the room, as were men. In most cases, a midwife, ideally strong, nimble, resolute, and virtuous, directed the childbirth preparations. Few materials were needed—warm water, a chair or stool, bedding for the recovery, linens to receive the newborn, a knife to cut the cord, and thread to bind.

The women retreated to a darkened or interior room where the laboring woman was relieved of all knots, laces, and buckles—a symbolic loosening of all hindrances. Customarily, she remained at least partially clothed and was encouraged to walk between contractions. She might adopt a variety of positions, including sitting, crouching, kneeling, or on all fours. The midwife would often manipulate and stretch the vulva, applying lubricants or using steam to soften the tissue. Massage or medicines were sometimes applied to tame a "wandering" womb if the labor seemed slow to progress. Little attention seems to have been devoted to the management of pain. Indeed, some Christian theories held that suffering was necessary as part of the legacy of Eve.

When the child was delivered, the newborn would be laid between its mother's legs. The cord was cut, longer for a boy, shorter for a girl, and tied. The afterbirth was extracted carefully since retention could lead to illness and the remains were thought to have the power of sympathetic magic. If complications arose, the midwife might baptize the newborn or see to the quiet burial of a stillborn.

After the birth, some of the women attended the mother, assisting her to the bed where she would rest for several hours or days. Her full recovery was thought to take a month or more and this "lying-in" was seen as a time when women visitors or "gossips" undermined the patriarchal order. Moralists argued that it was a mother's duty to nurse her own child but wet-nurses were sometimes employed by the upper classes.

European obstetrical texts drew on their ancient and medieval predecessors. Trotula of Salerno's advice continued to be frequently reprinted, although the Renaissance scholars Eucharius Roesslin and James Guillemeau

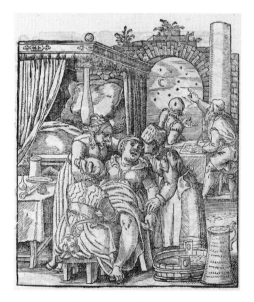

A Woman Gives Birth, 1587. A midwife and friends assist a woman giving birth while the men consult the heavens to draft the astrological birth-chart or horoscope. © HIP/Art Resource, NY.

produced illustrated guides to childbirth that were widely reprinted. However, few **midwives** had access to these books, learning most of their skills from other women. In some jurisdictions, such as England and Holland, authorities licensed midwives, but their concern was more for matters of virtue and good order than medical training. Few doctors involved themselves in the matter of birth, due to both the low esteem accorded childbirth as well as a concern for feminine modesty. Physicians might be called in to verify a death or to administer medications in a difficult recovery. A midwife, the laboring woman's female relatives, neighbors, and friends remained the customary childbed attendants and were often the subject of moralists' criticism for their secretive and presumably disorderly ways.

Many items and practices were thought to aid in labor. Natural abortifacents such as rue might be used to hasten the delivery. An "eagle-stone" or aetite was often hung around the expectant mother's neck to ease the birth. Traditional **Christianity** encouraged women to call on St. Margaret, the Virgin, or another local saint. Sometimes objects purporting to be the girdle, purse, or necklace of the Virgin were loaned out to childbearing women. The holy sacrament was also thought to help. Churchmen exhorted childbearing women to confess and receive the sacrament as their time drew near. During the Reformation, many of these aids were discouraged as superstitious custom and resort to prayer and meditation was prescribed. Even in Catholic regions, midwives sometimes found themselves under increasing scrutiny as their herbal medicines and practices brought suspicions of witchcraft. But, with the birthing process directed by women and few doctors seeking to intervene, the experience of childbirth for most women changed only in their access to customary comforts. It remained the leading cause of death for women of childbearing age during this time period. *See also* Childhood; Medicine; Obstetrical Manuals; Witches.

Further Reading: Cressy, David. *Birth, Marriage and Death: Ritual, Religion, and the Life-Cycle in Tudor and Stuart England.* Oxford: Oxford University Press, 1997; Gélis, Jacques. *History of Childbirth: Fertility, Pregnancy and Birth in Early Modern Europe.* Translated by Rosemary Morris. Boston: Northeastern University Press, 1991; Musacchio, Jacqueline M. *The Art and Ritual of Childbirth in Renaissance Italy.* New Haven, CT: Yale University Press, 1999.

Janice Liedl

CHILDHOOD. Childhood in the early modern period has been an area of intense interest over the last four decades—specifically since the publication in English of *Centuries of Childhood: A Social History of Family Life* (1962) by Philippe Ariès. Ariès not only asked a question that historians had not heretofore asked—what was the history of childhood?—but shaped the discussion over the next decades by posing certain powerful theses, two above all: first, that there was no real concept of childhood before the seventeenth or eighteenth century; second, that the high incidence of infant and child mortality resulted in parental indifference as evidenced in, among other indications, the absence of profound expressions of grief on the death of children. These claims were hotly debated by advocates and opponents, who raided archives and libraries for evidence in support of their positions. In the course of this debate, Ariès' principal point about the historicity of childhood, *and* the notion that childhood is subject to history, has been securely validated. What has resulted, then, from the Arièsan challenge is an extraordinarily rich episode of historical inquiry. It has taken many directions, outlined here.

HOUSEHOLD STRUCTURE. Beginning with the studies of the Cambridge Group of social scientists founded by Peter Laslett, who was often the sole or co-author of their publications, and continuing with independent investigations, it became clear that the experience of childhood varied according to household structure, which varied regionally and by class. Generally, in western and central (Germano/Latin) Europe (exceptions are mainly in southern France and Italy), and especially in the northwest, family size was small, the age of marriage was advanced, and marriage was neolocal. These patterns contrast with those evident in eastern Europe, India, China, and Islamic regions, where the continued authority of the patriarch over the married young, or the co-residence of adult brothers was more normal, as well as with many tribal societies. In Europe, consequently, young children received practical or formal instruction from mature parents who ran their own households. In some social strata, as among the artisans and burghers of Europe's several thousand cities, parental interest in children as heirs to parental skills, outlook, and fortunes could be intense.

That intensity was moderated, perhaps, in Europe as elsewhere, because the frequent remarriages of the male householder meant that a large number of siblings and half-siblings of a wide range of ages might at any time contend with each other. The remarriage of his widowed wife, who on remarrying left to join a new household, did not have the same impact. Alternatively, especially among property-less workers, household structure was simpler. Poor men might refrain from marriage altogether, or form small households with few children.

CHILDBIRTH AND RELATED THEMES. Essentially related to the study of childhood is the study of childbirth and the related matters of nursing and early infant care. Historians have studied the midwives who were, alone, and in the absence of male physicians until about the eighteenth century, the masters of the birthing chamber in Europe as in other contemporary civilizations. Midwives acquired their knowledge from older female mentors and from experience, and were highly valued by pregnant women. They, or a closely related group of female healers, also provided herbal remedies for women's illnesses and for birth control (unofficially, as its practice was illicit).

From the fifteenth century, university-trained males wrote advice manuals in the vernacular languages, implying the relatively high levels of literacy among practicing midwives, that recapitulated the obstetrical (and some pediatric) knowledge of ancient Greek physicians that had recently been recovered by the humanists. These professionals, as well as clerical and humanist experts, advised new mothers to nurse their own babies. Their advice, in Europe, was routinely ignored by women of the urban and noble elites among whom the employment of wetnurses was the norm—a situation conspicuously different from India and China, where wetnurses were generally employed only when the mother was unable to nurse. Beginning in seventeenth-century England, high-born women who began to nurse their own babies and encourage others to do so were the frontrunners in a new ideological surge that valued and valorized motherhood.

INFANTICIDE, ABORTION, ABANDONMENT. Whereas in ancient Mediterranean societies, India, and China, infanticide was widely practiced for population control (and gender selection), with male householders making the decision to "expose" unwanted newborns, in Christian Europe, infanticide was fairly rare and resorted to most often by the poor mothers of illegitimates. Prosecution of maternal infanticides was mild in the Middle Ages, but became serious in the sixteenth through eighteenth centuries. Other women, sometimes in concert with husbands or male companions, abandoned unwanted children at churches or hospitals. From the fifteenth century in Europe (earlier in Byzantium), specialized institutions for foundlings and orphans were established to receive them, and may even have encouraged the abandonment pattern which increased steadily into the eighteenth and later centuries. Abortion was forbidden and demonized, in Europe and in many other societies, seen variously as evidence of adultery (especially in ancient Rome), an assault on male authority, and an act of murder, as in Christian Europe and among Jews and Muslims.

THE CIRCULATION OF CHILDREN. Whereas in the extended families of some other societies children were raised to the age of marriage at home, in Europe, in many social and regional settings, they circulated out of the family for training, socialization, and sustenance. The children of nobles were often sent to other noble courts to acquire the skills of a knight or court lady. The children of merchants were dispatched to other members of the guild or company for training and for experience of remote places and languages. The children of artisans were apprenticed to another master, often of another trade. The children of the poor were dispatched at ages as young as seven, but more often around eleven or twelve, to become servants in the households of the wealthy. Other children were sent to monasteries as oblates, destined to become monks themselves, or as students, both male and female. From the fifteenth century, urban and landed elites dispatched their sons to the boarding schools of the humanists, the Protestant reformers, or the Jesuits.

HUMANISTS AND PEDAGOGUES. Humanists and other learned experts not only found schools, but engaged in a discussion of pedagogical goals and methods that launches an intellectual tradition reaching on to Jean-Jacques Rousseau and John Dewey. They advocated the study of the Greek and Latin classics, and defined the study of the liberal arts as the essential secondary curriculum that prepared young men for the university, for the professions, or for the life of a gentleman. Almost without exception, they opposed corporal punishment, its abuses eloquently denounced by such luminaries as Erasmus (for whom schools were "torture shops") and Montaigne (for whom they were prisons). The ideal of a liberal arts education at the secondary level, perhaps followed by university training, was uniquely European, although other systems of education flourished contemporaneously in Islam, India, and China. In China especially, where in this era the examination was the sole gateway to political and social advancement, an education in the Confucian classics was deemed invaluable.

RELIGIOUS DIMENSIONS. The religious turmoil that accompanied the Protestant challenge to the Catholic monopoly of the Christian church in western and central Europe is a central feature of the early modern period, and not surprisingly had an impact on the history of childhood. Although in those regions that became Protestant there seems to be no marked shift in household structure, two changes did take place. First, the abolition of the convents and the eradication of the notion of the superiority of virginity to marriage meant that nearly all women married, and that their role as mothers was valorized. Second, the doctrine that each believer was responsible for his own spiritual life—for Martin **Luther**, his own salvation—meant that each child, male or female, had to receive at least an elementary education so that he could read the Bible to understand God's will.

Although the goal of universal primary education was not realized, great progress was made in that direction. In addition, Protestants developed the first catechisms, simple instruction manuals in the basics of the faith organized in question-and-answer format. Later adopted (with changed content) also by Catholics, these represent an early genre of specialized literature for children. Radical religious sects (Anabaptists, Puritans, Quakers, Jansenists, Pietists, Lollards) were especially motivated to develop ways to rear children in the faith; their future survival depended on their ability to acculturate their offspring to be not merely loyal followers, but committed leaders. It is from this kind of milieu that the seventeenth-century pedagogue Jan Amos Komensky (Comenius) emerged, a bishop of the radical sect of Moravian Brethren, an advocate of universal male and female education, who concerned himself with learning in early childhood, especially the maternal role in that task.

In these efforts to acculturate young children to religious faith, pursued by persons with a variety of confessional allegiances, Europe is surely unique (although the Christian ventures described here resemble those of the European Jews, who in their segregated communities diligently educated their children in the Hebrew language and heritage). In other contemporary societies, as in Islam, there was no such religious multiplicity; where there was, as in India or China, there was no such premium placed on correct belief, and no need for the acculturation of the young to a distinct religious tradition.

THE UNIQUENESS OF THE WEST. The religious configuration of early modern Europe in its effects on childhood is certainly one area in which the uniqueness of the West may be seen. Others have already been noted. To these may be added, in closing, some other distinctive features. The absence (or pale presence) of an ancestor cult made possible a greater openness to cognate kin (kin on the mother's side), valorizing women and militating against the extreme gender bias characteristic of other civilizations. The relatively greater freedom enjoyed by women not only benefited female children, but allowed for the more powerful impress of maternal thought and attitudes upon sons. Notions of individual freedom and self-determination, moreover, which had diverse origins (in Christian thought; in small, nuclear, neolocal household structures) and reached a peak during the early modern period, encouraged those few children fortunate enough to be able to choose their destinies to seek their own self-realization. *See also* Abortion; Adolescents; Foundlings and Orphans; Infanticide; Luther, Martin.

Further Reading: Ariès, Philippe. *Centuries of Childhood: A Social History of Family Life*. Translated by Robert Baldick. New York: Random House (Vintage), 1962; Cunningham, Hugh. *Children and Childhood in Western Society since 1500*. 2nd ed. New York: Longman, 2005; Heywood, Colin. *A History of Childhood: Children and Childhood in the West from Medieval to Modern Times*. Cambridge: Polity Press, 2001.

Margaret L. King

CHINESE TREASURE FLEETS. Founded in 1368, the powerful Ming dynasty oversaw a period of transformation for China. Under the third Ming emperor, Zhu Di, known as the Yongle Emperor, who ruled from 1403 to 1424, China experienced an age of unprecedented economic expansion, most notably in the area of maritime trade. By the mid-fifteenth century, China was the world's premier maritime trading power. Supported by a superior seafaring technology, a powerful navy, and a strong economy, China sent out seven large trade armadas during the reign of the Yongle Emperor, who is often considered to be one of China's greatest rulers. Loaded with fine porcelain, silk, and other art objects, fleets of Chinese junks sailed from Korea and Japan throughout the Malay archipelago and along the coast of India to East **Africa** trading for gemstones, coral, cobalt, pepper, and other spices. By 1497, China's fleet was many times larger than that of the Portuguese, who, in that year, sent the first major European expedition into the Indian Ocean under Vasco da Gama.

The commander-in-chief of these voyages was Zheng He (Cheng Ho) (c. 1371– c. 1433), the Grand Eunuch of the Chinese Court, who commanded all seven journeys despite never having been to sea before. Each voyage comprised tens of thousands of men and hundreds of ships of various sizes. The first voyage consisted of almost 28,000 sailors and soldiers and 317 vessels, many of them the great nine-masted "treasure ships," which were among the largest wooden marine craft ever built. Over the seven expeditions, Zheng He led his men throughout Southeast **Asia** and into the Indian Ocean, establishing contact with India, East Africa, and the **Middle East**. Zheng He's efforts resulted in an expansion of China's tributary network, which soon reached from Indonesia to the coast of East Africa. The expeditions also rewarded the Chinese with knowledge and possession of foreign objects and animals. The contemporary reports of Zheng He's companion on his voyages, Ma Huan, a Muslim trader who acted as translator, claimed that as many as 36 countries came to acknowledge the emperor's lordship through their contact with the treasure fleet.

Besides trade, the voyages had serious political purposes. Because the Ming believed that all people on earth should submit to the Chinese emperor, the fleets were a means of enforcing Chinese hegemony throughout the regions visited. There is also some speculation among modern historians that the purpose of the fleets was to locate the vanished nephew whose throne the Yongle Emperor had usurped. The Ming emperors clearly viewed themselves as Sons of Heaven who, through their station, represented the population of the entire earth, and they therefore needed to establish their overlordship over the earth. If countries refused to submit, they were threatened with military force. If coercion was unnecessary, then the Chinese were lavish with their gifts, bestowing on the indigenous peoples many valuables, presumably with the desire to impress foreigners with China's power and wealth.

Zheng He's voyages began in 1405 and ended in 1433, when China ceased its long distance expeditions and focused on trade relations predominantly with Japan and the Philippines. The end of the voyages was due to a lack of political support for these expeditions from the Yongle Emperor's successors, who believed them to be extravagant and harmful to the Chinese state, a view promoted by the Yongle Emperor's minister of finance, Xia Yuanji. On a more philosophical level, the Chinese belief system was sufficiently anti-materialistic that the drive to collect wealth from other countries was not strong in Chinese culture. The Yongle Emperor was severely criticized for the cost of these journeys, which he took to heart when part of his new palace in Beijing, the Forbidden City, burned to the ground. He was also distracted by political and military problems along his northern border with the Mongols. He did stop the expeditions in the face of political pressure, but soon ordered them to resume.

The Yongle Emperor's immediate successor, the Hongxi Emperor (r. 1424–1425) brought the expeditions to a second halt in 1424. Zheng He made one more voyage in 1430–1433 under the Xuande Emperor, but then the expeditions ceased. Thus, China withdrew from any imperialistic activity and began its long retreat into isolation. It was the European nations of Portugal and Spain that became the great imperialistic powers of East Asia over the next century. By the early sixteenth century, the Portuguese had a stronghold in the Indian Ocean, against which China's now-inferior military could not compete. Unlike Christopher Columbus, Zheng He did not have successors; his were the sole maritime-expeditions ever sponsored, on a large scale, by a Chinese government.

Further Reading: Dreyer, Edward L. *Zheng He: China and the Oceans in the Early Ming Dynasty, 1405–1433*. London: Longman, 2006; Levathes, Louise. *When China Ruled the Seas: The Treasure Fleet of the Dragon Throne, 1405–1433*. Oxford: Oxford University Press, 1996; Menzies, Gavin. *1421: The Year the Chinese Discovered the World*. New York: Morrow/Avon, 2003.

Julie Sutherland

CHRISTIANITY. Christianity, during the early modern period, went through a tumultuous period of expansion, schism, reformation, and re-examination, entrenching its beliefs while undergoing a breathtaking revolution of belief, tradition, and structure. After the great schism of 1054, which split the Christian world between East and West, the state of Western Christianity remained more or less stable until the late Middle Ages, when the popes sought to gain and maintain political control of the Papal States in central Italy, and the office of the papacy itself experienced two crises in the fourteenth and fifteenth centuries. The first of these crises, was the so-called Babylonian Captivity (1305–1378), when a series of French popes dominated by the French crown moved the papal seat from Rome to Avignon, on the south eastern frontier of France. The second crisis, lasting from 1378 to 1417, was the emergence of two, and later three, competing lines of popes in Avignon and Rome. Each pope claimed to be legitimate, and each claimed the allegiance of differing states and kingdoms. These crises weakened the Western church, and left its reputation and authority open to question.

The early modern period in Europe is characterized by the rise of national monarchies. Everyday life changed from the theocentric (God-centered) medieval framework of earthly life as a passing-through of a valley of tears that would result in a better life in heaven to an anthropocentric (human-centered) worldview. In this new pattern, human beings, without casting God aside, became more self-reliant. They defined their current limitations as they expressed a characteristic notion of the self. The greater openness of the Renaissance did not evolve from the mistaken notion of "the dark ages"; rather, it was a re-invention of ancient Greece and Rome into the new mindset of humanism.

The Church throughout Europe owned much of the arable land, which meant that in the prevailing feudal system it controlled the greatest sector of the economy. Therefore, it held power among the peasantry, since it also controlled an enormous number of vassals. In this agrarian economy, the Church handed out benefices or "livings," the main source of income of a significant number of clergy. This economic power gave the Church political influence and brought it into conflict with national monarchies. The aristocracy exercised Church patronage out of a sense of *noblesse oblige*, self-interest, or genuine piety. From a practical standpoint, since only first-born sons inherited titles of nobility and property, sons not destined to royal service in political or military careers had access to a clerical career. Daughters entered convents for three respectable reasons: to fulfill a true religious vocation, to escape forced marriages, or because their families (whether aristocratic or upper bourgeoisie) could not afford the contractual payment of a substantial **dowry**. Sister Arcangela Tarabotti (1604–1652), the author of *Paternal Tyranny*, and Sister Bartolomea Riccoboni (1359–1436), the author of *Life and Death in a Venetian Convent*, represent opposite views of life as nuns. Increasingly, the early modern period saw women achieve a broader and stronger voice within religious life. In the case of the Republic of Venice—an example among many throughout Europe—women who created literature belonged to one of three groupings; they were **courtesans**, aristocrats, or religious.

Chronicles were not the only type of literature produced in convents. For example, *Dei Vergini Convent* (1519), the chronicle of the convent of Vergini in Venice, also served the purpose of publicizing the fame and virtue of the convent. It described in detail the state of holiness of the nuns that lived under the convent's roof.

Although historians, psychologists, anthropologists, and theologians over the centuries have pointed to the Church as a maternal institution, they have also invariably been aware that it had been, and was through the early modern period, a patriarchal institution that tolerated no dissent. The high regard for the Blessed Virgin Mary, mother of Jesus, generally did not help much to advance the way women were viewed in society or in the convent. Some priests may have been manly, others effeminate, but so long as there was no overt expression of **homosexuality**, they were accepted. They could move about with permission from their bishops, though such was not the case with female religious. Their modality of femaleness was to imitate the suffering mother of Christ or the valor of women martyrs. **Virginity** seems to have been a point of obsession, with the exception of widows who entered the convent late in life.

The Church sanctioned education in convents because nuns had to sing together the daily office (formal prayers throughout the day), and thus needed to learn to read so they could fulfill the mission of being good choir nuns. Convents were also the place where daughters of the nobility and high bourgeoisie went to obtain an education, and so at least a few nuns had to be able to write and to teach as well.

Early modern society saw a woman as a bride, a wife, and a mother. Alternate living patterns—with the exception of the convent—were considered inappropriate and dangerous to the virtue of men. Women not under the control of a husband could belong to three acceptable types: pious and celibate laywomen, religious women committed to their way of life (as described by Tarabotti), and truly holy women (as described by Riccoboni). Sisters and nuns pledged total obedience to God and to the Church in their role as brides of Christ. Upon entering the religious life, they made a series of vows witnessed by the bishop or his delegate.

In the early modern period, the guilds formed in the Middle Ages continued to support local parishes and contributed funds for the only organized means of social welfare available, for example, to orphanages and hospitals. The emerging bourgeoisie—university-trained professionals and merchants—saw support of the Church as a genuine duty, while there is also evidence that at times social advancement was relevant to some.

The Church in the West referred to itself as Catholic (universal), while the Church in the East called itself Orthodox, although it certainly believed it had a genuine claim to catholicity (universality) as well. Unlike the strongly centralized Roman church, the Byzantine branch of Christianity continued the tradition of the autocephalous (self-headed) church. It was led by Patriarchs, such as the Patriarchs of Constantinople and Alexandria, who presided over a number of bishops and, at the same time, directly over the faithful. The Bishop of Rome—the office to which the College of Cardinals formally elects the pope—is also a Patriarch who has the same authority as any other bishop. The pope is accorded the additional mark of respect in the West because he is seen as the direct successor to Saint Peter the Apostle, founder of the Church of Rome. Other than when faced with the imminent threat of attack from the Muslim Ottoman Empire, which conquered Constantinople and overthrew the Byzantine Empire in 1453, the Eastern Churches wished no contact with the West.

Using a term borrowed from the former Roman Empire, the Church survived the fragmentation of the early Middle Ages in isolated monasteries or abbeys and in the dioceses. A diocese is the fundamental administrative unit headed by a bishop who reports directly to Rome. Several parishes make up a diocese. A priest heads a parish, his official title is pastor (from the Latin *parochus*), and other priests serving the same parish would be subject to his authority. Properly speaking, the clergy consist of men who have received holy orders. In the early modern era, deacons, priests, and bishops received major orders. Minor orders, such as lector, porter, and sub-deacon, also existed in the early modern Church, but no longer do so today. Laypersons carry out their former functions. Archbishops were in charge of metropolitan dioceses, to which other dioceses and their bishops had to report. Cardinals were papal electors.

Priests could be diocesan, also called secular (i.e., from the world), or regular, as those who belonged to orders such as the Franciscans or Dominicans. Diocesan priests were attached to the bishops who ordained them and remained incardinated (permanently based) in a diocese. Priests regular could serve under the authority of a local bishop; they may have lived in a community or in small groups carrying out the specific apostolate, i.e., type of ministry, of their particular order. These were called friars or monks if they lived in an abbey or a monastery. Among friars, as is the case with modern Dominicans and Franciscans, most were priests but others were brothers; priests are properly called clerics and are members of the clergy. However, brothers and sisters (nuns technically lived isolated from the world) were called religious but, according to canon law (Church law), are not clerics but a special type of layperson. The Dominican and Franciscan families had congregations for women and men. Nuns and brothers professed vows, but did not receive holy orders.

In 1517, Martin **Luther**, an Augustinian monk in Germany, initiated the movement that would become known as the **Reformation**. As a reaction to the criticisms of Luther and other reformers, the popes convened the Council of **Trent** (1545–1547, 1551–1552, and 1562–1563) to review and revise Church doctrine and practice. The issue of salvation—intertwined with sociopolitical and economic realities—became the defining test as to who was seen to belong to the "true" Church. Sometime during Trent, Rome and the Papal See began to favor the use of the term Catholic (with a capital C, as opposed to a lowercase c, which in the original Greek of the New Testament means "universal"). Various national or quasi-national churches found the term Protestant an adequate marker to distinguish themselves from Rome. The Church of Rome throughout Europe underwent what we now call the Catholic Reformation, which was once termed the "Counter-reformation."

Contact with the New World in 1492 resulted in a near-immediate spread of Roman Catholic Christianity by Franciscans, Dominicans, and Augustinians. The Society of Jesus, the Jesuits, established by Ignatius of Loyola in 1540, soon followed. These missionaries worked under the sponsorship of Spain, Portugal, and, eventually, France. But they had a supranational vision of Christianity, which soon caused the Spanish Crown to seek to reduce the power of the religious orders in New Spain (Mexico) by appointing bishops directly and by favoring priests secular over priests regular. Protestant Christianity arrived in other parts of North America and the Caribbean in the late sixteenth and seventeenth century through English and Dutch exploration and colonization.

The missionary effort—Protestant and Roman Catholic—to bring the Christian faith to Africans, Amerindians (whom many of them saw as "noble savages"), and Asians became a global phenomenon with the technological breakthroughs of Portuguese navigation in reaching India, China, Japan, and the Philippines, although evangelization in the Far East proved to be a difficult task.

The Councils of Nicaea (325 and 787) and Constantinople (381, 553, and 680–681) defined the basis of Christian doctrine in the Creeds with further clarifications. Belief in a triune God—the Trinity as mystery of God the Father, the Son, and the Holy Spirit; the centrality of baptism to finding salvation in the life, death, and resurrection of Jesus Christ; the idea of the Church as the Body of Christ on earth; and the real presence of Christ in the Eucharist are the principles that united and divided Roman

Catholic and Protestant Christians in the early modern period. Unfortunately, for reasons other than theology, which is the attempt to understand as much as humanly possible of God, nations fought fiercely to crush slightly different ways of seeing the same realities.

After the Diet of Worms in 1521, considerable pressures prevented Emperor Charles V (r. 1519–1556) from halting the spread of Protestantism in Germany. The Diet of Augsburg in 1530 required his attention to continue his exercise of supreme authority over the German Electors. At this point, Charles heard Luther's position. Who would follow what religion was summarized by the formula *cuius regio, eius religio*; a nation would follow the religion of its ruler. Thus, we find the Augsburg Confession as the foundation of the "Evangelical Church"—Luther's followers did not use the term "Lutheran" until they arrived in the United States. The Church of England also came into being in the sixteenth century as the result of a complex process far greater than the sexual desire of **Henry VIII** for a new wife. The Portuguese phrase *auto da fe* ("act of faith") came into frequent use among Roman Catholics. An *auto da fe* was a public act of penance undertaken by condemned heretics and apostates. In its mildest form, people were ridiculed in public as punishment for their sins; at its cruelest, they were burned at the stake. By definition, a heretic is someone who—while professing to hold the faith of his or her church's organizational framework—willfully and stubbornly goes against Church teaching. Heretics, moreover, tend to start trouble by causing others to follow beliefs that contradict such teaching; seen this way, sin is pernicious to the individual, the state, and humankind because it is an open insult against God.

The Tribunal of the Inquisition, or Holy Office, established in Italy in 1233, spread to all Christian nations. Its chief original purpose was to excommunicate—to cast out from the Christian community—people, by denying them the ability to attend mass and receive communion and other sacraments. They could come back if they showed repentance, gave alms to the poor and the church, performed acts of humility, and did good works. In a sense, eternal damnation was potentially the fullest extent of the judgment of excommunication. On this point, Luther disagreed with Rome squarely. In his view, a person was justified (or saved) by faith alone.

When the Spanish monarchs Ferdinand and Isabella defeated Boabdil, the last Moorish king of Granada, in 1492, the unification or so-called *Reconquista* of Spain was complete. The symbolic and geopolitical rise of Castile as the central power of Spain led to the expulsion of Jews and Muslims who refused coerced mass-conversion in 1492. Within a year of the Spanish Semitic Diaspora, Portugal pronounced and enforced a similar decree. The Inquisition was also extended to the newly established archdiocese of Mexico-Tenochtitlan in New Spain during the tenure of founding Franciscan bishop Juan de Zumárraga after the conquest of Mexico (1519–1521). *See also* Celibacy; Remarriage/Widows.

Further Reading: Bellitto, Christopher M. *The General Councils: A History of the 21 Church Councils from Nicaea to Vatican II*. New York: Paulist, 2002; Dwyer, John C. *Church History: Twenty Centuries of Catholic Christianity*. New York: Paulist Press, 1998; Evans, G. R. *A Brief History of Heresy*. Malden, MA: Blackwell, 2003; González, Justo L. *The Story of Christianity*. 2 vols. New York: HarperCollins, 1985; Halsall, Paul. Compiler. Fordham University. *Internet Modern History Sourcebook:* http://www.fordham.edu/halsall/mod/modsbook.html; Jones, Cheslyn, et al., eds. *The Study of Liturgy*. Rev. ed. New York: Oxford University Press, 1992; Livingstone, Elizabeth A. *The Concise Oxford Dictionary of the Christian Church*. New York: Oxford University Press, 1996; Riccoboni, Bartolomea. *Life and Death in a Venetian Convent: The*

Chronicle and Necrology of Corpus Domini 1395–1436. Edited and translated by Daniel Bornstein. Chicago: University of Chicago Press, 2000; Tanner, Norman P., et al. *Decrees of the Ecumenical Councils.* 2 vols. Washington, DC: Georgetown University Press, 1990; Tarabotti, Arcangela. *Paternal Tyranny.* Edited and translated by Letizia Panizza. Chicago: University of Chicago Press, 2004.

Nicolás Hernández, Jr.

CHURCHING. The churching of women in early modern England was a customary practice involving the blessing of women after recovery from childbirth. Immersed in a history of powerful religious theory and symbolism, churching reflected the Catholic belief in the rite of purification for the new mother, who had completed her private matter of giving birth and now entered the public domain of the church community. The biblical background for churching is found in Leviticus 12.1–5, where a woman who recently gave birth to a son was regarded as ritually unclean. After forty days, the new mother brought the required offerings to the temple where the priest would cleanse her of her impurity. As a rite of purification, churching cleansed a woman from the pollution of intercourse and from the dangers related to the bloody process of childbirth. In the medieval church, churching was regulated by ecclesiastics, who developed this rite for properly married mothers. A purpose of the rite was not only to augment the role of wife and mother, but also to promote conformity with the Catholic Church's interpretation of marriage. Prior to the Reformation, a woman wore a white veil, carried a white candle, and met the priest outside the church where he sprinkled holy water on her. She entered the church with female family members and friends, the midwife, the nurse carrying the new baby, and sometimes the husband and male relatives.

Churching remained a female-centered event despite the transformations it underwent under the Anglican Church. In the 1549 Book of Common Prayer, the ritual of churching changed to reflect the new faith's interpretation of this religious rite by moving the location of the ceremony from outside the church door to inside, where the woman could kneel at a place near the altar. Instead of a ritual of purification, churching became a rite of thanksgiving for members of the established church. Revising Catholic practice, Anglicans did not mandate holy water or candles, and wearing a veil became optional. In the 1552 prayer book, the association with purification was dropped and the rite was renamed "The Thanksgiving of Women after Child-birth." The churching of women officially ended in 1645 when the prayer book was replaced by the Directory of Public Worship. Diaries and family histories, however, continued to provide evidence of the practice of churching, particularly among the royalist gentry. Anglican women, like Lady Mary Verney, in the mid-1600s, were able to find ministers to perform the rite and families recorded the event as a matter of routine in their writings. Puritans were adamant in their opposition to churching, and believed this ecclesiastical ceremony reflected Jewish, popish and superstitious practices. Without any formal ceremony, Puritan women privately were thankful for a safe delivery and acknowledged God's divine hand. *See also* Childbirth; Christianity; Mikveh.

Further Reading: Cressy, David. *Birth, Marriage and Death: Ritual, Religion, and the Life-Cycle in Tudor and Stuart England.* Oxford: Oxford University Press, 1997; Coster, William. "Purity, Profanity and Puritanism: The Churching of Women 1500–1700." In *Women in the Church*, edited by W. J. Sheils and Diana Wood, 377–87. Oxford: Blackwell, 1990; Knödel, Natalie.

"Reconsidering an Obsolete Rite: The Churching of Women and Feminist Liturgical Theology." *Feminist Theology* 14 (1997): 106–14; Rieder, Paula M. *On the Purification of Women: Churching in Northern France, 1100–1500.* Hampshire, England: Palgrave Macmillan, 2006; Thomas, Keith. *Religion and the Decline of Magic. Studies in Popular Belief in Sixteenth and Seventeenth Century England.* London: Penguin, 1971.

Patricia Nardi

CONCUBINES. A concubine is a woman living with a man in a relationship that is, usually, socially accepted and conjugal. Nevertheless, concubines were secondary to ceremonially married consorts, and concubinage was inferior to legal wedlock in the early modern period. The position of concubines relative to wives and the status of their children varied considerably from region to region during this time, and the concubines could be anything from noblewomen to slaves or war captives.

Concubinous relationships were licit or tolerated in many early modern regions either as an alternative or a supplement to matrimony. Concubinage usually presupposed unilateral sexual exclusivity only on the part of concubines—their unfaithfulness could constitute **adultery**, while men could usually terminate the arrangement at will. Thus, as the position of concubines was seldom protected by law or custom, the duration of such relationships often depended on male whims.

In western Europe during the latter half of the sixteenth century, Counter-Reformation Catholic and Reformation authorities intended to weed out not only the sexual sins of clerics, but also those of the laity, which included concubinage. In the Catholic world, this new attitude was applied especially to priests, who had to remain celibate, but who had families with *de facto* wives despite official bans and occasional counter-campaigns. In other parts of the Christian world, where clerical matrimony was permitted, this was considered hypocritical and punishable, **marriage** being a remedy for sin even for priests. However, concubinage remained a viable alternative if a marriage impediment or social inequality prevented wedlock.

Islamic law not only allowed men four concurrent wives, but also an unlimited number of their own female slaves as concubines, while being forbidden to keep several sisters as concubines or wives simultaneously. In the Islamic world, matrimony was constituted by a marriage contract, specifying the dower (*mahr*), and by consummation. Thus, the *mahr* and the wedding festivities were significant in distinguishing marriage from concubinage. While wives were not required to share their dwellings with co-wives, they could be obliged to reside with their husband's concubine(s). All children born of these acknowledged concubinous unions were legitimate and free. Slave-concubines, mothers of their master's recognized children (*umm walad*), were automatically manumitted at their master's death. Gifts and contracts promising financial support to concubines could be made, but were voluntary only. In Jewish law, marriage contracts also separated wives from concubines.

Concubines (*qie*) were commonplace in prosperous Chinese families. A concubine's status was between a maidservant's and a wife's, as she was usually either purchased or hired. Theoretically this destiny could even befall daughters and wives of impoverished but honorable families. A concubine entered the household without rituals, was obliged to obey her mate or "master" and his wife, and be disciplined by her "mistress." A concubine's and her mate's families did not become related other than through the banning of further intermarriage for reasons of consanguinity. Her children were, nevertheless, equal to the wife's offspring. When concubines died, their demise only necessitated limited ancestral mourning obligations and, unlike wives, the law left concubines unprotected after the deaths of their mates. In this period, however, widowers were allowed to marry their concubines under certain conditions, and the position of concubines improved slightly. Rich or noble early modern Japanese kept concubines in addition to wives.

In post-Conquest Latin America, the scarcity of white women caused practically all Spaniards and Portuguese to take local women as concubines. While some of these relationships were voluntary, others were based on force, especially in the conquest era. Concubines were usually baptised and given Christian names. The most famous of these was Malintzin, or Marina, the concubine of Hernán Cortés and mother of his son, who was married off to another Spaniard after a five-year liaison (see **La Malinche**). While matrimony between high-ranking native women and lower-ranking Spanish men was initially possible, such legitimate unions were increasingly considered dishonourable, especially after 1560 when Spanish women started to arrive. Concubinage remained an option for socially or racially disparate couples. It was also common among slaves and the poor, despite pressure from the Church. The old Andean custom of trial marriage or cohabitation before finally deciding to marry was disapproved of by the secular and religious authorities, but never totally abolished. See also Americas (North and South); Bastardy; Celibacy; Christianity; Islam; Judaism; Mistresses; Polygamy/Polyandry.

Further Reading: Ebrey, Patricia Buckley. *Women and the Family in Chinese History*. London: Routledge, 2003; Socolow, Susan Midgen. *The Women of Colonial Latin America*. Cambridge: Cambridge University Press, 2000; Tucker, Judith E. *In the House of the Law: Gender and Islamic Law in Ottoman Syria and Palestine*. Berkeley and Los Angeles: University of California Press, 1998.

Mia Korpiola

CONFUCIANISM. Confucianism takes its name from the ancient philosopher Confucius (Kong Qiu [551–479 BCE]); it is one of the great indigenous religious/philosophical traditions of Chinese civilization. For most of Chinese history Confucianism, Buddhism (which arrived in China from India c. 100 CE), and Daoism were the three most influential cultural traditions in the empire. Among these three, Confucianism took pride of place as the officially sanctioned ideology of virtually all imperial governments. Confucianism provided the philosophical underpinnings of the imperial state and laid the guidelines for selection of government personnel. Beyond this, the prevailing basic mores of both elites and common folk throughout the Chinese empire bore the heavy imprint of Confucian teaching.

From its earliest foundations Confucians expressed complex attitudes toward sexuality. On the one hand sexual feelings were fraught with danger, as their power and intensity could lead individuals to transgress the normative order of the family or the state. Female sexuality was particularly suspect. A preoccupation with female beauty and sexual pleasure could cause men to abdicate their proper patriarchal authority or neglect their social and political duties. Overindulgence fueled by lust was even considered a health hazard, leading to a depletion of male (*yang*) energies that sapped vitality and curtailed longevity.

Even as they acknowledged these pitfalls of human sexuality, however, Confucians celebrated sex as a natural and necessary element of the human condition. The Confucian moral order begins with the family, and Confucians were acutely aware that without sex and the ties that sexuality forges there would be no family upon which to found the larger society. Sexuality was associated with life and creativity, the sexual impulses that moved within the human being were correlated to the dynamic cosmic processes that caused the world to regenerate and revitalize with each new spring.

This productive tension regarding sexuality is embodied in Confucius's famous dictum in *Analects* 15: "I have never seen one who loved virtue as much as he loved female beauty." Though this obviously implies that love of virtue is generally deficient, it does not necessarily mean that sexual feelings are too prevalent or too intense. Rather it could, and was often taken to, mean that one's desire for virtue should intensify until it acquires an erotic quality. In other words, sexuality can provide a template for the passion with which one should pursue moral conduct and moral self-improvement.

An example of this dynamic is found in a Confucian exegetical text discovered at Ma Wangdui Tomb Number Three (interred 168 BCE) in south-central China. In a commentary to a text known as "The Five Conducts," the author invokes the "Guan ju," the first poem of the Confucian canonical text *The Book of Odes*. The "Guan ju" is a love poem expressing the intense yearning of a man for his lover. The commentary asks the reader to imagine being in the grips of such passion and in the presence of one's lover. The urge to act on such desires would be almost irresistible. Then, instructs the author, imagine your parents walk in upon the scene. The irresistible impulse would evaporate. This demonstrates that our spontaneous sexual impulses are at least minimally imbued with ethical sensibilities. Procreation is an individual's first and foremost filial duty to one's parents. The fact that the impulse to procreate can be short-circuited in this manner proves that the rules of ritual propriety that guide social conduct are just as intrinsic to human nature and just as organically necessary to the propagation of human life and vitality as sexuality itself.

One can see in these writings a perspective that diverges sharply from the attitudes toward sex expressed in many writings of the Abrahamic religious traditions. For Confucians there was nothing intrinsically immoral in sexual desire or sexual activity. Quite the contrary, sexuality was a bridge connecting the human realm to fundamental sources of value and redemption. Sex only becomes "wrong" according to the particular context in which it transpires.

Even as this is true, one must acknowledge that sexuality exposes a provisional "blind spot" in the Confucian orientation toward the human condition. Though the forms and manifestations of Confucianism have been very diverse over time, most Confucian teachings have been rooted in a program of "learning to be human" through interaction with other people and the artifacts of human culture. The basic Confucian faith (to the extent that such can be articulated) is that we can overcome our selfish limitations and harmonize our relationships with one another through concerted refinement and effort. Such imperatives incline Confucian thinkers toward an emphasis on those aspects of the human condition that are most common and shareable. Much Confucian ambivalence toward sexuality thus arises from a sensibility that the sexual dimension of the human persona houses the greatest potential for idiosyncrasy and individuation. Each individual is more distinct from others in his or her sexual tastes and preferences than in perhaps any other regard, thus sexuality represents a potential "danger zone" for the socially redemptive Confucian project of "learning to be human." This has not led Confucians to stigmatize sexuality as inherently wicked or degenerate, but has generally imposed discernable limits on the depths to which Confucian writers are willing to explore the terrain of human sexual psychology.

An example of this phenomenon can be seen in expressed Confucian attitudes toward **homosexuality**. The earliest writings of the Confucian tradition acknowledge the existence of homoerotic feelings and practices. Most recorded instances of homosexuality are criticized, not because homosexual feelings or acts are themselves deemed "evil," but because of the social consequences of homosexual attachment. Homosexual desire necessarily transpired outside of the parameters of marriage, and in the case of male homosexuality could intrude into relations in the public realm. Thus most instances of same-sex attachment were critiqued for arousing partial feelings that led the individual to act against obligations to the family or state. This occasional engagement with **homoeroticism**, however, did not lead Confucian writers to speculate as to the origins of this realm of human sexuality or its intrinsic logic. Confucians were never inclined to view homosexuality as an inherent "problem" requiring fundamental solutions. At the same time, though later sources acknowledge that same-sex love could be very enduring and intense, Confucian writers did not explore the possibility that a same-sex couple could form a family bond akin to marriage or speculate as to what the larger social consequences of such a phenomenon might be. As was true of many particular aspects of human sexuality, Confucian thinkers were aware of the human potential for homoeroticism but largely ignored it.

During the Ming Dynasty (1368–1644 CE) Confucianism was institutionalized in a number of fundamental organs of the imperial government. Most important of these was the exam system, a complex of regional, provincial, and capital exams by which virtually all government personnel were accredited and recruited. Confucianism formed the entire curriculum of the imperial exams. Examinees were asked to write essays on an authoritative canon established by the scholar Zhu Xi (1130–1200 CE). This officially sanctioned "Neo-Confucianism" viewed the human being as divided between a material "*qi* nature" that was the source of passions and feelings and a metaphysical "Dao nature" that was the seat of morality and reason. It thus stressed control of the more volatile dimensions of the human condition, such as sexuality, through diligent study with teachers and of ancient texts.

Outside of the official exam curriculum, however, the Ming saw the rise of innovators within the Confucian tradition whose disposition toward sexuality was less adversarial. Chief of these was Wang Yangming (1472–1529 CE), who propounded a new interpretation of the Confucian tradition that exclusively emphasized human beings' inborn moral capacities. Wang asserted that knowledge and action were unified and that moral cultivation consisted only of activating the mind's original goodness in conduct. Spontaneous impulses such as sexual desire thus acquired new salience and moral efficacy within Wang's Confucian synthesis. His disciples and latter-day followers (especially those of the notorious "Taizhou School") explored new forms of teaching, writing and social action that dealt candidly with love and human sexuality. Under the influence of Wang Yangming's teachings leading Ming scholars rejected the bifurcation of the human being into material and metaphysical aspects and insisted that if moral guidance was to be found at all it would have to be rooted firmly in the material nature and conditions of the individual and society.

In social and economic terms the Ming was ripe for such new cultural trends. Broadening and deepening international trade networks brought Chinese farmers and craftsmen into contact with consumers as far away as Europe and the Americas. The resulting influx of silver fostered the burgeoning of the domestic commercial economy and the integration of the entire empire into an expansive and diverse market system that brought an ever-widening variety of consumer goods to all levels of urban and rural society. Though trade never approached the social primacy of scholarship and official service, merchants and other prominent urbanites enjoyed increasingly elite status and contributed to shaping prevailing cultural priorities and tastes.

A new mass market for the written word created an explosion of new genres of literary production. Short stories, novels, popular songs, poetry, and all forms of drama and performing arts were created to fill an ever-expanding demand for the written and spoken word. As commerce became more and more central to the daily life of the Chinese people, merchants spontaneously hit upon the eternal verity that "sex sells." All aspects of the new consumer market became laden with erotic content both overt and subliminal, and erotica accounted for an increasingly large share of published commodities.

Confucian-trained scholars were naturally possessed of literary skills that could be profitably employed in this new economy. Even so, many Confucians lamented an emerging world in which ordinary people were barraged with constant stimuli to their material and sexual desires in the absence of any moral instruction as to how those feelings should be correctly channeled, a trend to which they were reluctant to contribute. Countervailing forces worked to overcome Confucian resistance to the literary mass market, however. An expansion of literacy (itself driven by the widening accessibility of learning materials facilitated by the market) made competition in the imperial exam system increasingly intense. Individuals whose training might have guaranteed them a lucrative government career in earlier eras were forced to translate their skills into economic sustenance through other channels. At the same time, the new Confucian synthesis of Wang Yangming afforded Ming intellectuals motive and justification to engage the emergent market culture on its own terms. In this spirit many set out to create literature that satisfied both the eroticist imperatives of the mass market and the morally redemptive goals of the Confucian humanist program.

One example of such literature is "The Pearl Sewn Shirt," a popular short story by Feng Menglong (1574–1646) based on earlier sources. The story concerns a merchant whose wife is tempted into infidelity while he is away on business. He learns of the adulterous affair when in his travels he encounters his wife's lover in possession of his pearl-sewn shirt, which the wife had given to her lover as a gift. The merchant divorces his wife and winds up remarried to the lover's widow, which coincidence is discovered because the widow has inherited the self-same pearl-sewn shirt from her departed husband. The merchant eventually winds up afoul of the law because of an accident that transpires because of an argument over some pearls he was attempting to purchase. The magistrate before whom he is tried happens to be his former wife's new husband, and out of love for the merchant she pleads with her new husband to spare him. The magistrate does so, and, seeing their intense mutual love, allows the two to be reunited as man and wife.

"The Pearl-Sewn Shirt" is thus not only a love story but an allegory about the new social economy of Ming times and the eroticism that it engendered and by which it was animated. Sensual impulses drive merchants about the world in search of rare commodities, dividing families and causing strife between individuals. Those same impulses, however, draw men and women together and inspire them to redemptive acts of clemency and mutual love. The story does not categorically reject the present age as degenerate, therefore, but cautions that a moral mindfulness is required to harness the positive energies of this new society and to avoid its destructive pitfalls. Many writers of Ming erotica and romantic fiction such as Li Yu (author of the novel

The Carnal Prayer Mat), Tang Xianzu (playwright of *The Peony Pavilion*) and the anonymous author of *The Plum in the Golden Vase* wove similar Confucian themes into their prose. *See also* Daoism.

Further Reading: Birch, Cyril, trans. *Stories from a Ming Collection*. New York: Grove, 1958; De Bary, William Theodore, ed. *Self and Society in Ming Thought*. New York: Columbia University Press, 1970; Hinsch, Bret. *Passions of the Cut Sleeve: The Male Homosexual Tradition in China*. Reprint ed. Berkeley and Los Angeles: University of California Press, 1992; Wawrytko, Sandra A. "Prudery and Prurience: Historical Roots of the Confucian Conundrum Concerning Women, Sexuality, and Power." In *The Sage and the Second Sex: Confucianism, Ethics, and Gender* edited by Chenyang Li, 163–97. Chicago: Open Court, 2000.

Andrew Meyer

CONTRACEPTION. See Abortion and Contraception

COUNCIL OF TRENT. See Trent, Council of

COURTESANS. A highly educated and exclusive prostitute characterized by physical beauty, artistic virtuosity, and learning, the courtesan enjoyed a level of mobility and independence unknown to most Renaissance women. Whether a *cortigiana* in Italy, a *tawa'if* or *ganikā* in India, a *ji* in China, an *oiran* in Japan, or a *gisaeng* in Korea, the courtesan was particularly recognized for a high level of education, which almost universally included music, dance, poetry, and the art of conversation. In precolonial India, courtesans were considered to be the keepers of culture, while in China, Korea, and Japan they were thought of as bearers of their respective society's artistic traditions. The courtesan's role, however, remained also a sexual one, and her profession a venal one, illuminating not only the philosophical link between body and mind that these societies shared, but also the fact that the idea of selling the body was perhaps commonplace for her contemporaries. Although usually from the lower classes, the courtesan's erudition and talent allowed her to cater exclusively to the highest echelons of male society, with whom she was frequently able to interact almost as an equal, whether in the patron's home, her own salon, or an urban pleasure quarters. Because her trade was ultimately independent from reproductive systems that required female purity for the maintenance of the paternal line, the courtesan offered both the intellectual stimulation and sexual gratification that patriarchal societies habitually barred sheltered wives from providing.

While dating back to the third or fourth century BCE in **Europe** and **Asia**, courtesanship was primarily an early modern phenomenon, its zenith coinciding with the Renaissance of the fifteenth through seventeenth centuries. Such timing can be ascribed across both continents to specific, shared social realities. Firstly, in these societies male adulthood was reached rather late in life, delaying **marriage** and often forcing men to find female companionship and sexual release outside the marriage bed. The desire for extramarital companionship was exacerbated by the nature of early modern matrimonial systems that separated **love** and sex from the institution of matrimony and from procreation. Secondly, these societies were in a process of economic modernization that challenged traditional, highly stratified social hierarchies by offering increased opportunities for social mobility and for the adoption of leisure and luxury. However, the same economic trends increasingly excluded women from the work force, forcing some into the sex trade as a means of survival. Thirdly, economic

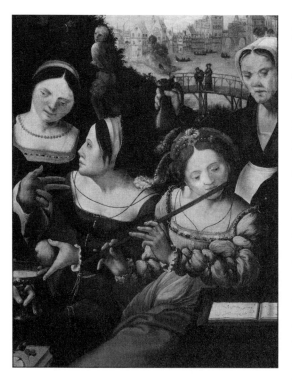

Woman playing flute, courtesans, and servant, detail from *L'enfant Prodigue chez les Courtisanes* (*The Prodigal Son with Courtesans*), sixteenth century. © The Art Archive/Musée Carnavalet Paris/Dagli Orti.

changes coincided with the flourishing of new, broadly circulated cultural forms. Erudition and the mastery of the new cultural forms became symbols of status, and were thus equally important to upwardly mobile men and the women they sought for company. The courtesan, in whose profession sex and the arts were interdependent, served both as a substitute for the matrimonial bed and as a symbol of a man's heightened social standing.

For that reason, courtesans were widely sought after. Their allure enabled them to arrange relationships granting them a significant degree of mobility, both physical and social, as well as an unusual and often problematic independence. Whether kept by several patrons who offered indirect financial support, like in Italy and China, or supported by the state, as in India and Korea, the courtesan escaped the financial misfortune of being fully dependent on a father, husband, brothers, or sons, and unable to own her home or even her own clothes. Rather, some courtesans came to be quite wealthy, and many were able to maintain luxurious lifestyles for themselves and their dependants. In fact, courtesans came often to be indistinguishable from upper-class women in dress and manner. Their mobility was also a social one for, although they could not regularly rise to the highest echelons of the hierarchy, they did operate at the elite level, where they had direct access to those in power.

Courtesans' independence, however, at least in Europe, often led to ambiguous feelings on the part of contemporaries, who not only attempted to curtail courtesans' mobility in an effort to neutralize their influence, but even blamed them in times of plague, for example, as having brought the wrath of God upon society. Such sentiments frequently led to virulent and even violent attacks against courtesans, making their profession, while financially attractive, a hazardous one. The courtesan's success could also have a very limited shelf life, as beauty and youth were generally a prerequisite. Once either was lost, the courtesan could turn to a natural or adopted daughter, whom she would train to follow in her footsteps, continuing the traditions of what some scholars have termed an almost hereditary **caste**.

The courtesan was replaced in nineteenth-century Europe by opera singers and actresses, while in Japan the *oiran* was displaced by the geisha in the eighteenth century. In both cases, the greater visibility and accessibility to the public of the new figures rendered them generally more attractive. In places like Korea and North India, where the height of courtesanship was during the early centuries of the Joseon Dynasty (1392–1910) and the centuries prior to Indian Independence (1947), respectively, the courtesan has survived into the twentieth-first century. However, the development of modern sex industries and the canonization of traditional arts have made her almost obsolete. The Renaissance courtesan nevertheless continues to fascinate scholars and learned audiences, who persistently attempt to explain her allure and rescue her traditional arts from oblivion. *See also* Prostitution.

Further Reading: Brackett, John K. "The Florentine Onestà and the Control of Prostitution, 1403–1680." *Sixteenth Century Journal* 24, no. 2 (Summer 1993): 273–300; Contogenis, Constantine, and Wolhee Choe, eds. "Introduction." In *Songs of the Kisaeng: Courtesan Poetry of the Last Korean Dynasty*, 11–24. Rochester, NY: BOA Editions, Ltd., 1997; Feldman, Martha, and Bonnie Gordon, eds. *The Courtesan's Arts: Cross-Cultural Perspectives.* New York: Oxford University Press, 2006; Lawner, Lynne. *Lives of the Courtesans: Portraits of the Renaissance.* New York: Rizzoli, 1986; Pinch, Vijay. "Gosain Tawaif: Slaves, Sex, and Ascetics in Rasdhan, ca. 1800–1857." *Modern Asian Studies* 38 (2004): 559–97; Robin, Diana. "Courtesans, Celebrity, and Print Culture in Renaissance Venice: Tullia D'Aragona, Gaspara Stampa, and Veronica Franco." In *Italian Women and the City: Essays*, edited by Janet Levarie Smarr and Daria Valentini, 35–59. Cranbury, NJ: Rosemont Publishing & Printing corp., 2003; Rosenthal, Margaret F. *The Honest Courtesan: Veronica Franco, Citizen and Writer in Sixteenth-Century Venice.* Chicago: University of Chicago Press, 1992; Seigle, Cecilia Segawa. *Yoshiwara: The Glittering World of the Japanese Courtesan.* Honolulu: University of Hawaii Press, 1993; Stortoni, Laura Anna, and Mary Prentice Lillie, eds. *Women Poets of the Italian Renaissance: Courtly Ladies and Courtesans.* New York: Italica Press, 1997; Widmer, Ellen, and Kang-I. Sung Chang, eds. *Writing Women in Late Imperial China.* Stanford, CA: Stanford University Press, 1997.

Maritere López

THE COURTIER. See *The Book of the Courtier*

CROSS-DRESSING. Early modern and Renaissance persons dressed in the clothing of the opposite sex for many pragmatic reasons exclusive of sex and gender identity. The best-known Renaissance example of a woman who cross-dressed to assume a male role was **Joan of Arc**. Whatever her specific motivation, dressing as a man helped her assume the traditionally male role of military leader and cross-dressing was one of the crimes for which she was eventually condemned to death, although ecclesiastical condemnations of female-to-male cross-dressed persons were usually much milder. (There had even been a medieval tradition of female-to-male cross-dressed saints.)

Cross-dressed females, escaping the limits and perils of the female role, were common in Renaissance literature. The disharmony between outward seeming and inward reality was almost always resolved, either through the re-assumption of female garb, as in the case of *Twelfth Night*'s Viola and several other Shakespearean heroines, or (much more rarely) through a magical or miraculous transformation into a male, as in the Elizabethan playwright John Lyly's *Gallathea*. A female-to-male cross-dresser in Chinese culture was the legendary Mulan, whose story continued to attract interest in the early modern period. Unlike Joan of Arc, Mulan donned male garb to actually pass as a man. These literary heroines reflect the reality of an unknown population of women who cross-dressed and passed as men, temporarily or permanently, to assume more lucrative careers than were ordinarily available to women or to enhance personal security in societies where unaccompanied women were often subjected to sexual violence.

Motivations for men to cross-dress were fewer, given the many advantages men held over women in early modern societies. In many theatrical traditions, including those of Europe and East Asia, women's appearance on the stage was forbidden, and young men or boys took female parts. A common plot device in European Renaissance literature, inherited from the Middle Ages, was for men to dress and pass as women for sexual access to females, as does Riciardetto in Ariosto's *Orlando Furioso*. Male-to-female cross-dressing was also found in Carnivals as part of the general practice of disguise and social inversion. In other cultures, men such as the *bissu* of the Bugis people of south Sulawesi in modern Indonesia dressed in female or gender-mixed clothing as a way of asserting religious or ritual power. Involuntary cross-dressing could be used as a form of humiliation—both the Aztec and Inca empires forced the warriors they defeated to wear female clothing.

Despite the existence of a limited space for socially sanctioned cross-dressing in European culture, Europeans in the Americas were frequently shocked by the existence of **berdaches** or two-spirit people and other socially accepted cross-dressers in Native American cultures. Spanish writers invoked cross-dressing along with **homosexuality** as evidence of Satan's rule over America before the Spanish invasion and as justification for the conquest. *See also* Hinduism; Shakespeare, William; Theater.

Further Reading: Bullough, Vern L., and Bonnie Bullough. *Cross-Dressing, Sex and Gender*. Philadelphia: University of Pennsylvania Press, 1993; Wiesner-Hanks, Merry E. *Christianity and Sexuality in the Early Modern World: Regulating Desire, Reforming Practice*. London and New York: Routledge, 2000.

William E. Burns

CUPID. *See* Eros

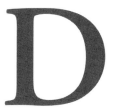

DAOISM. Daoism is one of the great indigenous religious traditions of China. It takes its name from the "Dao" or "Way," a term that denotes the cosmic ultimate. Daoist lore attributes the tradition's founding to Laozi (or Lao Dan), the archivist of the state of Zhou, who in the sixth century BCE purportedly instructed Confucius (551–479 BCE) and authored the *Daode jing*. Most historians agree that this tale is legend, however, and would accept that Daoism originated no later than the Warring States Period (450–221 BCE). At that early stage Daoism was a narrowly elite tradition exemplified by texts like the *Daode jing* and the *Zhuangzi*. In the Later Han Dynasty (25–220 CE), with the appearance of groups like the Yellow Turbans and the Celestial Masters, there first emerged a popular Daoist Church that claimed thousands of adherents and evinced the institutional structures conventionally associated with organized religion.

The Daoist Church, or perhaps more accurately, Churches (as to this day the Daoist devotional community has never been wholly practically integrated), have remained a fixture in Chinese society until the present day. The parameters of Church and Daoism, however, have never been completely identical. Throughout Chinese history a vast array of texts, ritual traditions, medical practices, art forms, macrobiotic regimens, and occult sciences have (with varying degrees of justification) come under the rubric of "Daoism." Though it is an intensely broad and overused generalization, it can basically be said that where Confucianism set the cultural patterns of Chinese elite and official society, Daoism (along with Buddhism, with which Daoism was often syncretized) laid the basis of popular culture and provided much inspiration for various countercultures.

The earliest classical texts of Daoism have little explicit to say on the subject of human sexuality. The *Zhuangzi* advocates stripping away the accrued cognitive and emotional layers of the self to arrive at a mystical state it calls "clarity"—a perfect fusion with and embodiment of the Dao. Arriving at this state requires relinquishing attachment even to life itself. Sexual desire would thus logically impede one's progress toward attaining "clarity." The *Zhuangzi* does not contain diatribes about the dangers of sexual desire, however, and it portrays the putative author of the text, Zhuang Zhou (fl. c. 300 BCE) as having been happily married.

The Daoist Church established the ideal of becoming an "immortal (*xian*)" as a religious goal for individual practitioners of the tradition. Various paths were charted to this end, but most entailed a profound personal transformation that was both psychic and physiological in nature. From its earliest inception Daoism conceived of the human being as a dynamic energy system uniting mind and body. No permanent change could be effected in one's mental state that did not simultaneously entail a shift in one's physical well-being, and vice-versa. As sexuality was a realm that implicated a broad range of cognitive, emotional, and physical responses within the dynamic energy system of the human being (and was thus perceived to be deeply implicated in the most critical vital processes), it attracted much interest and attention from Daoist theorists of self-cultivation. One of the earliest extant texts of the Celestial Masters Church, the *Xiang'er Commentary* to the *Daode jing*, gives detailed prescriptions to regulate the sexual life of the laity, dictating the frequency with which male parishioners are to have intercourse on the basis of their age.

Though the *Xiang'er Commentary* condemns such practices, it provides evidence that other early Daoist communities beyond its provenance practiced various forms of sexual yoga (generally called "the methods of the bedchamber"), a tradition that persisted throughout the history of Daoism up to the present day. Such sexual yogas were instrumental to the goal of becoming an "immortal" in two ways. On a physiological level, it was believed that one could increase and refine one's reserves of energy (*qi*) through controlled sexual contact. This type of advice was usually directed toward and composed for men. Men were instructed to engage in sex approaching but never arriving at the point of ejaculation. This technique of "semen retention" was thought to foster expansive reserves of male *yang* energy within a man's mind-body energy matrix, as semen was considered the quintessence of the *yang* force intrinsic to male sexual differentiation. Ideally the male yogin was advised to bring his female partner to orgasm, as this was understood to release *yin* energies that were vitalizing to the male form. The goal of the male yogin was thus to withhold the *yang* energies that would be of benefit to his female partner while simultaneously inducing her to release the *yin* energies that would nurture his own health and vitality. Though this theory was undeniably and callously instrumental and explicitly sexist, it did inspire a great deal of candid exploration of female sexual physiology that was wholly absent in other similarly patriarchal cultures.

On a cognitive level, sexual yoga was practiced as a form of meditation aimed at achieving psychic union with the Dao. The theory behind this practice was congruent with the various tantric traditions of India. Yogins were enjoined to engage in sexual contact in a state of mindful detachment, remaining focused on breath control and the maintenance of undisturbed consciousness. Such meditative practice was thought to aid the practitioner in breaking the powerful hold that lustful feelings may exert over the conscious mind, thus removing an intractable obstacle to spiritual perfection. Such conceptualizations were in no way incommensurate with the practice of sexual yoga as an aid to health and longevity; as mind and body were assumed to be inextricably intertwined in the same dynamic energy-system.

These forms of meditation and yoga were of course among the more esoteric dimensions of the Daoist tradition. They were an integral part of Daoism from its earliest origin, yet a variety of more prosaic concepts and practices informed many laypersons' experience of Daoism as it impacted daily sexual life. A whole complex of spells, curses, charms, amulets, and potions developed within the purview of Daoist culture that could be harnessed to sexual or procreative ends. The Daoist Church came to worship an array of gods and spirits, many of whose help could be enlisted in sexual matters. The most prominent of these was the Princess of the Azure Clouds (*Bixia yuanjun*), also know as the Sacred Mother or the Lady of Taishan. The cult of this goddess has been very popular throughout Chinese history. She is enshrined at most Daoist temples and her help is customarily sought by women requiring assistance with all aspects of childbirth.

During the Ming Dynasty (1368–1644 CE) many varying manifestations of Daoism influenced Chinese society. In major market towns, urban centers, and at sacred mountains there existed a network of officially sanctioned Daoist temples, shrines, and monasteries. The ordination of Daoist priests at these "orthodox" centers was regulated by official bureaus of the Ming imperial government. Though religious life at orthodox temples was somewhat sanitized, the officially sanctioned Daoist Church still preserved and disseminated knowledge about sexual yogic practices. The Jiajing Emperor (r. 1522–1566 CE) employed a Daoist priest, Tao Zhongwen (c. 1481–1560 CE) to teach him the arts of vitality and longevity. Tao's instruction included an intensive regimen of sexual yoga, for which he enlisted a stable of over eight hundred young virgin girls to aid in strengthening the emperor's *yang* energies.

In rural society a vast and diverse Daoist community existed beyond the realm of the state-sanctioned Daoist Church. At this social level Daoism was often very heavily syncretically mixed with Buddhism, and there was great variation in doctrine and practice from region to region. These rural Daoist devotional communities created their own vernacular sacred texts, known as *bao zhuan* or "precious volumes." Though there was much overlap between the teachings of these writings and those of the official Daoist canon, these vernacular texts most often eschewed the esoteric practices of sexual yoga and stressed more traditionally conservative values like chastity, moderation, and marital fidelity.

The Ming saw a great burgeoning of the commercial economy, lucrative market networks tied together producers and consumers in all parts of the empire and beyond. Mass-consumable commodities proliferated throughout rural and urban society, among which all manner of erotic art and literature were prevalent. Daoism left its mark on this new market culture in several ways.

Manuals were printed to instruct the purchaser in all aspects of sexual life, many of them illustrated. Some of these were narrowly focused on teaching the reader how to increase their own or their partner's sexual pleasure. Other texts made generally accessible the teachings of Daoist sexual yoga. *The Marvelous Discourses of the Plain Girl* gives practical advice on sexual performance and hygiene in the form of a dialogue between "the Plain Girl" and the Yellow Emperor, the legendary ancestral ruler of high antiquity. *The True Classic of the Complete Union* and the *Explanation of the Meaning of Cultivating the Genuine* describe regimens aimed at achieving mystical transcendence through the practice of sexual yoga. All of these texts were purchasable on the open market during the first half of the Ming, and all are informed to one extent or another by the theories of human physiology and mind-body energy dynamics developed within the long Daoist cultural tradition. During the last half of the Ming dynasty a wave of official censorship clamped down on these mass-market books, a trend that intensified during the subsequent Qing Dynasty (1644–1911). By the twentieth century most of these sexual manuals no longer survived in China and could only be found in extant printed editions in Japan.

The new literary mass market also produced a huge corpus of fiction and drama for public consumption. Novels, short stories, and plays frequently dealt with romantic or erotic themes, and Daoism provided much of the iconography and many of the themes that animated this popular literature. Novels like *The Journey to the West*, *The Romance of the Three Kingdoms*, or *The Canonization of the Gods* portrayed Daoist figures, practices, and ideas even as they influenced the religious imagination of society at large. Some of the most popular Daoist gods worshipped in temples throughout China today are figures (such as the Monkey King Sun Wukong or General Guan Yu) that were invented or made prominent by Ming era novels. *See also* Confucianism.

Further Reading: Overmyer, Daniel. *Precious Volumes: An Introduction to Chinese Sectarian Scriptures from the Sixteenth and Seventeenth Centuries.* Cambridge, MA: Harvard University Asia Center, 1999; Robinet, Isabelle. *Daoism: Growth of A Religion.* Stanford, CA: Stanford University Press, 1997; Van Gulik, R. H. *Sexual Life in Ancient China.* New ed. Leiden: Brill Academic Publishers, 2003; Wile, Douglas. *The Art of the Bedchamber: The Chinese Sexual Yoga Classics Including Women's Solo Meditation Texts.* Reprinted. Albany: State University of New York Press, 1992.

Andrew Meyer

D'ARAGONA, TULLIA (c. 1510–1556). Tullia d'Aragona was one of the more famous Italian **courtesans** of the sixteenth century. During the Italian Renaissance, many beautiful women of intelligence, refined taste, and education offered eroticism in an atmosphere of culture to rich and powerful lovers, both clerical and lay. In the process, some of these women attained fame and fortune and a measure of independence. Tullia was born in a small town near Rome between 1505 and 1510. Her mother, Giulia Campana, was an established courtesan, but it is not known whether her father was Costanzo Palmieri d'Aragona or Cardinal Luigi d'Aragona, the illegitimate grandson of King Ferdinand of Aragon. Like many other courtesans, Tullia's claim to noble birth helped to enhance her image as a courtesan, distinguishing her from a common prostitute.

Giulia Campana groomed her daughter to be a successful courtesan, and even though Tullia did not have classic good looks, her wit and accomplishments in music made her a great success, capturing the attention of many of the great literary figures of her day and using her connections with them to establish herself as a poet. Evidence shows that although she was mostly based in Rome where the tragic Filippo Strozzi was the most renowned of her lovers, she also sojourned in Siena, Florence, Ferrara, Bologna, and Venice at various times in her life. It was in Ferrara that she met Girolamo Muzio, who encouraged her writing career and became her literary mentor and editor. In 1543 in Siena, she married Silvestro Guicciardi of Ferrara but nothing else is known about him. Nevertheless, he proved useful to Tullia, for when the Sienese authorities ordered her to wear the distinguishing emblem of a prostitute, she was able to successfully appeal on the grounds that she was a married woman. Once again, in her subsequent move to Florence in 1547, she was denounced to the Office of Decency as a prostitute and ordered to wear the required yellow veil. This time she appealed for exemption to Duke Cosimo de'Medici through the intercession of his wife, Eleanor of Toledo. Cosimo recommended that the Office of Decency "be merciful to her as a poet."

In Florence, Tullia was really able to attain status as a poet; through the help of the writer Benedetto Varchi, she published a volume of her *rime*, or lyric poetry, that same year. Her book of poems included forty-nine of her own poems as well as poetry either dedicated to her or in which she featured. Following up on this success, she published her *Dialogues on the Infinity of Love*, a Neo-Platonism debate, which she dedicated to Duke Cosimo in gratitude for his intervention on her behalf. The literati of the day frequented her literary salon, but, mysteriously, at the height of her newly established career, she unexpectedly left Florence for Rome where she lived in seclusion and poverty until her death in 1556. During this time she wrote her last work, an unfinished epic poem, *Il Meschino, altremente detto il Guerrino*, which was published posthumously in 1560. In this work, her hero Guerrino, in the tradition of the heroic quest, journeys far and wide on a personal odyssey to find his parents. D'Aragona's lyric poetry represents a genre through which women became increasingly accepted as writers in the late Renaissance. *See also* Prostitution.

Further Reading: Masson, Georgina. "Tullia d'Aragona, Intellectual Courtesan." In *Courtesans of the Italian Renaissance*, edited by G. Masson, 91–131. London: Secker and Warburg, 1975; Pallitto, Elizabeth A., ed. and trans. *Sweet Fire: Tullia d'Aragona's Poetry of Dialogue and Selected Prose*. New York: George Braziller, 2006; Russell, Rinaldina. "Tullia d'Aragona." In *Italian Women Writers*, edited by R. Russell, 26–34. London: Greenwood, 1994.

Mary Hewlett

DIANE DE POITIERS (1499–1566). As the mistress of King Henry II of France (r. 1547–1559), Diane de Poitiers, the daughter of minor nobility, was a figure of great influence at the French court, where she often held the balance of power between political factions. Although her position depended solely on the favor of the king, Diane, through her beauty, wit, and sexuality remained Henry's most trusted advisor and confidant for over twenty years.

In 1514, Diane, then only fifteen, married Louis de Brézé, the seneschal of Normandy, by whom she had two daughters. After the death of her husband in 1531, Diane remained at the notoriously licentious court of Francis I (r. 1515–1547), where her exceptional beauty made her the subject of many rumors, including claims that she was sexually involved with the king and with various prominent courtiers. Because most of these rumors emanated from the circle surrounding the royal mistress, Anne d'Heilly, duchess of Etampes, it is now difficult to determine how much truth they contained. At some time in the 1530s, Diane formed a close connection with Henry, the king's second son, who became dauphin (heir to the French throne) upon the death of his elder brother in 1536. Although several court observers, including the Venetian ambassador, Marino Cavalli, claimed that Henry's attachment to Diane was platonic, other evidence suggests that the couple began a sexual relationship in about 1538, when he was nineteen and she thirty-eight.

Upon Henry's accession to the throne in 1547, Diane immediately replaced Etampes as the nexus of favor and influence at court. Besides the lands and jewels confiscated from Etampes, Diane received numerous other gifts of titles and property, including the royal château of Chenonceaux. In October 1548, the king granted Diane the highest dignity available to nonroyal ladies, creating her duchess of Valentinois, which title allowed her to stand with the women of the royal family at the 1549 coronation of Henry's wife, Catherine de'Medici. Although the duchess was astute enough never to openly challenge the queen's position—she even nursed the queen when Catherine was ill and encouraged the king to sleep with his wife—Diane's political influence was far greater than that usually exercised by a royal mistress. In 1547, an envoy of the duke of Ferrara reported that the king spent a third of each day with Diane, to whom he gave a full account of any state business he had transacted. On one occasion, Henry sat on Diane's lap and fondled her breasts while encouraging the

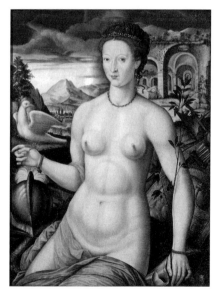

Diane de Poitiers in *Allegory of Peace*, by Giovanni Capacin, c. 1568–1570. © The Art Archive/Musée Granet Aix-en-Provence/Dagli Orti.

assembled courtiers to remark upon her beauty. The extent of the duchess's influence was most fully symbolized by the rebuilding of Anet, an ancient manor that had belonged to her husband's family and that she transformed into one the glories of French Renaissance architecture.

The duchess sought to disguise the sexual nature of her relationship with the king by encouraging her identification with Diana, the chaste goddess of the hunt, a policy that resulted in Jean Goujon's *Diana the Huntress*, the most famous of many artworks, including several nude depictions, which took Diane as their subject. The duchess was also the subject of much laudatory poetry, and a group of court poets, known as the Pléiade, sought and won her patronage. Diane's influence came to a complete and abrupt end in July 1559, when Henry died of wounds received during a royal joust. Kept from the king's deathbed by the queen, Diane left court before Henry's death, which resulted in her own and her daughters' banishment from court. Forced to return the jewels given to her by Henry and to sell Chenonceaux to the queen, Diane lived quietly at Anet until her death in 1566. *See also* Mistresses.

Further Reading: Baumgartner, Frederic J. *Henry II, King of France, 1547–1559*. Durham, NC: Duke University Press, 1988; Cloulas, Ivan. *Diane de Poitiers*. Paris: Fayard, 1997 (French-language work); Ffolliott, Sheila. "Casting a Rival into the Shade: Catherine de Medici and Diane de Poitiers." *Art Journal* 48 (1989): 138–43; MacRae, Margaret J. "Diane de Poitiers and Mme de Clèves: A Study of Women's Roles, the Victim and the Conqueror." *Papers on French Seventeenth Century Literature* 12, no. 23 (1985): 559–73; Strage, Mark. *Women of Power: The Life and Times of Catherine dé Medici*. New York: Harcourt Brace Jovanovich, 1976.

John A. Wagner

DÍAZ DEL CASTILLO, BERNAL (c. 1495–1584).

Bernal Díaz del Castillo, a soldier, conquistador, and chronicler of the Spanish conquest of the Aztec Empire of Mexico, was born and educated in Medina del Campo, Castile, Spain. The son of María Díez Rejón and Francisco Díaz del Castillo, a *regidor* or city councilor, Díaz del Castillo came from a respectable but not a moneyed family. Little is known about the childhood of Díaz del Castillo who had an elder brother whom he admired. In 1514, Díaz del Castillo left Spain to seek adventure and fortune in the New World. After serving under Pedro Arias de Ávila in present-day Cuba, Díaz del Castillo joined two early explorations of the coast of Mexico, then known as New Spain. On both expeditions, in 1517 and 1518, attacks by native inhabitants forced the explorers to return to Cuba, from where Díaz del Castillo decided to sail with Pedro de Alvarado and Hernán Cortés on their 1519 expedition to Mexico. In spite of the losses they suffered at the hands of hostile natives, the explorers decided to march inland, to Mexico-Tenochtitlán, the Aztec capital, in search of the legendary riches of Montezuma, the Aztec ruler.

Arriving in Mexico-Tenochtitlán, Díaz del Castillo was greatly impressed by the beautiful cities, towns, temples, palaces, and waterways that graced the majestic Aztec capital. Díaz del Castillo, who was one of the soldiers who jailed Montezuma, was present throughout the siege of Mexico-Tenochtitlán, which ended in August 1521 when the city was captured by the Spaniards. After the fall of Mexico-Tenochtitlán, Díaz del Castillo traveled with Cortés to Honduras before returning to Mexico. In 1539, he wrote a sworn declaration of his services to the Crown of Spain. This affidavit, or "*Información de Servicios y Méritos*," was the beginning of Díaz del Castillo's monumental work on the discovery and conquest of Mexico, the *Historia verdadera de la conquista de la Nueva España* (*True History of the Conquest of New Spain*).

Díaz del Castillo fathered numerous illegitimate offspring by Indian women in both Mexico and Guatemala, where he settled about 1541. In Guatemala, where he became a *regidor*, he married Teresa Becerra, a Castilian widow with whom he had nine sons. Assumedly in an attempt to gain favor from the Crown and earn a better fortune for himself, Díaz del Castillo began writing his chronicle of the Conquest of Mexico, which he became determined to complete after reading the misrepresentations in the account of the Conquest that was written by Francisco López de Gomara, whose work Castillo criticized as being erroneous and unworthy of belief.

In 1575, Díaz del Castillo sent a version of his manuscript to Madrid, where it was later altered by Friar Alonso Remón of the Order of Mercy. First published in Madrid in 1632, other editions and translations of the book followed. In 1904, the Mexican historian Génaro García published an authentic version of the chronicle based on Díaz del Castillo's original manuscript, which had been uncovered in Guatemala. Completed in 1572, Díaz del Castillo's *True History of the Conquest of New Spain* focuses mainly on the conquest of the Aztec Empire, 1519–1521. It is an exciting eyewitness account of intrigue, adventure, war and conquest. In spite of its inaccuracies, it is considered to be the most reliable source of information on the history of the Conquest of Mexico. Díaz del Castillo, who emphasized in his chronicle that he was writing the sacred truth, died in Guatemala City, Guatemala, and is believed to be buried in the Cathedral of Santiago de Guatemala. *See also* Americas (North and South).

Further Reading: Cerwin, Herbert. *Bernal Díaz: Historian of the Conquest.* Norman: University of Oklahoma Press, 1963; Díaz del Castillo, Bernal. *The Discovery and Conquest of Mexico, 1517–1521.* Reprint ed. New York: Da Capo Press, 2004; Thomas, Hugh. *Conquest: Montezuma, Cortés, and the Fall of Old Mexico.* New York: Simon and Schuster, 1993.

Ronna S. Feit

DIVORCE. There were few changes in attitudes toward and the practice of divorce in the non-European world in the fifteenth and sixteenth centuries. In **Europe**, however, the Protestant **Reformation** led to changes in the law and practice of **marriage** and divorce that paved the way to cultures of mass divorce that appeared later in the millennium.

Among the social and theological issues taken up by critics of the Church in the fifteenth century, and pressed more forcefully by reformers who broke with the Catholic Church in the sixteenth century, were the canon laws relating to marriage and divorce. Although various Church councils and authorities had permitted divorce under limited circumstances (for example, in 465 CE, the Council of Vannes allowed **remarriage** after a divorce for reason of **adultery**), canon law had effectively banned divorce by 1300. The only remedy permitted for marital offenses was a separation, which allowed spouses to live apart, but prohibited sexual relationships with others or remarriage.

Arguing that the Bible should be interpreted as allowing divorce, various sixteenth-century reformers legalized divorce in those parts of Europe where Protestant churches were established. The most important models were put forward by John **Calvin** (who was most influential in Switzerland, the Netherlands, and Scotland) and Martin **Luther** (Germany and Scandinavia). Calvin was relatively restrictive, arguing that the prime offense justifying divorce was adultery, although he included desertion on the ground that a man or woman who deserted a spouse would almost certainly commit adultery while away. Luther also started with adultery and desertion, but expanded the list of grounds for divorce to include behavior such as a wife persistently refusing her husband intercourse, because, he thought, it placed the husband in danger of committing adultery.

Other sixteenth-century reformers adopted more liberal positions. The most liberal was Martin Bucer, whose teachings on divorce became law in the city of Strasbourg. Starting from the view that marriage was essentially an emotional relationship, Bucer argued that a marriage that lacked love or sexual fidelity could be dissolved by divorce because there was no true marriage. Bucer's teachings effectively recognized divorce by mutual consent, but he also allowed divorce for a range of specific matrimonial offenses that included marital violence and witchcraft.

Divorce laws reflecting the teachings of the most influential reformers were enacted throughout Protestant Europe from the 1520s, and courts (some secular, some ecclesiastical, some mixed) were established to grant divorces. The number of divorces was small, however, and the success rate of divorce petitions was generally low. The judges of Zurich granted twenty-eight of eighty petitions between 1525 and 1531 (an average of five a year), while in Basel between 1550 and 1592, 125 of 226 petitions succeeded (three a year).

The major exception to the legalization of divorce in Protestant Europe was England. Ironically, because the break with the Church of Rome came about because the pope refused to allow **Henry VIII** an **annulment** so he could marry again, the Church of England refused to permit divorce. With that exception, the early modern period saw divorce gain a foothold in much of Europe in a manner that provided the basis for its liberalization and later legalization in other countries. *See also* Witches.

Further Reading: Ozment, Steven. *When Fathers Ruled: Family Life in Reformation Europe.* Cambridge, MA: Harvard University Press, 1983; Phillips, Roderick. *Putting Asunder: A History of Divorce in Western Society.* New York: Cambridge University Press, 1988.

Roderick Phillips

DOMESTIC VIOLENCE.   Only in the last quarter of the twentieth century has the term "domestic violence" come into being; the early modern period did not require such a term because what twenty-first-century readers recognize (and criminalize) as domestic violence would then have been understood as relatively normal behavior. Physical and non-physical acts, which now would be understood as abusive, were often used in the early modern period by the head of the household to maintain proper obedient behavior from any subordinate, be it his wife, child, or servant of either gender.

Despite this, there were limitations on male heads of households. While Christian commentators, for example, always upheld the supreme authority of the father/husband, who demanded absolute obedience from his subordinates, these writers also set limits on corporal punishment by advising husbands not to discipline a subordinate in a rage or to use overly harsh punishment for a minor fault. English conduct books and sermons of the late sixteenth century register a growing concern about a husband's unlimited use of physical violence to "correct" or "chastise" his wife's behavior. In *The Homily of the State of Matrimony* (customarily read at Anglican weddings c. 1563–1640), the anonymous author takes up the issue of what modern readers would consider domestic violence by advocating that men find other means than wife-beating to keep women subordinate. Although *The Homily* never says that men do not have the right to use physical violence, it advocates that a husband resist using it because it does not achieve the desired effect (a wife's subordination). While sermons and conduct books signal a change in attitude toward using corporal discipline to correct wives, they do not express the same concern about the use of physical correction with the other common members of the domestic household, such as servants and children. By the end of the early modern period, men still had the legal right to use physical force against their subordinates, as long as it was not lethal. Status seems to have had a greater impact than gender in terms of who might be the victim of domestic violence. While wives might be the object of physical correction from their husbands, some women were also authorized to use physical correction with other household subordinates.

Scholars find it difficult to judge the extent of domestic violence in the period because most cases only made it to court when severe injury, disturbance, or death had taken place. In the case of lethal domestic violence, status also played an important role in terms of punishment; when men killed their wives they were guilty of murder, but women who killed their husbands and servants who killed their masters were charged with petty treason and punished as such. Social historians debate whether or not there was more domestic violence than there is now, but surviving evidence, including numerous examples from imaginative literature, suggest that marital violence was a topic of interest, and perhaps debate, rather than taken for granted as the norm. *See also* Divorce; Rape.

Further Reading: Amussen, Susan Dwyer. "'Being Stirred to Much Unquietness': Violence and Domestic Violence in Early Modern England." *Journal of Women's History* 6 (1994): 70–89; Brundage, James. "Domestic Violence in Classical Canon Law." In *Violence in Medieval Society*, edited by Richard W. Kaeuper, 183–95. Rochester, NY: Boydell Press, 2000; Detmer-Goebel, Emily. "Civilizing Subordination: Domestic Violence and *The Taming of the Shrew.*" *Shakespeare Quarterly* 48 (1997): 273–94; Dolan, Frances E. *Dangerous Familiars: Representations of Domestic Crime in England, 1500–1700.* Ithaca, NY: Cornell University Press, 1994; Gowing, Laura. *Domestic Dangers: Women, Words, and Sex in Early Modern London.* Oxford: Clarendon Press, 1996; Hanawalt, Barbara A. "Violence in the Domestic Milieu of Late Medieval England." In *Violence in Medieval Society*, edited by Richard W. Kaeuper, 197–214. Rochester, NY: Boydell Press, 2000; Hunt, Margaret. "Wife Beating, Domesticity and Women's Independence in Eighteenth-Century London." *Gender and History* 4 (1992): 10–33; Salisbury, Eve, Georgiana Donavan, and Merral Llewelyn Price, eds. *Domestic Violence in Medieval Texts.* Gainesville: University Press of Florida, 2002; Walker, Gathine. *Crime, Gender, and Social Order in Early Modern England.* New York: Cambridge University Press, 2003.

Emily Detmer-Goebel

DONA MARINA. *See* La Malinche

DOWRY. In early modern Europe, a dowry comprised the money, goods, or property that a woman brought to her husband at the time of **marriage**. Since a woman's dowry in most cases represented her share of her family inheritance, the dowry system limited a daughter's claims to her family's wealth. However, payment of a dowry also permitted the woman's family to forge social, political, or economic bonds with her husband's family, connections calculated to increase the wealth or power of both families.

Regulations for the handling of dowries are found in the Code of Hammurabi from the second millennium BCE, and dowries were a common part of Greek and Roman marriages. The practice lapsed during the early Middle Ages, but by the twelfth century had been revived and become an important facet of marriage throughout most of Europe, particularly among the propertied classes. By the sixteenth century, daughters who were not their father's heirs, and thus could bring no landed property to their marriages, were expected instead to bring a large sum of cash known as a "portion." In England and elsewhere, the portion went directly to the groom's father, who often used it to provide dowries for his own daughters. Upon receipt of the dowry, the groom's father promised to provide the bride, should she outlive her husband and remain unmarried, an annuity known as a "jointure," which freed the bride's family from supporting her in widowhood. In this way, early modern marriage, especially among the upper classes, involved a significant transfer of real or personal wealth.

When a dowry came in the form of land, it technically remained the wife's property for life, although the husband had the managing of it during his lifetime. At her death, such real property passed on to her heirs, male or female (if local practice permitted the latter to inherit), and not to any children her husband might have by other wives. Depending on local customs, the wife might also possess other property, usually left to her by her father, outside the dowry; such property, again depending on prevailing tradition, might be devisable by will to heirs of the woman's choosing. Among the non-propertied classes, whether the poor of the towns or the peasantry, dowry arrangements might be less formal, but women were still expected to bring some tangible property to the marriage, even if only furniture, jewelry, or cooking utensils and other household items.

The dowry system had a number of important consequences for propertied society in early modern Europe. Because only husbands from families of a similar social or economic status were suitable recipients of the dowry payment and had fathers of sufficient means to provide an acceptable jointure, marriages to persons outside one's economic class were socially unacceptable and quite rare. Also, the system gave great power to male heads of families in controlling the marriages of their children, younger sons as well as daughters, who were dependent upon their fathers for dowry and jointure arrangements. Marriages were largely arranged by parents, mostly fathers, and not by the children themselves. Dowry arrangements were often settled by the parents before the prospective bride and groom had even met one another. Early modern society made no distinction between a marriage based on interest—e.g., for money, power, or social status—and one based on love or sexual attraction. Love and romance were held to be irrational grounds for marriage, which instead was considered a means by which the family as a whole could increase its wealth, social standing, or political influence. Finally, while daughters could be a financial drain on a family, useful mainly for cementing political or social connections, wealthy wives for sons, and especially rich widows, were much sought after valuable commodities. Families seeking a suitable wife for a son often employed a marriage broker to commence negotiations with the woman's family.

Dowry systems also existed outside Europe in the early modern period, particularly in China, where, by the sixteenth century, the practice was quite ancient. Traditional Confucian society prevented women from inheriting property, so the dowry system allowed Chinese families to provide some support for daughters. Because it was considered shameful for a man to have to rely for support on his wife's property or income, a Chinese husband usually had less control over his wife's dowry than did his European counterpart. However, custom often limited what the wife could do with her dowry, stipulating the best uses for such funds, primarily the education or livelihood of the eldest son. In India where the practice of giving dowries was common under British rule, the dowry system did not exist prior to the beginning of the British ascendancy in the eighteenth century. *See also* Confucianism; Remarriage/Widows.

Further Reading: Basu, Srimati, ed. *Dowry and Inheritance*. London: Zed Books, 2005; Macfarlane, Alan. *Marriage and Love in England 1300–1840*. Oxford: Blackwell, 1993; Molho, Anthony. *Marriage Alliance in Late Medieval Florence*. Cambridge, MA: Harvard University Press, 1994; Stone, Lawrence. *The Family, Sex and Marriage: In England 1500–1800*. New York: Harper and Row, 1977.

John A. Wagner

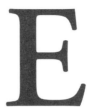

ELIZABETH I, QUEEN OF ENGLAND (1533–1603). The daughter of **Henry VIII** and Anne Boleyn, Elizabeth I, the last Tudor monarch of England, was one of the most successful female rulers in history. Coming to the throne in an age when women were considered unfit to govern a kingdom and queens were expected to take a husband to exercise power on their behalf, Elizabeth remained unmarried. By encouraging creation of a secular political cult celebrating her **virginity**, Elizabeth made her gender and **celibacy** the focus of devotion and service for the men through whom she ran her kingdom. In doing this, she presided over an age of advancement in English government, trade, exploration, and literature, and made herself one of England's most effective and beloved monarchs.

Because she never in adult life made mention of her mother, some historians argue that Elizabeth was psychologically scarred by the knowledge that her father had ordered her mother's execution. However, being not yet three at her mother's death, Elizabeth can have had few memories of Anne. Of far more importance, especially for the development of Elizabeth's attitudes toward **marriage** and sex, were the inappropriate sexual advances directed to her when she was in her middle teens by the handsome and charming Thomas Seymour, Lord Seymour, her half-brother's maternal uncle. After the death of Henry VIII, Seymour married the Henry's last queen, Katherine Parr, who had taken Elizabeth into her household. A reckless and provocative man who was engaged in various plots to increase his influence, Seymour often entered Elizabeth's bedchamber in the early morning while she was still in her nightclothes. On one occasion, during a romp in the garden, Seymour cut the princess's gown to ribbons while Katherine held her fast. In 1548, Katherine, having caught her husband and her ward in a compromising embrace, sent Elizabeth to live elsewhere. However, when Katherine died in **childbirth** in September 1548, Seymour proposed marriage to the princess. Although clearly attracted to Seymour, Elizabeth was wise enough to reject the marriage suit. When Seymour was executed in 1549, Elizabeth saved herself from being implicated in his treason by steadfastly refusing to admit any wrongdoing. One modern historian has argued from this episode that Elizabeth would today be considered a victim of child sexual abuse and a candidate for psychological counseling.

After Elizabeth's accession in 1558, following a dangerous period during the reign of her half-sister Mary I, her marriage became an important political issue. Because a woman was thought unable to lead armies—the oldest function of a monarch—and unable, because of mental incapacity, to exercise the full authority of a man—one

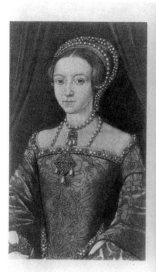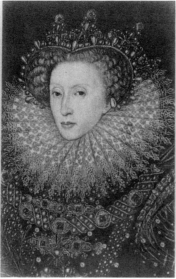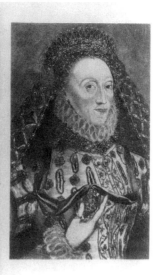

Undated portraits of Elizabeth I. Courtesy of the Library of Congress.

Elizabethan minister thought diplomatic dispatches "too much for a woman's knowledge" (Haigh, 9)—Elizabeth was universally expected to marry, and her ministers and Parliament frequently urged her to do so. It was believed that a queen needed a male consort to help her rule and, even more important, that Elizabeth needed a (preferably male) heir to secure the succession. Many suitors presented themselves, including Philip II of Spain, Erik XIV of Sweden, various Austrian archdukes, and the future **Henry III** of France and his brother the duke of Alençon, but all were eventually rejected for various political or religious reasons. Although she had promised to marry, Elizabeth seemed in no hurry to do so.

Were she not a queen for whom marriage was such a complicated undertaking, Elizabeth would likely have married Robert Dudley, future earl of Leicester, the great love of her life. In January 1559, only weeks after her accession, Elizabeth named Dudley Master of Horse, a position that gave him access to the queen and made him a regular companion when she rode or hunted. By April of 1559, Dudley was in such high favor that gossip concerning the nature of their relationship was beginning to spread throughout the court and the country. Rumors began to circulate that Dudley planned to poison his wife, Amy Robsart, and so free himself to marry the queen. When scurrilous rumors about Elizabeth and Dudley were heard at foreign courts, Elizabeth's reputation both at home and abroad began to suffer. Although most contemporaries assumed that the queen and Dudley were involved in a sexual relationship, Elizabeth later denied it and it is now impossible to determine the truth.

On September 8, 1560, at the height of these fears and rumors, Dudley's wife was found dead at the foot of her stairs. The timing of this event was devastating to Dudley's ambitions and the queen's good name. Although a careful investigation led to an official verdict of accidental death, a verdict accepted by most modern historians, rumors that Dudley was involved in murder, or at least some sort of cover-up, continued to dog him for the rest of his life. The queen lessened the intensity of her relationship with Dudley after October 1560, but he remained the royal favorite until his death in

1588, and Elizabeth was clearly attracted more to him than to any other man. Although Dudley thereafter tried in various ways to convince the queen to marry him, including scheming with foreign ambassadors, creating a domestic political following, and commissioning plays and entertainments that set forward his merits as a husband, Elizabeth had decided that even though she loved Dudley, she was unwilling to share her throne with him.

By 1580, with the queen past the age of forty and her childbearing years ending, the cult of the Virgin Queen, which celebrated Elizabeth's celibacy, began to be developed. In 1578, a series of plays and masques performed during Elizabeth's annual progress praised the queen's virginity by making frequent reference to the Virgin Mary and the chaste goddess Diana. In 1579, the poet Edmund Spenser employed allegorical imagery that did the same in his *Shepheardes Calender*. During the 1580s, a series of portraits appeared showing Elizabeth holding a sieve, the symbol of the Roman vestal virgins, who were renowned for their **chastity**. Where the knightly ideal of chivalry had dedicated itself to the Virgin Mary and the devotion and protection of chaste femininity, Elizabethan courtiers dedicated themselves to the service and protection of a ruler who was not only a woman, but a virgin. The cult of the Virgin Queen allowed Elizabeth to identify herself with the state and to channel the touchy pride and ready violence of her courtiers away from disorder and into controlled competition for her favor. Beginning with an element of romance between the queen and favored courtiers like Dudley, the cult of the Virgin Queen became, by Elizabeth's later years, almost a form of worship, with the name and idea of Elizabeth, England's Gloriana, inspiring men to fight, write, and explore.

Elizabeth's last intimate relationship was with a man more than thirty years her junior, Robert Devereux, earl of Essex, and Robert Dudley's handsome stepson. The queen's relationship with Essex was based on his connection with Dudley and on the pleasure his lively company gave an aging woman. Although rumor claimed a sexual relationship for the couple, this is less likely to be true than in Dudley's case. In any event, by the end of the reign, assumptions about the basis of Dudley's special position, and the queen's open use of sexual byplay to show favor, led most male courtiers to play the public role of Elizabeth's ardent suitor. Essex achieved the status of favorite by playing this role more fully than most; nonetheless, in 1601, when he rose in rebellion against the political limits Elizabeth placed on him, she consented to his execution. *See also* The Reformation; Shakespeare, William.

Further Reading: Erickson, Carolly. *The First Elizabeth*. New York: Summit Books, 1983; Haigh, Christopher. *Elizabeth I*. 2nd ed. London: Longman, 2000; Haynes, Alan. *Sex in Elizabethan England*. Stroud, England: Sutton Publishing, 1999; Johnson, Paul. *Elizabeth I*. New York: Holt, Rinehart and Winston, 1974; Levin, Carole. *The Heart and Stomach of a King: Elizabeth I and the Politics of Sex and Power*. Philadelphia: University of Pennsylvania Press, 1994; MacCaffrey, Wallace. *Elizabeth I*. London: Edward Arnold, 1993; Neale, J. E. *Queen Elizabeth I*. Chicago: Academy Chicago Publishers, 1992; Wagner, John A. *Historical Dictionary of the Elizabethan World*. Phoenix: Oryx Press, 1999.

John A. Wagner

EROS. Also referred to as Cupid or *Amor*, Eros, the god of **love** and desire, is a figure from classical Greek and Roman mythology. Defining Eros was a difficult task in the Renaissance, since ancient sources did not agree concerning his exact genealogy. In his *De Natura Deorum* Cicero identified at least three different Cupids: one is the son of Mercury and Diana, another the child of Mercury and Venus, and the third is the offspring of Mars and Venus. This ambiguity was registered in the Renaissance; it carried over into Boccaccio's *Genealogie Deorum Gentilium*, one of the most complete and commonly-referred-to Renaissance compilations of ancient myth.

Eros is, foremost, the embodiment of all attractions that provoke love. He is young and beautiful, and usually described as having wings, a bow, and arrows. As in Raphael Sanzio's *Loggia of Cupid and Psyche* (Rome, Villa Farnesina), Eros is often accompanied by a number of infantile *putti*. These "spirits of love," however, are distinct from Eros; they are not figures in ancient mythology, but arose from a distinctly Renaissance formulation of erotic desire.

There are two distinct Renaissance conceptualizations of Eros; the poetic and the philosophical. On the one hand, the poets were primarily concerned with exploring the destabilizing psychological effects of Eros upon the lover, underlining the deceptive power of love and the conflicting nature of the lover's desire; on the other hand, philosophers sought to understand Eros as an abstraction, a cosmic force that animated all of creation with passion and desire.

The personification of Eros was integral to the rise of vernacular poetry in the late medieval period. Cupid played a central role in French Provençal poetry, the *dolce stil novo*, and the later poetry of Petrarch and Boccaccio. Following the characterization of Eros set forth in many ancient texts, particularly the *Greek Anthology*, Renaissance poets envisioned Cupid as a cruel adolescent, intent upon widely spreading the pain of unrequited love.

Love, as it was understood in the Renaissance, was caused by excessive meditation (*immoderata cogitatione*) on the image of the beloved: it was a physical malady that sickened both the body and the soul (*see* **Love Sickness**). In response to the perturbations of love there arose a tradition of polemical writing attacking Eros. Thinkers such as Baptista Mantuanus, Battista Fregoso, and Pietro Edo, advised their readers to avoid Eros in order to preclude the mental perturbations that accompany erotic desire. This train of thought finds a visual counterpart in the iconography of the crucified cupid, showing victims of Eros who, having turned upon the adolescent god, now torture him.

To counter this negative understanding of Eros, others attempted a recuperation of Eros by regarding Love as a unitary principle, a power that animated creation with a desire (*voluptas*) that is essential to all living beings. This divergent conception of Eros was drawn out of the tradition of the Orphic Hymns (and Lucretius's *De Rerum Natura*), offering a "natural," demiurgic understanding of Eros, as in Mario Equicola's 1525 treatise *De natura de amore*; alternatively Eros could be understood as a Platonic manifestation of Divine Love, as in Marsilio Ficino's *Commentary on Plato's Symposium* from 1469.

A number of Renaissance commentaries on Eros took the form of Platonic dialogues, presenting arguments *in utramque partem*; the most famous examples of the dialogue format are Pietro Bembo's *Gli Asolani* (1505) and Baldassare Castiglione's **The Book of the Courtier** (1528).

According to Renaissance mythography Eros also had a brother, Anteros. It is often wrongly assumed that they symbolize the diametric opposition between sacred and profane Love, respectively. While this reading of Anteros was put forward by a number of authors including Hedo, Fregoso, and Andrea Alciati, it was forcefully countered Celio Calcagnini, who argued that Anteros was not the god of sacred Love, but rather love-returned: Eros symbolizes the initiation of the desire, while Anteros represents its reciprocation. Artistically this reading can be seen in countless representations of the infants Eros and Anteros who are shown playfully wrestling with one another, as in Annibale Carracci's frescoed ceiling in the Galleria Farnese in Rome.

Further Reading: Beecher, D., and M. Ciavolella, eds. *Eros and Anteros: The Medical Traditions of Love in the Renaissance.* Toronto: Dovehouse, 1992; Campbell, Stephen J. *The Cabinet of Eros: Renaissance Mythological Painting and the Studiolo of Isabella d'Este.* New Haven, CT: Yale University Press, 2006; Dempsey, Charles. *Inventing the Renaissance Putto.* Chapel Hill and London: University of North Carolina Press, 2001; Merril, Robert V. "Eros and Anteros." *Speculum* XIX (1944): 265–84; Nelson, John Charles. *Renaissance Theory of Love: The Context of Giordano Bruno's Eroici Furori.* New York: Columbia University Press, 1958; Randolph, Adrian. *Engaging Symbols: Gender, Politics, and Public Art in Fifteenth-Century Florence.* New Haven, CT: Yale University Press, 2002.

Christopher J. Nygren

EUNUCHS. Castrated males, or eunuchs, played many roles in the Renaissance. In many polities, particularly in China, Islamic lands, and Byzantium, they exercised great political influence through their connections to courts.

The Ming dynasty in China made extraordinarily heavy use of eunuch royal servants as generals, admirals, arms manufacturers, trade supervisors, mining superintendents, engineers, and judges. The eunuch admiral Zheng led the massive Chinese expeditions in the Indian Ocean in the early fifteenth century (*see* **Chinese Treasure Fleets**). Self-castration became a common strategy for desperate men seeking Imperial employment, despite Imperial prohibitions. The Ming dynasty's heavy reliance on eunuchs was condemned by Confucian scholars and officials, who always suspected prominent eunuchs of being unprincipled tools of Imperial power. The fourteenth-century founder of the Ming, Hongzi, had promised not to employ eunuchs in politically sensitive roles, a promise he quickly broke.

In Islamic societies, the keeping of **harems** was traditionally entrusted to eunuchs. Following the conquest of Constantinople in 1453, the Ottoman sultans adopted the Byzantine tradition of entrusting powerful court offices to eunuchs. The chief harem-keeper of the Ottoman Empire was the Lord of the Black Eunuchs, while contacts between the Sultan's court and the outside world were regulated by the Lord of the White Eunuchs. Eunuch officials were not restricted to the court and harem, but served as military leaders and administrators throughout the Islamic regions. In both Islamic societies and China, eunuchs were often members of peripheral or foreign ethnic groups. Much of the Indian Ocean African slave trade was devoted to supplying courts with eunuchs. The Caucasus was another source of slave-eunuchs.

Although Latin Europe lacked court eunuchs and eunuch officials, eunuchs played an important role in music as castrati. To become castrati, talented boys would be castrated as youths, before their voices changed. The singers, as adults, were able to combine high vocal registers with masculine force. Castrati were particularly associated with Italian church music because Italian choirs excluded female singers, and the Renaissance saw a growing use of castrati because they displaced boy singers and falsettists from the papal choirs. Castration was supposedly forbidden by church law (and eunuchs were barred from the priesthood), but continued anyway.

Some societies accorded eunuchs a sacred status. In the Indian *hijra* community, males (not all of whom were castrated) who adopted female garments were associated with a particular Hindu goddess, Bahucarah Mata, although some *hijra* were Muslim. The sacrifice of the male organs was interpreted as a powerful act of ascetic self-denial that brought spiritual power. The *hijra* functioned as a **caste** in India's corporatist society and supported themselves partly as entertainers during family celebrations. In **Islam**, the traditional guardians of Mohammed's tomb in Medina were the Eunuchs of the Prophet, a group whose origin dates back to the twelfth century. The Eunuchs of the Prophet were the only ones allowed to enter the tomb. *See also* Castration; Christianity; Confucianism; Hinduism.

Further Reading: Marmon, Shaun. *Eunuchs and Sacred Boundaries in Islamic Society*. New York: Oxford University Press, 1999; Tsai, Shih-Shan Henry. *The Eunuchs in the Ming Dynasty*. New York: State University of New York Press, 1996.

William E. Burns

EUROPE.   Amidst war, famine, disease, and religious conflict European civilization in the early modern period became increasingly urban, literate, and stratified. The early modern period of European history is marked by dramatic upheavals and, at the same time, continuities that reach back to medieval and classical traditions. This new age of the **printing** press, was also the age of exploration and conquest, as well as the age that saw the formation of nation states, and soon-to-be empires, out of principalities and republics. Governments and churches aimed to control and censor the people in an effort to sustain and enhance themselves. Through the first decades of the sixteenth century, all parties, except Jewish communities, worshipped at the Catholic Church. Protestants like Martin **Luther** offered their criticism and forged new Christian churches for society. The religious divide and turmoil of the Protestant **Reformation** and the Catholic Counter-Reformation menaced Europe for centuries to come.

Culturally, there was a divide, too. When scholars refer to a Renaissance, they are describing a renewal of ancient Greek and Roman letters that humanists recovered and revitalized. This important intellectual movement was conducted by wealthy men (and a few women) and sponsored by elite patrons. The elite, middling kind, and poor experienced the Renaissance in extremely different ways because of their differing means and access to books, art, antiquities, theater, and opera.

*S*TUDIA *H*UMANITATIS**.**   The *studia humanitatis* was an academic program that included the study of history, poetry, rhetoric, moral philosophy, and logic in Latin and, sometimes, Greek. Through this intellectual program, scholars reexamined a multitude of themes including the dignity of humankind, the worth of women, and the possibility of free will. In their answers, Renaissance writers displayed a new attitude toward life and the human condition. Scholars such as Pico della Mirandola found that "man" or human beings were the measure of all things—capable, even, of experiencing the divine and carrying out divine works. In sum, humanists and Renaissance philosophers did not take the tradition of knowledge for granted; they looked at matters critically and often amended heretofore accepted doctrine.

Begun in Italy and soon spread north of the Alps, humanism served governments, churches, and powerful individuals to help enhance images and create persuasive messages to the governed, or the faithful. Even science found a renewal in old traditions: Copernicus, Kepler, Galileo, and Newton among others, used Greek and Roman mathematics and concepts to forge a new astronomy and physics. Debates about heliocentrism began in the sixteenth century and very nearly cost Galileo his life in the seventeenth century. It would be several centuries before medicine made tangible advances, but Renaissance physicians were taking steps toward understanding diseases and healing. Still, the bubonic plague and other diseases ravaged the population and left everyone mystified as to how and why. Almost everyone agreed that the Black Death must have been a demonstration of divine displeasure. Prayer seemed their only hope.

Patriarchy. In the home, patriarchy reigned, supported by the churches and governments. Men were full citizens, whereas, in most areas, women were dependents with very limited access to political, economic, or legal arenas. While boys often went to school to be trained for a profession or apprenticed to a tradesman, schools and apprenticeships for girls were much less common. In fact, in this age of religious strife, most schools for secular girls were opened to train them in religious orthodoxy so that they would be transmitters of religion in the home as they grew to be mothers and wives.

Marital matters were often arranged by families for economic and political reasons, especially at the highest levels of society. A bride's **dowry** was expected by the groom and his family. This "portfolio" of wealth was often made up of cash, real estate, chattels, jewelry, and other valuable household items. The dowry was intended for the groom's use, and in the event of his death, it would revert to the widow. **Marriage** was intended to produce children, who would become heirs to their families' estates. The transmission of the family patrimony to the rightful heir was central. Therefore, in marriage, female **adultery** was less tolerated than male promiscuity. **Divorce** was extremely rare, while desertion was more prevalent, especially in poorer circles.

As patriarchy was the main organizing structure for society, how did female rulers manage to wield power in this period? In short, the concept of the royal bloodline was paramount in most early modern European kingdoms. France followed the Salic law, which denied women the right to rule. In other countries, a woman could rule only after the line of male heirs was exhausted. If a female was the next in line for the throne, the hope was that she would marry early and her husband would join her in ruling, and they would produce a male heir to secure the future. Clearly, this did not always happen. The case of **Elizabeth I** of England (1533–1603) is the most illustrious example. A learned and wise woman, Elizabeth employed a number of strategies to maintain her position as queen. She described herself as having manly qualities so that her people would have more faith in her ability to rule. As a young queen she entertained marriage proposals, but always maneuvered out of these political entanglements. Still, despite her able rule, there was vociferous resistance to her, as a woman, heading a country. In 1558, the very year Elizabeth I ascended to the throne, John Knox wrote ***The First Blast of the Trumpet Against the Monstrous Regiment of Women***, which was an attack upon the government of Elizabeth's predecessor on the English throne, her Catholic half sister, Mary I (1516–1558). In *The First Blast*, Knox argued from biblical and patristic sources that female rule was not pleasing to God, and, in fact, it endangered society. Among other things, this misogynistic tract repudiated women's rationality, a most desirable characteristic in a head of state. Nevertheless, Knox's rant did not remove Mary from the throne nor prevent her sister from succeeding her, although it did prompt an angry Elizabeth to ban Knox from returning to England. He went instead to his native Scotland, where he became a strong opponent of another female ruler, Mary Queen of Scots (1542–1587), who had been crowned as an infant after her father's death.

The People: Urban and Rural. In the urban centers, the underclass crowded cities as beggars and criminals, while the elite, dispensing charity as it saw fit, enjoyed the bounty of country villas and city houses. Concepts of the "deserving" poor and "undeserving" poor were used to determine which of the unfortunate ought to get alms. The deserving poor were "good" Christians who had fallen on hard times, while the "undeserving" were errant types who took too much drink and did not attempt to live a proper Christian life. In Catholic countries, mendicants, like the Franciscans, congregated in the cities tending to the poor and the sick. Hospitals were erected to house unwed mothers, abandoned children, along with the sick and dying. These hospitals were typically staffed by a few physicians and a cadre of religious men and women. Sometimes funded by the state, and sometimes by private patrons, the hospital was an early modern phenomenon.

The rural rubric of the early modern period revolved around ownership of land. While there were some small landowners, increasingly, wealthy and powerful landowning families dominated the terrain. Ordinary farmers leased land and owed rents that were paid in cash more than goods. The enclosure movement, best known in England, re-appropriated the Commons (fields that people living in the areas used for pasture and planting) to an individual landowner and thereby made communal space private property. This movement had devastating effects on families living at the subsistence level and contributed to famine and food riots.

LOVE, MARRIAGE, AND FAMILY. In the early modern period, divine **love** was considered much more important than earthly love. Love of God was the highest and most respected form of love. According to Christian teaching, by serving one's fellow, one demonstrated love of God. While different sects would debate the merit of service to others in terms of whether it made a difference in one's salvation, most agreed that service to others was a good practice.

Earthly love or secular love did not necessarily correspond with marriage. Coming out of the medieval courts was the courtly notion that love outside of marriage, an unobtainable love, was especially moving (called courtly love). The early modern period, with all of its rhetoric of chastity, constancy, and fidelity, witnessed untold numbers of extramarital affairs and fornication (sexual relations outside of wedlock). The legal record is especially rich in matters of promised engagements, and illegitimate children. Most ordinary couples married when the woman was in her twenties and the man was in his thirties with an established profession. The recurrence of plague and the ravages of war checked the population, as did a high rate of infant and maternal mortality. Parents did not expect all of their children to survive into adulthood, but this knowledge did not prevent them from establishing intimate bonds with their offspring.

Mothers were encouraged to nurse their own babies, but if families could afford to do so, they typically hired wet-nurses. When the child returned from the nurse, he or she received the first lessons in the home, most often from the mother. It was a mother's particular responsibility to inculcate Christian precepts and insist upon moral behavior, particularly in Protestant households. If the mother could read and/or write, she typically passed those important skills onto her children. Many Europeans of the period sent their children "out" to other households to be apprenticed or act as maids. In turn they would receive other children into their homes and train them accordingly. The hope was that the children would not be coddled in a relative's or associate's home, as they might be in their own homes. A stricter upbringing, people hoped, would produce more capable adults.

EXPLORATION AND CONQUEST. In this age of exploration and conquest, sailors were needed, and many men went to sea looking for wages and adventure. In the early modern period a significant commercial shift occurred, where the Mediterranean Sea, after centuries of centrality, became a less lucrative site for business with the introduction of trans-Atlantic trade. The Portuguese and Spanish led the way in the fifteenth and early sixteenth centuries; they were soon followed by the Dutch, English, and French. The new European nation states aspired to have empires overseas. Laden with guns and microbes, Europeans immediately dominated the indigenous peoples of the Americas and enslaved Africans to accomplish the work of the *hacienda* and plantation. Their theories of government, natural and divine order, as well as their desire to produce Christian converts helped them to justify their actions, which co-mingled with atrocities.

OCCUPATIONS. Those who remained in Europe worked in many different occupations: farmers, day laborers, artisans, bakers, smiths, weavers, masons, etc. Women tended to work in textiles but were often blocked from the more lucrative jobs in the field. Other women assisted their husbands with a range of businesses, and in some cases, in the event of the death of the spouse, widows were permitted to continue their husband's trade. Some were even members of guilds in their own rights. Guilds were extremely powerful professional associations that set standards for the professions, set prices, and took care of its members in times of crisis. More than that, membership in a guild was an important part of one's identity, along with one's parish, neighborhood, and clan.

SEXUALITY. During the early modern period, the model of two sexes was generally accepted by all, and heterosexuality was touted as the appropriate sexual orientation. For maidens, **virginity** was expected. If there was any question about a young woman's chastity when her marriage was being contracted, it jeopardized her future and could dissolve prenuptial arrangements (*see* **Betrothal**). While young men were also supposed to be virgins before marriage, their sexual history was not scrutinized in the same way as their female counterparts. Women's honor and the honor of the family were bound up in female **chastity**, whereas that was not the case with men. Unmarried men could find partners at **brothels** and elsewhere, and increasingly, sexually active people would find themselves with **venereal disease**, also known as the "French disease."

Sexual and romantic themes abounded in European society. Within Europe's cultural complexity, contradictions about these themes are apparent. On the one hand, secular law and churches condemned lust and fornication, and on the other, these "sins" were celebrated in art, pageantry, poetry, literature, and pornography. Even within religion, Christ's Church was known as His Beloved, His Spouse, and erotic imagery featured in mystical unions between Christ and some believers. Painters and sculptors expressed erotic notions through images from Greek and Roman mythology. In this way, Venus graced both private homes and public places with her symbolic figure, almost ubiquitous in this period. *See also* Christianity; Mystics.

Further Reading: Grantham, James, ed. *Sexuality and Gender in Early Modern Europe: Institutions, Texts, Images*. Cambridge: Cambridge University Press, 1993; Trinkaus, Charles Edward. *In Our Image and Likeness: Humanity and Divinity in Italian Humanist Thought*. Notre Dame, IN: University of Notre Dame Press, 1995; Wiesner, Merry E. *Women and Gender in Early Modern Europe*. Cambridge: Cambridge University Press, 2000.

Victoria L. Mondelli

EXPLORATION AND COLONIZATION, EUROPEAN. Exploration of the East Indies, **Africa**, and the **Americas** by early modern European explorers was facilitated by the opening up of overseas trade routes and an improvement in shipbuilding and navigation. The reasons for the curiosity and interest in expansion, particularly of the Portuguese, English, French, and Spanish, grew out of more than the simple desire for trade, being driven also by the desire for economic and political dominance and a desire to bring the benefits of **Christianity** and European civilization to the rest of the world. In the process, Europeans also spread their sexual attitudes and practices to other peoples and were in turn influenced by the sexual views and practices of the other religions and societies they encountered.

ECONOMIC AND POLITICAL EXPANSION AND DOMINANCE. In the fifteenth and sixteenth centuries, the development of the caravel and better navigational and other seafaring methods by the Portuguese and Spanish precipitated the European expansionism that came to dominate the seas and eventually create or influence the cultures and borders that exist throughout much of the world today. The prime figure in popularizing trade through his financial support and development of seafaring vessels was Prince Henry the Navigator (1394–1460) of Portugal, whose enthusiasm prompted voyages that eventually led to the unprecedented exploration of Africa and the establishment of sea routes to the East Indies.

Colonial enterprise had as much to do with dominating people as it did with controlling land, and its dominance was commonly justified by feminizing the landscape and people the colonists encountered. The analogy between colonization and the domination of women was typical in early modern writing and the conflation of woman and land was expressed as the penetration of virgin territory, and the land itself was depicted as a virgin. The trade (and its corollary, plunder) and domination and hybridization (and their corollaries, enslavement and genocide) that took place were the result of a desire for increased economic capital and better access to such valuable commodities as silk, cotton, spices, timber, and slaves, among others. Expansion to both the eastward and the westward was pioneered by the Portuguese, but westward explorations grew to be dominated by the Spanish, who were, in the later sixteenth and early seventeenth centuries, joined by the French, English, and Dutch. The domination of European military methods, facilitated by firearms, over those of the indigenous peoples of Africa, the Americas and the East Indies, along with, in many cases, the disastrous impact of European-borne diseases, such as smallpox, left the indigenous people subject to European domination.

THE EVANGELISTIC/CIVILIZING MISSION. Shocked by the lack of the knowledge of Christ that they encountered in Africa, **Asia**, and the Americas, and moved by the biblical exhortation to go out to the four corners of the world and spread the Gospel, Europeans undertook an overt mission to civilize the "savage"—or the "Other,"—proselytizing and evangelizing Christianity to the indigenous peoples they encountered. The first expression of this sense of responsibility to evangelize was the redirection of the Order of Christ, a medieval military order, to the Christianizing of new lands opened up by Portuguese exploration. At the request of the king of Portugal, the pope named Prince Henry the Navigator grand master of the order in 1417. The king granted the order a 5 percent levy on all merchandize coming into Portugal from the new Africa trade, and Prince Henry used this money to built and expand his navigation school *Sagres*, from which the great Portuguese trade expeditions of the late fifteenth century set forth to Africa, India, and Southeast Asia.

Outside of the Order of Christ, missionaries travelled to all the newly discovered lands with intentions of converting the "heathens." The Jesuits, members of the Society of Jesus, which was founded by the Spaniard Ignatius Loyala in 1534, were active in the New World and China. In particular, St. Francis Xavier (1506–1552), considered one of the most active missionaries since the early Church, focused his attention on Japan and China.

The pure motives that these missionaries professed to have often went hand in hand with extreme brutality. Partially to counter this brutality, Pope Paul III, in 1537, declared "that the Indians are truly men and that they are. . . . capable of understanding the Catholic Faith." While still highly problematic, this pronouncement was an improvement over Pope Nicholas V's bull of 1452, which gave permission to the Portuguese to "capture, vanquish, and subdue" the heathens, and to make them slaves. The self-created image of civilized Europeans taming the "savages" was, at times, a defensive reaction to the fact that the indigenous peoples of the New World were differently accomplished, with ceremonies, rituals, agricultural practices, and delineated class and gender roles (e.g., **berdaches**) that often made little sense to Europeans. In their defense, European colonists in North America often created the illusion, for people back in Europe, that the Native Americans were dependent on the superior knowledge of the Europeans, when, in fact, the European colonists, particularly the first English colonists in the seventeenth century, were highly dependent for survival on the native Americans' food and knowledge of the resources and geography of their land.

INDIVIDUAL EXPLORERS. European expansionism began in earnest after 1400 in Spain, Portugal, France, and England, countries that sought to expand their spheres of power, trade, and influence beyond the boundaries of Europe. It is impossible to entirely celebrate the manner in which early modern European explorers colonized the New World, Africa, and the East Indies. Regardless, they remain an essential part of world history and development. The following are among the most important individual early modern European explorers.

Christopher Columbus (1451–1506). An Italian who secured Spanish support, Columbus is regarded as the first individual to explore uncharted seas to the west in an effort to find a western route to China. As a reward, the Spanish rulers Ferdinand and Isabella appointed him governor of all the lands he "discovered," a region that eventually included parts of Central and South America, as well as the West Indies. In 1492, his inaugural voyage to what is now the Americas secured for him the title "Admiral of the Ocean Seas," despite his error in believing that he had reached Asia, a contention he never withdrew. Despite his expressed desire for the "natives to develop a friendly attitude toward us because I know that they are a people who can be made free and converted to our Holy Faith" (log entry for October 12, 1492), his incompetent governorship and the rapacious desire for gold and treasure on the part of the Spanish led to the destruction of the Arawak Indians and the enslavement and cultural destruction of other Caribbean peoples. In 1998, in a mock trial carried out on the 506th anniversary of Columbus's first landing in the Americas, he faced ten criminal charges, including **rape**, slave-trading, and genocide against the hemisphere's indigenous peoples. The trial concluded with his conviction and condemnation to execution.

John Cabot (c. 1450–c. 1498). An Italian who sailed in the service of Henry VII of England, Cabot sailed from Bristol in 1497, leading a northern expedition (i.e., away from Spanish-held territory) that aimed to discover a western route to China. En route he arrived at what is now Newfoundland, Canada, thus named because Cabot was certain he had found an Asian island that he hailed as the "new found land." Henry VII gave Cabot license to "set vp our [English] banners and ensigns in euery village, towne, castle, isle, or maine land. . . . newly found." Cabot's explorations gave England an eventual claim to North America, which later English colonizers, such as Sir Walter Raleigh, who was active in the 1580s during the reign of Elizabeth I, used to establish

English settlers on the eastern coast of the continent. According to Lorenzo Pasqualigo, an Italian merchant living in London in 1497, Cabot planted the banners of England and St. Mark on his new discovery, as well as a large cross, which was presumably a mark of the English intent to evangelize in these "regions or prouinces of the heathen and infidels" (Henry VII, Letters Patent to John Cabot). On his second voyage in 1498, John Cabot disappeared, and his body was never found.

Ferdinand Magellan (1480–1521). A Portugese explorer under the Spanish flag who is said to have executed the first circumnavigation of the earth by sea, Magellan did not in fact return to Europe; he was killed in the Philippines and his crew returned without him. His voyage (1519–1522) was fraught with internal struggle, and Magellan faced several attempted mutinies. He most famously discovered a strait to the west side of South America, which was later named after him (the Straits of Magellan). Eventually, one ship, badly damaged and filled with starving and sick (predominantly of scurvy) men reached Guam, where the crew finally found some nourishment. Shortly after, they sailed to the Philippines where Magellan was killed in battle by Filipino soldiers led by Chieftain Lapu-Lapu.

Hernán Cortés (1485–1547). The Spanish adventurer Hernán Cortés is remembered for seizing what is now Cuba, becoming mayor of Santiago, Cuba, in 1511, and then conquering the Aztec Empire of Mexico in a series of expeditions beginning in 1518. Hungry for Aztec gold, Cortés led his men into what is now Mexico, gaining some power and dominance because the indigenous peoples mistook him for a divinity. Further, the sailors carried smallpox, which spread to the Aztecs, killing them by the thousands. Cortés' own letters suggest that the Spaniards' initial meetings with the Aztecs were peaceful, and that the Aztecs communicated to them that "we [the Aztecs] will obey you and hold you as our lord" (from the second letter). In 1519, Cortés marched with his men into the Aztec capital, Tenochtitlan, securing his position by taking hostage the Aztec emperor Montezuma. Despite this step, the Aztecs revolted, possibly stoning Montezuma himself, and forcing the Spanish and their allies out of the city.

Although forced to retreat, Cortés, in 1521, regained control of the capital, which he destroyed and rebuilt as Mexico City. Thus ended the great empire of the Aztecs. Cortés spent the next seven years in Mexico developing mines and farmlands before returning home in 1528. However, he later returned to Mexico as a military commander. Before his death in Seville in 1547, Cortés was responsible for extending Spanish rule in Mexico and Central America. Private Spanish investors and the Spanish king gave contracts to Spanish colonists who oversaw their conquered lands in Mexico and South America, while simultaneously working to subject the indigenous peoples to religious conversion and Spanish-controlled labor.

Francisco Pizarro (c. 1474–1541). A Spaniard sailing for Spain, Pizarro was the illegitimate and poorly educated son of a nobleman. However, the conquest of the Inca Empire in Peru eventually earned him the title of Governor of Peru from the Spanish Crown. Being illegitimate and having achieved no status in his home country, Pizarro settled in Panama in 1519, where he began to prosper. He led three expeditions in 1522 to the vast Inca Empire, which he succeeded in overthrowing in no small part due to divisions and weaknesses in the realm caused by civil war, a large-scale smallpox pandemic—which killed the emperor Huayna Capac and his heir—and fractured tribal loyalties.

By 1532, Pizarro and his cavalry had laid claim to the Inca lands through the assassination of the emperor, Atahualpa, and they continued to expand Spanish hegemony in the Andean region. Pizarro's influence and control spread south, where he established the capital of Lima in 1535. Divisions in his own ranks led to weaknesses that would result in his own assassination, by the family of his original ally, Diego de Almagro, in 1541. *See also* Chinese Treasure Fleets; La Malinche; Slavery.

Further Reading: Fritze, Ronald H. *New Worlds: The Great Voyages of Discovery, 1400–1600*. Westport, CT: Praeger, 2003; Fernandez-Armesto, Felipe. *Pathfinders: A Global History of Exploration*. Oxford: Oxford University Press, 2006; Morison, Samuel Eliot. *Admiral of the Ocean Sea: A Life of Christopher Columbus*. 2 vols. New York: Time Inc., [1942] 1962; Morison, Samuel Eliot. *The European Discovery of America: The Northern Voyages A.D. 500–1600*. New York: Oxford University Press, 1971; Morison, Samuel Eliot. *The European Discovery of America: The Southern Voyages A.D. 1492–1616*. New York: Oxford University Press, 1974; Quinn, David B. *North America from Earliest Discovery to First Settlements: The Norse Voyages to 1612*. New York: Harper and Row, 1977; Sauer, Carl Ortwin. *Sixteenth-Century North America*. Berkeley and Los Angeles: University of California Press, 1971.

Julie Sutherland

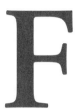

FATHERHOOD. Early modern men took the getting and rearing of children seriously. Fatherhood encompassed affection, education, and ambition in men of all social ranks. Fathers were intimately involved in their children's lives into adulthood. The father's role mirrored the authority of the ruler and ensured the good order of the community.

All men were expected to want children, and sons in particular, to carry on their family legacy. Aristotelian science, still widespread in Renaissance Europe, held that the unborn child combined the father's creative force with the mother's passive material to create, under ideal conditions, a close replica of the sire. Adoptive fatherhood was not universally recognized, especially in regards to inheritance of property or position, but a spiritual ideal of fatherhood flourished in the Christian church as a mentoring relationship between celibate clergymen and their flock. Roman legal tradition enshrined a father's authority in the family in the tradition of the *pater familias*, although, by the fifteenth century, the power of the father over his family was far more limited than it had been in Roman times. In cases of **marriage** breakdown, fathers customarily won custody of children who were deemed to be their property and exercised a range of rights in tradition and under law to determine their offspring's education, employment, and marriage.

Fathers were to protect and direct their children toward a proper and productive maturity. While mothers traditionally oversaw the first seven years of childrearing, according to the classical model popular in Renaissance Europe, fathers still influenced important aspects of early childcare, including choosing wet-nurses, inculcating good behavior, and administering discipline. Moralists cautioned against the excesses of coddling (thought to be the mother's fault) and overly harsh discipline, especially of very young children. Fathers were expected to administer corporal punishment, but only as appropriate, all the while ensuring that their children received a fitting education for their gender, rank, and expectations.

Fathers were particularly interested in the education and advancement of their sons. Well-off fathers secured tutors and schooling for their sons that would enable their children to follow in their footsteps. Under partible inheritance, fathers could divide their property among several sons. Under primogeniture, only the eldest son succeeded to his father's real holdings and other privileges of rank. Nevertheless, in all cases, fathers attempted to provide for all their children. In the lower ranks, fathers also strove for their sons' betterment, negotiating apprenticeships in trades or professions. Ambition did not end there. Many fathers negotiated advantageous marriages for their sons and daughters. Fathers also had to provide dowries or bride-prices of land, money, or movable property on the marriage of their children.

Fathers expected obedience and attention from their children; something that law and custom supported. The Ming moralist, Wang Yang-Ming, celebrated the transcendent virtue of filial piety in "The Identification of Mind and Principle." A French royal edict of 1556 allowed fathers to disinherit children who married without permission and set the age of marriage without consent at thirty for men and thirty-five for women. Well into adulthood, filial duty demanded obedience and respect from children to their fathers.

Contrary to some historians' arguments, affection bonded early modern fathers to their offspring. Writing in the early fifteenth century, Florentine humanist Leon Battista Alberti marveled at "how great and intense is the love of a father towards his children." Diarists such as Gregorio Dati recorded heartfelt sentiments of grief at the death of their children and endless gratitude when a child survived illness or injury. Fathers would be surrounded by their wives and children for eternity in the funerary monuments of the wealthy.

Many advice books explained how to be a good father or sought to pass on a father's wisdom to his sons. Alberti advised on the proper conduct of a man as father and head of the household in *Della Famiglia*. Barthélemy Batt's sixteenth-century treatise, *De oeconomia Christiana*, directed fathers on maintaining godly discipline in their households. Scotland's James VI wrote *The True Law of Free Monarchies* in 1598 to prepare his son and heir, Prince Henry, for manhood and monarchy. In many of these cases, the authors drew upon their own experiences in prescribing effective and affective modes of fatherhood. Metaphors of fatherhood threaded through the culture; as a father was to his family so was a king to his country. Fatherhood was the guiding metaphor for the social order. *See also* Childhood; Dowry; Masculinity; Motherhood.

Further Reading: Haas, Louis. *The Renaissance Man and His Children: Childbirth and Early Childhood in Florence, 1300–1600*. New York: St. Martin's Press, 1998; Ozment, Steven. *When Fathers Ruled: Family Life in Reformation Europe*. Cambridge, MA: Harvard University Press, 1983.

Janice Liedl

THE FIRST BLAST OF THE TRUMPET AGAINST THE MONSTROUS REGIMENT OF WOMEN (John Knox, 1558).

Published in Geneva in 1558, *The First Blast of the Trumpet Against the Monstrous Regiment of Women* (in modern English, "Against the Unnatural Government of Women") was written by Scottish Protestant reformer John Knox (c. 1514–1572). The pamphlet was a virulent attack on Mary I (r. 1553–1558), the Catholic queen of England. By denouncing the very idea of a woman ruler and then sanctioning the overthrow of a divinely ordained female monarch, Knox shocked contemporary public opinion and laid himself open to charges of sedition and treason. The pamphlet so outraged **Elizabeth I**, Mary's Protestant successor, that she banned its author from ever again entering England. *First Blast* also caused Knox to be seen as a radical revolutionary by contemporaries and as a rabid woman-hater by posterity.

Around 1544, living in Scotland, Knox was converted to Protestantism by George Wishart, whom Knox then followed until Wishart's execution for heresy in 1546. When a group of disaffected gentlemen, seeking to avenge the death of Wishart, murdered Cardinal David Beaton and seized his castle, St. Andrew's Knox became chaplain to Beaton's murderers. When the French, allies of the Scottish throne, subsequently captured St. Andrew's, Knox was confined aboard a French galley until the English government arranged his release in 1549. Knox then came to England, where the Protestant Edward VI (r. 1547–1553) licensed him to preach and appointed him royal chaplain.

After Mary's accession in 1553, Knox, like other Protestants, fled England. In Geneva, he began writing a series of works that attacked the Marian regime in England and the Catholic government of Marie de Guise, mother of the then underage Mary, Queen of Scots, in Scotland. Knox probably wrote *First Blast* while resident in the Huguenot (French Protestant) community of Dieppe in late 1557. Knowing that the pamphlet would cause him trouble, Knox arranged for it to be published anonymously in Geneva without the knowledge or permission of John **Calvin** or the city authorities. To protect the printer, the title page gave no publishing information, only the title and date.

Most of *First Blast* is an attack on the English queen, whose government was then engaged in burning Protestants as heretics. Mary is denounced as "a wicked woman, yea, . . . a traitress and bastard" (Ridley, 269), and Englishmen are urged to overthrow her. Knox then condemns rule by women as against the laws of God and nature and denigrates women as a sex, calling them "weak, frail, impatient, feeble and foolish . . . unconstant, variable, cruel and lacking the spirit of counsel and regiment" (Ridley, 271). Because leading armies into battle was still considered one of the chief duties of a monarch, and because male superiority was considered divinely ordained, Knox's opinion largely accorded with accepted tradition and popular prejudice. What outraged contemporaries found to be truly radical was Knox's passage exposing the illogic of a society that denied women access to every public office except head of state. Mary as a woman could not sit as a judge in the legal system over which she as queen was head. While other theologians urged men to obey a divinely ordained queen, Knox refused to do so, thereby weakening the mystique of sixteenth-century monarchy.

Despite his harsh denunciation of women in *First Blast*, Knox had shown no particular animosity toward the sex in his previous writings. In his personal life, he seems to have preferred the company and friendship of women to that of men. Many of his letters are addressed to women and many praise women as important, if subordinate, members of Christ's congregation. Knox also married twice. In 1563, when he was near fifty, Knox opened himself to much Catholic ridicule by taking as his second wife seventeen-year-old Margaret Stewart.

Prevented from returning to England, Knox, in 1559, went to Scotland, where he became a leading spirit in the Scottish **Reformation** and a strong opponent of the Catholic queen, Mary of Scots. By encouraging the Protestant lords of Scotland and rousing the Protestant majorities in Edinburgh and other towns, Knox's preaching helped ensure the success of the Scottish Reformation. Although heartened by Mary's deposition in 1567, Knox, who died in 1572, was thereafter robbed of his political voice by the need of subsequent Scottish governments to stay on good terms with Mary's captor, Elizabeth of England, who never forgave the author of *First Blast*.

Further Reading: Knox, John. *The First Blast of the Trumpet Against the Monstrous Regiment of Women*. Edited by Edward Arber. London, 1878. Reprint ed. New York: AMS Press, 1967; Marshall, Rosalind K. *John Knox*. Edinburgh: Birlinn, 2000; Reid, W. Stanford. *Trumpeter of God: A Biography of John Knox*. New York: Scribner, 1974; Ridley, Jasper. *John Knox*. Oxford: Oxford University Press, 1968.

John A. Wagner

FONTE, MODERATA (1555–1592). Moderata Fonte is the pen name for the protofeminist Venetian writer Modesta Pozzo. Orphaned at age one and raised by her maternal grandmother, Fonte's parents both belonged to the privileged elite group of the Venetian *cittadini originari* ("original citizens"). Fonte received an elementary education in a convent and returned at age nine to the home of her grandmother, whose second husband, a lawyer, encouraged her literary interests. According to Giovanni Niccolò Doglioni, her one-time guardian, relative by marriage, and biographer, Fonte largely fashioned her own education by convincing her elder brother Leonardo to repeat to her the material he had learned in school each day. Fonte decided to publish her work under a pseudonym for, as an unmarried girl, she was well aware of the need to protect her reputation as a decent woman, as most prior female Venetian authors were either married or widowed.

Married in 1583 to Filippo Zorzi, a Venetian lawyer and civil servant, Fonte attracted modern attention as a respectable mother from a comfortable background who was also a writer. Published posthumously in 1600, *The Worth of Women* (*Il merito delle donne*), Fonte's most substantial work, was completed in 1592 shortly before her death at age thirty-seven, following the birth of her fourth child. Written in dialogue form, the work emphasizes women's exclusion from education and men's failure to recognize their value, and suggests possible solutions to men's disregard for and hostility toward women. The intellectual scope of *The Worth of Women*, which combines the humanistic tradition of defenses of women with insights into the realities of the daily lives of early modern women, showcases Fonte's wit and encyclopedic knowledge.

Her earlier published works include the *Floridoro* (*Tredici canti del Floridoro*, or *Il Floridoro*, 1581), an incomplete chivalric romance consisting of thirteen *canti* of the fifty that Fonte intented to write; the dramatic dialogue *Le feste* (*Celebrations*, 1582); and the verse narratives *La passione di Christo* (*The Passion of Christ*, 1582) and *La resurretione di Christo* (*The Resurrection of Christ*, 1592). In these narrative poems, the Fonte pays particular attention to both the Virgin Mary and Mary Magdalene, the Biblical female protagonists of the Gospel stories.

Fonte's work differs markedly from conventional women's writing of the period, because her chivalric romance and literary dialogue are written in genres that are traditionally considered masculine. From the 1580s, Fonte, whose poetry was included in a volume of verse published in Venice in 1583, was included in the guidebook *On the Notable Features of the City of Venice* and was listed as an important living Venetian writer. After the middle of the seventeenth century, her work received scant critical attention, but was once again brought to the public eye in the 1970s by the feminist movement. Scholarship on Fonte, whose writings merit broader recognition, is increasing as her work is reaching a wider audience through translation.

Further Reading: Cox, Virginia. "The Single Self: Feminist Thought and the Marriage Market in Early Modern Venice." *Renaissance Quarterly* 48 (1995): 513–81; Malpezzi Price, Paola. *Moderata Fonte: Women and Life in Sixteenth-Century Venice*. Madison and Teaneck, NJ: Fairleigh Dickinson Press, 2003; Malpezzi Price, Paola. "A Woman's Discourse in the Italian Renaissance: Moderata Fonte's *Il merito delle donne*." *Annali d'Italianistica* 7 (1989): 165–81.

Ronna S. Feit

FOOTBINDING. Footbinding is a form of body alteration widely practiced in late imperial China. Very tight bandages were applied to a girl's feet in childhood so as to constrict their normal growth. This application aimed to produce a foot shape known as the "three inch golden lotus," though such an ideal was rarely achieved. The practice was unknown in ancient and medieval times, but there is some evidence that it originated with dancers during the tenth century CE. It began to spread through elite society during the twelfth century and became increasingly popular in subsequent eras.

To bind the foot, a bandage three meters long and two inches wide was wrapped around the ball of the foot, beginning at the instep. The small toes were wrapped and forced inward toward the sole; the large toe was left unbound. The bandage was then drawn around the heel of the foot so tightly that the toes were drawn inward toward the heel, causing the arch of the foot to warp so that the foot was drastically shortened. The initial binding process was very painful. Even after the foot achieved its new shape (generally after two years) the bindings had to be worn in order to walk, as the foot lacked the structural integrity required to bear a woman's weight in the absence of the bindings. Bindings had to be cleaned and replaced regularly. If the binding was skillfully done a woman could walk short distances without pain once the foot began to grow into its new shape. If the binding had been poorly done a woman could be effectively crippled. Complications like gangrene and the loss of toes were common. Even under the best of circumstances a woman's mobility was curtailed by the footbinding process, as bound feet would invariably experience pain from walking any considerable distance.

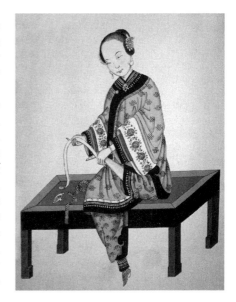

Undated illustration of a young Chinese girl binding her feet. © The Art Archive/Private Collection/Marc Charmet.

Footbinding was done within each family by the female members of the household. A woman's feet would generally be bound between the ages of three and six by her mother or grandmother, though poorer families might bind daughters' feet later. The more elite a family's status the more likely it was to bind its daughters' feet. Families that were poor enough to depend on their daughters' hard labor would generally leave their daughters' feet unbound, though it was not uncommon for poor families to sell daughters into the sex trade, for which purpose their feet would have to be bound.

The bound foot was a highly erotic object within the culture of late imperial China. The "golden lotus" foot was celebrated as a hallmark of female beauty and the most arousing feature of the female anatomy. Once married, only a woman's husband could view her unbound feet. Husbands reportedly derived great pleasure from unwrapping their wives' feet, kissing and fondling them. A fetishistic lore grew up around the bound foot and its supposed beautifying properties. The distinctively restricted gait that the bound foot imposed upon women was said to perfect the tone and shape of the legs and buttocks and to tighten the muscles of the vagina, heightening a man's sexual pleasure in intercourse.

Some scholars have posited that footbinding was an instrument of patriarchal control imposed upon women. Whether this was a self-conscious intention behind footbinding is in some sense moot, as its practical effect was indisputably to severely curtail women's freedom. Even while acknowledging this as the case, it is important to view footbinding in the larger context of global cultural attitudes toward the human body. Various societies have at different times practiced cranial elongation, scarification, male and female circumcision, tooth extraction, and many other forms of radical body alteration. In today's society, men and women elect to undergo painful and sometimes dangerous plastic surgical procedures in order to change their bodily appearance. Though footbinding was an egregiously cruel practice, history demonstrates that there are very few lengths to which human beings will not go to make the body conform to prevailing standards of beauty and sexual allure.

The practice of footbinding ended in the early twentieth century. "The liberation of the foot" was one of the first and most successful "modernizing" mass movements to achieve broad popularity in China. Chinese families entered into local compacts in which all swore not to bind their daughters' feet or allow their sons to marry women whose feet were bound. In the last decades of the twentieth century, one occasionally encountered a very elderly woman whose feet had been bound before the practice was eradicated; that generation has now almost entirely passed away.

Further Reading: Greenhalgh, Susan. "Bound Feet, Hobbled Lives: Women in Old China." *Frontiers: A Journal of Women Studies* 2, no. 1 (Spring 1977): 7–21; Ko, Dorothy. *Every Step a Lotus: Shoes for Bound Feet*. Berkeley and Los Angeles: University of California Press, 2001; Wang, Ping. *Aching for Beauty: Footbinding in China*. Reprint ed. New York: Anchor, 2002.

Andrew Meyer

FORNICATION. *See* Premarital Sex

FORTEGUERRI, LAUDOMIA (1515–c. 1555). A native of the Italian town of Siena, Laudomia Forteguerri was an important poet and muse, whose poems are possibly the earliest examples of "lesbian" poetry in the Italian literary canon.

Born into the Sienese nobility, Forteguerri married twice, both times into important families of her city (the Colombini before 1535 and the Petrucci in 1544). She had three children by her first husband, composed sonnets (of which only six are extant), and disappeared from the records sometime around 1555. In 1538, Marc'Antonio Piccolomini used her as one of the two principal interlocutors in his dialogue on whether Nature produces a physically and spiritually perfect woman by chance or by design. From 1539 to 1544, his cousin, Alessandro Piccolomini dedicated several of his works, both literary and scientific, to her. In his dialogue *On the Nobility of Women* (1549), Ludovico Domenichi described her as beautiful, virtuous, and learned. A few years later, in his *Images in the Temple of Lady Joanna of Aragon* (1556), Giuseppe Betussi praised her as one of the twelve most beautiful women in Italy and made her an emblem of "true fame." However, she is today remembered mostly as one of the three "women of Siena" who, in 1553, led a troupe of 3,000 women in building a defensive bastion in anticipation of an imminent siege by Florentine troops, an episode first narrated by Marco Guazzo in his *Chronicle* (1553) and then popularized by Blaise de Monluc in his *Commentaries* (1592).

Five of Forteguerri's six extant sonnets are dedicated to Margaret of Austria, duchess of Parma and Piacenza. In his *Dialogue on the Beauty of Women* (1548), Agnolo Firenzuola mentions them as an example of women who are attracted to other women, but then points out that they love each other "in purity and holiness," not lasciviously as the ancient poet Sappho or as the contemporary Roman courtesan Cecilia the Venetian loved other women. His "outing" of Forteguerri and Margaret was not news, however, among the literati of northern Italy, for several years earlier Alessandro Piccolomini had already described the two women's first meeting and their mutual, irresistible attraction for each other in terms that are clearly passionate and erotic. According to the published version of his *Lettura* (Bologna, 1541), they first met in 1536 at a *festa* in honor of Margaret and, "as soon as Laudomia saw Madama, and was seen by her, suddenly with the most ardent flames of Love each burned for the other, and the most manifest sign of this was that they went to visit each other many times."

Forteguerri's sonnets to Margaret of Austria are firmly set within the Petrarchan tradition and recount her anguish at the absence of her beloved. Because there is no attempt on the part of the poet to hide the sex or name of the beloved, the sonnets can be read as unmitigated expressions of same-sex affection, if not love, between women.

Further Reading: Eisenbichler, Konrad. "Laudomia Forteguerri Loves Margaret of Austria." In *Same-Sex Love and Desire Among Women in the Middle Ages*, edited by Francesca Canadé Sautman and Pamela Sheingorn, 277–304. New York: Palgrave, 2001; Eisenbichler, Konrad. "Poetesse senesi a metà Cinquecento: tra politica e passione." *Studi rinascimentali* 1 (2003): 95–102.

Konrad Eisenbichler

FOUNDLINGS AND ORPHANS. The large public institutional shelters of western Europe dedicated solely to orphans and foundlings first emerged in the Renaissance and early modern periods. Foundlings were usually illegitimate infants abandoned anonymously, while orphans were legitimate children who had lost one or both parents. Demographic pressures and social conditions dramatically increased the numbers of both in this period, straining earlier informal means of surrogate care. Care for orphans and foundlings both inside and outside of the new institutions demonstrates that 'family' was as much a deliberate social construct as a natural biological entity.

Few single women had the economic or social resources to raise a child on their own, and this often triggered abandonment of foundlings. The mothers of illegitimate children might be servants assaulted by their masters or their masters' family members or friends; young women who consented to intercourse on the promise of marriage; prostitutes, nuns, or women in adulterous unions. Yet it was the father's decision to withhold recognition or support that triggered abandonment, usually within a few days or weeks of birth. Girls were more frequently abandoned than boys.

Early moderns described as "orphans" those who had lost fathers, and possibly mothers as well. Widows frequently lacked financial resources to care for all their children. If they remarried, new husbands were not obligated to assume care of children who were not their own. As a result, the death of one parent could trigger the abandonment of children. Since up to a fifth of women died of complications related to childbirth, and since many women married older men and so were likely to be widowed young, many children were abandoned and raised outside their birth family. By the eighteenth century, poverty in rapidly expanding cities drove married couples to also abandon children in increasing numbers.

Most orphaned and abandoned children were absorbed into family networks, fostered informally, or contracted out as domestic servants or apprentices. Fears of inadvertent incest and of adoptees stealing family patrimonies made formal adoption difficult and, in France, illegal. Yet informal fostering was common. Almost all the girls apprenticed in Lyon were orphans, with contract terms longer than those for boys. Employers gave shelter and training and, in the case of girls, often undertook to find a husband for their wards at the end of the contract period.

Before the fifteenth century, small numbers of orphaned and abandoned children entered monasteries as oblates, or found shelter in general civic hospitals like Siena's S. Maria della Scala, or religious homes like Paris' Couche. Large dedicated foundling homes like Florence's Ospedale degli Innocenti expanded from the fifteenth century, and everywhere aimed explicitly to prevent infanticide. Parents preserved anonymity by depositing infants in fonts located outside foundling hospital doors, or in boxes and turntables set into the walls. Most infants were dropped off in dark of night and within hours or days of birth. Infants usually spent their first years with rural wetnurses and foster parents before returning to the institution aged four to seven. Overcrowding and malnutrition frequently pushed up death rates. Homes with many hundreds of children offered basic education, care in gender-divided wards, and the surname that they would take back into society (e.g., "Esposito" in Naples, "Columbo" in Milan). This ensured that the stigma of their birth would never be erased.

Orphanages for older legitimate children emerged from the sixteenth century, and aimed to preserve social standing and honor together with life. Amsterdam opened an institution for citizen orphans (1520s) long before its shelter for poor children (1664), and offered the former a better diet, jobs, care, and clothing. Cities like Bologna, Augsburg, and London placed boys in trades, crafts, or the military, and used service and textile piecework in proto-factory workrooms to allow girls to save for their own dowries. They were intended as temporary homes, but in some parts of Europe girls who did not marry, enter service, or return to family remained in the orphanage till death.

Formal and informal care was seen as a charitable duty and was framed in terms of symbolic kinship. Guild and confraternal brotherhoods provided a model that allowed the language of parent and child to be adapted to relations between masters and apprentices, guardians and wards, administrators and orphans. Orphans and foundlings thus gained through contracts and institutions a constructed family to take the place of the one they had lost or, in the case of illegitimates, the one that contemporary legal, social, and religious restrictions would never allow them to have. *See also* Childhood.

Further Reading: Gager, Kristin. *Blood Ties and Fictive Ties: Adoption and Family Life in Early Modern France*. Princeton, NJ: Princeton University Press, 1996; Gavitt, Phillip. *Charity and Children in Renaissance Florence: The Ospedale degli Innocenti*. Ann Arbor: University of Michigan Press, 1990; Manzione, C. K. *Christ's Hospital of London, 1552–1598: A Passing Deed of Pity*. Selinsgrove, PA: Susquehanna University Press, 1995; McCants, Anne E. *Civic Charity in a Golden Age: Orphanage Care in Early Modern Amsterdam*. Urbana: University of Illinois Press, 1997; Safley, Thomas M. *Charity and Economy in the Orphanages of Early Modern Augsburg*. Atlantic Highlands, NJ: Humanities Press, 1996; Terpstra, Nicholas. *Abandoned Children of the Italian Renaissance: Orphan Care in Florence and Bologna*. Baltimore: Johns Hopkins University Press, 2005.

Nicholas Terpstra

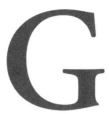

GANYMEDE. The myth of Ganymede was very familiar in the Renaissance and in the other cultures of Europe influenced by Italian philosophy and literature. The first account of this myth was in the work of the ancient Greek poet Homer, in which Ganymede, the son of Tros and Callirhoe and the most beautiful of mortals, was carried off by the gods to fill the cup of Zeus and live forever among them. Later writers added that he was taken from Crete or from Mount Ida in the Troad by the eagle of Zeus or by Zeus himself, disguised as an eagle. There were two interpretations of this story: that it was about the love of boys—as suggested by the cockerel that Ganymede often held, a gift in Greece bestowed on boys by older men seeking their sexual favors—or that it was a spiritual allegory, representing the ascent of the pure soul toward the full knowledge of the divine. A final episode to the story came to be added: that after his years of service, Ganymede was spared old age and transported to the constellation of Aquarius, the water carrier, to live out his old age.

All this was known in the Middle Ages, but it was in the work of the great Italian writers Petrarch and Boccaccio that the full story was restored, whether to justify pederasty or, as in neo-Platonism, to say that Ganymede referred to the idea of divine and perfect inward beauty, outwardly celebrated in flesh. The most famous representation of the myth was in a drawing by Michelangelo, done in 1530, and presented to his friend Tommaso Cavaliere, together with one of Tityos, eternally punished for his attempted seduction of Leto. The image of Ganymede spoke of the mystical union of love; Tityos of its tortures. Several other images of Ganymede appeared in the sixteenth century, especially in the courts. One, by Correggio, was in a set of the loves of the Gods done for the Gonzaga family in Mantua; another was executed by Giulio Romano for a room there in the Ducal Place. A further image is one of a series of scenes from his life by Parmigianino for the court of Parma.

In all these it was seemingly the homoerotic significance of the myth that was expressed, especially since it could be said that Zeus, in using Ganymede to replace his daughter Hebe as his servant, was responding to an idea that the relationship between men was superior, spiritually and intellectually, to that between men and women. The strictures of the Council of **Trent**, promulgated in the 1550s and 1560s, however, were not sympathetic to any such suggestions. And if still, beyond adaptations of Michelangelo, there were occasional representations of this myth, these were now found only in more private spaces, as in the decorations by Annibale Carraci in Rome at the Palazzo Farnese between 1596 and 1600 or in those in the 1640s by Pietro da Cortona on the piano nobile of the Palazzo Pitti in Florence. The end to all this was

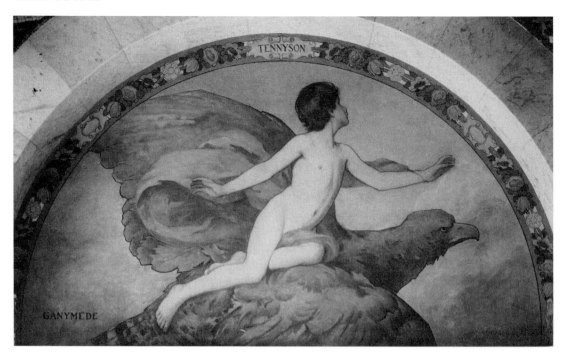

Ganymede, by H. O. Walker, c. 1899. Courtesy of the Library of Congress.

near as shown in two examples of this theme by Peter Paul Rubens and Rembrandt where then the humorous or even scatological details included suggest that Ganymede was forever bound to earth rather than safe in the pure realm of the gods. *See also* Homoeroticism; Pederasty.

Further Reading: Panofksy, Erwin. *Studies in Iconology: Humanistic Themes in the Art of the Renaissance.* New York: Oxford University Press, 1939; Saslow, James M. *Ganymede in the Renaissance: Homosexuality in Art and Society.* New Haven, CT: Yale University Press, 1986.

David Cast

GILLES DE RAIS (c. 1404–1440). Gilles de Laval, baron de Rais (or Retz), was one of the richest landholders in the western Loire Valley and surrounding regions. He kidnapped and married his cousin in 1420, and had a daughter with her in 1429. That same year, as one of the commanders of the troops under **Joan of Arc**, he assisted in raising the English siege at Orléans. He played an important part at the coronation of Charles VII, who named him Marshal of France. He established a religious collegium dedicated to the Holy Innocents in 1435, and he staged *The Mystery of the Siege of Orléans* with hundreds of performers. His prodigality was such that he was obliged to alienate many of his landholdings or offer them as security for loans. His suzerain, the duke of Brittany, acquired several of them and named him Lieutenant General of Brittany. De Rais also, in 1432, began sodomizing and murdering children and adolescents.

During this time, de Rais reportedly employed alchemists and demon-conjurers in the hope of obtaining wealth and power. In 1440 he seized a priest attending mass at

Saint-Etienne-de-Mermorte, and in seizing the fortress there, wronged his suzerain, to whose agent he had legally transferred ownership. Subsequently the ducal court imposed a heavy fine on de Rais, but he did not pay it. Soon afterward, he was investigated, arrested, and put on trial. The judges at the canonical hearing pronounced him guilty of heresy, sodomy, sacrilege, and violation of the immunity of the Church, for which he was excommunicated, but the sentence of excommunication was immediately lifted after de Rais expressed remorse for his crimes. At his sentencing in the civil trial later the same day, the court imposed a large fine to be paid in lands and other possessions to the duke of Brittany, and it sentenced him to hanging and burning for homicide. His public execution by hanging, along with that of two accomplices, took place the next day, and his partially consumed body was interred in a church in Nantes.

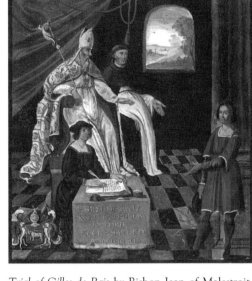

Trial of Gilles de Rais by Bishop Jean of Malestroit, 1440. © Snark/Art Resource, NY.

For details of Gilles de Rais's violent sex crimes, the reader is referred to the works listed below, but there is strong evidence that he was a sadistic pedophile, serial murderer, and necrophile. Testimony in his trials indicated that several procurers provided him with victims, mainly the sons of petty merchants, artisans, laborers, farmers, shepherds, and beggars. Young male accomplices were observers and active participants at the scenes of his crimes. Gilles and his accomplices confessed that victims were of both sexes, but the sentencing in the civil trial refers only to males, and the reports of specific incidents and missing youths named only males. Victims numbered around 140, according to the prosecutor in the canonical trial, but the estimate in the civil trial amounted to over 200. Theories about the motivation for Gilles's crimes of sexual violence abound. Gilles himself attributed his sexual excesses to idleness, excessive consumption of rich foods and warm wines, and his luxurious, permissive upbringing (commonplaces of medieval and Renaissance religio-moral discourse). Abuse of strong wine, at least, seems consistent with the delirious nature of the criminal scenes—e.g., beauty competitions among severed heads and limbs—which extreme inebriation might explain in part. Gilles displayed considerable affection for a young Tuscan conjurer in his service and the accomplices who died with him, one of whom he had sodomized many years earlier.

Gilles de Rais has long been identified in the popular imagination with Bluebeard, or *Barbe-Bleue*, the serial wife-murderer of Charles Perrault's tale. Tourism publicity in the *pays de Retz* today evokes ogrish Bluebeard in the gloomy ruins of de Rais castles. In the early twentieth century, around the time of Joan of Arc's canonization, a few scholars attempted, unconvincingly, to rehabilitate Gilles by casting doubt on the reliability of the trial documents, and in 1992 legal scholars, historians, and writers met in Paris to examine the question of his guilt; pleading judicial error, they called upon the then French president to reopen the case. Others have claimed that de Rais was part of a long-surviving Dianic cult and died as a witch, or as part of a conspiracy on the part of the Church to acquire his lands. Since the publication over a century ago of the minutes of the trials, Gilles de Rais's criminal passions and aesthetic sensibility have inspired high-cultural imaginings of international playwrights, novelists, and composers. *See also* Pederasty; Sodomy.

Further Reading: Bataille, Georges. *Le procès de Gilles de Rais. Les documents.* Paris: J.-J. Pauvert, 1965; Bossard, Eugène. *Gilles de Rais, maréchal de France, dit Barbe-Bleue (1404–1440), . . . d'après les documents inédits réunis par M. René de Maulde.* 2nd ed. Paris: H. Champion, 1886; Hyatte, Reginald, trans. *Laughter for the Devil. The Trials of Gilles de Rais, Companion-in-Arms of Joan of Arc (1440).* Rutherford, NJ, and London: Fairleigh Dickinson University Press and Associated University Presses, 1984.

Reginald Hyatte

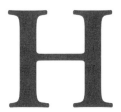

HAREM/SERAGLIO. The word "harem" (ùarïm, ùaramgäh, zanäna) is derived from the Arabic root ù-r-m, which denotes something that is sacred or protected. Within Muslim societies, the term "harem" was adopted to refer to the section of a house to which entrance is forbidden, particularly the women's quarters. The cloistering and seclusion of women from having contact with males outside their immediate families has been a long-standing practice throughout the Middle East, central Asia, and south Asia among Muslim populations. **Islam** allows polygamous **marriage**s with up to four wives.

Polygamous marriages are allowed under Islamic law only on the condition that the husband can provide for all of his wives equally. Due to this requirement, polygamous marriages among the poor and middle class were financially limited by the number of wives that they could afford to maintain. Among the rich and the aristocracy, polygamy was much more prevalent. In a number of instances where large extended families lived together, the area of the home reserved for the harem could be quite extensive.

While Islam limited the number of wives, it allowed for an unlimited number of **concubines**. Among the ruling class and wealthy this necessitated the establishment of large and specialized areas of their palaces to be established for the women. This additionally required the employment of attendants, eunuchs and guards. These arrangements varied from region to region, from Indonesia to Africa. Western imaginations from an early date became obsessed with oriental sensuality and took a particular interest in the harems of the Ottoman Empire. Consequently, the word *saräy* designating the separation of men's and women's quarters in the Ottoman court produced several loan words in European languages such as *seraglio* in Italian and *ser' ail* in French.

The harems of the sixteenth and seventeenth-century Ottoman courts provide a good example of the prevailing practices in *harems* throughout the Muslim world. The segregation of women within the *harems* at the highest level of society did not subordinate women, but rather created a parallel hierarchy that mirrored the one maintained by the males. It can be divided into three strata. The first and highest level consisted of the mother of the sultan, the queen mother or *Valide Sultan*, who was in charge of the harem, consorts and concubines, as well as unmarried or widowed royal princesses.

The sultan's mother exercised close control of all sexually active women of childbearing age within the harem. Female elders within the harem controlled the younger women and the harem was the major arena of family politics. Sex took on

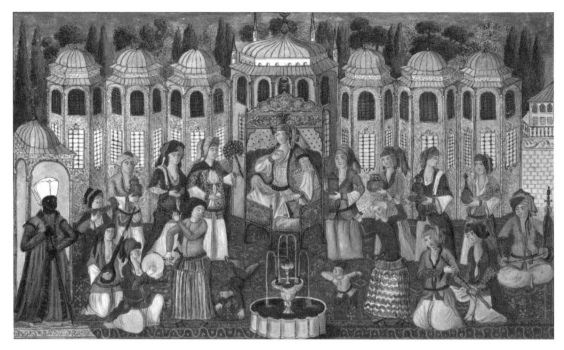

A Turkish miniature depicts the ceremony given to the Sultan's wife in the seraglio. © Giraudon/Art Resource, NY.

a very significant political meaning within this highly complex family dynamic. As a result of the complications and political obligations entailed in interdynastic marriages, the sultans found it easier and less restrictive to prefer concubines. In turn, motherhood endowed concubine mothers with political roles.

The term *haseki* was used for the favorite concubine of the sultan. She possessed a high degree of power and was not a blood relation. Her status was higher than that of the sultan's sisters, aunts, or other royal princesses. Childless concubines were married off and left the harem. Below the harem elite came the administrative and training staff, who were all women.

The harem stewardess (*ketkhuda khatun*) was in charge of the administration and managers within the harem at midlevel. Training activities were extensive and encompassed the training of new concubines who were specially trained and selected for their roles as well as the training of an army of servants that were required to maintain services within the harem. Servants and slaves comprised the lowest level and worked in the laundry, the pantries, the kitchens and performed an extremely large number of varied and specialized services. The harem was truly a complex institution. It paid daily stipends and maintained harmony within the palace(s). It should also be noted that an all male inner harem was also maintained for those who attended to the sultan and accompanied him throughout his daily routine.

The death of a sultan initiated the need to retire the existing harem. They were moved out of the royal palace to another location. Continuity could be maintained at the administrative level, when the elites were replaced by a new cohort of women. One unsettling aspect of dynastic change within the Ottoman Empire was the common practice of executing all other sons of the sultan and then expelling the women from the harem. *See also* Polygamy/Polyandry.

Further Reading: Bon, Ottaviano. *The Sultan's Seraglio, an Intimate Portrait of Life at the Ottoman Court (From the 17th Century Edition of John Withers)*. London: Saqi Books, 1996; Peirce, Leslie. *The Imperial Harem: Women and Sovereignty in the Ottoman Empire*. New York: Oxford University Press, 1993.

Mark David Luce

HENRY III, KING OF FRANCE (1551–1589). The sixth child and fourth son of Henry II and Catherine d'Medici, Henry III, the last Valois king of France, saw a reign (1574–1589) marked by economic distress and religious upheaval end in assassination and civil war. Faced with intense political and religious opposition, Henry became the target of a vicious propaganda campaign that branded him a sexual deviant unworthy of the throne, a charge that destroyed his contemporary reputation and also colored most subsequent portrayals of him by writers and historians.

Christened Édouard-Alexandre, but known as Henry since his confirmation in 1564, Henry, who was his mother's favorite, became duke of Angoulême in 1551, duke of Orléans in 1560, and duke of Anjou in 1566. In 1573, his mother engineered his election to the throne of Poland, a crown he assumed with reluctance and which he readily abandoned upon succeeding his childless brother, Charles IX, as king of France in 1574. An intelligent youth with some military ability, Henry, acting as lieutenant-general of the realm, was nominal commander of the royal armies that defeated the Huguenots (French Protestants) at the 1569 battles of Jarnac and Moncontour, victories that made Henry a hero of the Catholic faction. In the late 1560s, Henry, then duke of Anjou, was mentioned as a possible husband for **Elizabeth I** of England, but the duke, who was devoutly Catholic and almost twenty years Elizabeth's junior, denounced the Protestant queen as "a whore" (Knecht, 140) and refused all his mother's attempts to promote the match. In 1572, Henry was implicated in the St. Bartholomew's Day Massacre, the bloody destruction of thousands of Huguenots that was probably ordered by his mother and brother.

Two days after his coronation in 1575, Henry married Louise de Vaudémont, but the couple remained childless, and after the death of his younger brother, Francis, duke of Anjou, in 1584, Henry's heir was his Protestant cousin Henry of Navarre. A weak man with autocratic tendencies, a sensitive nature, and refined artistic and intellectual tastes, Henry as king was caught in the increasingly violent conflict between the Huguenots, led by Navarre, and the extreme Catholics, led by Henry, duke of Guise. In 1576, Henry, who was known for his intense Catholic piety—he founded several religious orders—made himself head of the Holy League, an ultra-Catholic group later identified with Guise. However, by the late 1580s, continual civil war, high bread prices, and the hostility of the increasing ambitious Guise made Henry widely unpopular with both Huguenots and Catholics.

Fond of fine clothes and court pageantry and surrounded by his *mignons*, young male favorites from families of little social prominence, Henry opened himself to a series of vituperative polemical attacks by his enemies, who characterized him as a bisexual cross-dresser whose increasingly gross perversions made him unfit to rule. In 1589, one pamphleteer, writing in terms characteristic of most anti-Henry literature, addressed the king as "Henry of Valois, buggerer, son of a whore, tyrant" (Crawford, 513). These increasing prurient denunciations so destroyed the king's reputation that, in May 1588, Henry was driven from Paris by a pro-Guise mob. In December 1588, in an effort to restore his authority, Henry ordered the assassination of Guise and his brother, acts that led to Henry's own murder at the hands of a fanatical monk in August 1589.

The disorders of Henry's reign and the success of his opponents' propaganda made him an infamous figure in French history. Although modern historians dismiss most of the sexual charges as gross distortions or outright lies, many descriptions of the king written prior to the twentieth century portrayed him as promiscuously bisexual or homosexual and much given to dressing in women's clothes. In film, this image still persists. Patrice Chéreau's *La Reine Margot* (1994) shows Henry as driven both by an attraction to his young male friends and by an incestuous passion for his sister Marguerite. And, although the real Henry never visited England, Shekhar Kapur's *Elizabeth* (1998) depicts him as a flamboyant cross-dresser who, while in London, destroyed his chances of marrying Elizabeth by displaying a greater preference for the royal clothes than for the royal person. *See also* Cross-Dressing; Homosexuality; Incest.

Further Reading: Cameron, Keith. "Henri III—The Anti-Christian King." *Journal of European Studies* 4 (1974): 152–63; Cameron, Keith. *Henry III: A Maligned or Malignant King?* Exeter: University of Exeter Press, 1978; Crawford, Katherine B. " Love, Sodomy, and Scandal: Controlling the Sexual Reputation of Henry III." *Journal of the History of Sexuality* 12, no. 4 (October 2003): 513–42; Knecht, R. J. *Catherine de' Medici*. London: Longman, 1998; Potter, David. "Kingship in the Wars of Religion: The Reputation of Henry III of France." *European History Quarterly* 25 (1995): 485–528; Teasley, David. "The Charge of Sodomy as a Political Weapon in Early Modern France: The Case of Henry III in Catholic League Polemic, 1585–1589." *Maryland Historian* 18 (1987): 17–30.

John A. Wagner

HENRY VIII, KING OF ENGLAND (1491–1547). In an effort to produce a male heir and thus avoid a female succession, Henry VIII (r. 1509–1547), second king of the House of Tudor, initiated the English **Reformation** and fostered the development of Parliament. However, in sexual terms, Henry is best known for his six marriages, two beheaded wives, and supposed contraction of syphilis.

Henry's first wife, Catherine of Aragon, was the youngest daughter of Ferdinand and Isabella of Spain and the widow of Henry's elder brother, Prince Arthur. Although the couple had been betrothed in 1503, the fluctuating state of Anglo-Spanish relations delayed the **marriage** until shortly after Henry's accession in 1509. Initially, the couple's relationship seemed close and affectionate, with the chivalric young king writing Katherine songs and poems and often turning to her for diplomatic advice. By contemporary royal standards, Henry was also a faithful husband. He had only two known sexual liaisons, one with Elizabeth Blount, who gave birth to the king's only acknowledged bastard, Henry, duke of Richmond, and the other with Mary Carey, the sister of Anne Boleyn. However, modern historians argue over the reasons for this apparently restrained sexual appetite. Was it due to morality, affection, or physical problems resulting in an occasional inability to perform sexually?

Some evidence of the latter is found in the couple's sad reproductive history. After miscarrying her first child, Catherine gave birth to a son in 1511, but the infant died shortly thereafter, and four subsequent pregnancies—the last in 1519—resulted in only one living child, a daughter, Mary, born in 1516. By the 1520s, Catherine, who was almost six years older than her husband, was in her mid-thirties and almost beyond childbearing. Fearful of what might happen to a kingdom ruled by a woman, Henry became increasingly preoccupied with having a son.

In about 1526, Henry began pursuing Anne Boleyn, the daughter of a prominent courtier. Attractive, intelligent, and witty, Anne knew how to entertain the king, who was probably seeking only to initiate a brief sexual relationship similar to the one he had enjoyed with Anne's sister. Although Henry had long been troubled by doubts about his marriage—the Book of Leviticus condemned to childlessness any man who married his brother's widow—Anne's apparent rejection of Henry's advances coincided with his decision to seek an **annulment** of his marriage, and made her begin to seem a divinely inspired choice as a second wife. Because the pope, for political reasons, refused an annulment, Henry and Anne were not married until January 1533, by which time Anne was pregnant. To obtain a separation from Catherine, who fiercely opposed any dissolution of her marriage, Henry, through his chief minister Thomas Cromwell, orchestrated the parliamentary abolition of papal authority in England. The English Church, with the king newly placed at its head, now granted Henry his annulment.

Henry and Anne's relationship remained strong throughout the long annulment battle, but weakened when Anne's reproductive record began to mirror Catherine's. Anne gave birth to a daughter, the future **Elizabeth I**, in 1533, and then suffered two miscarriages over the next three years, the last of a son. Although one recent theory holds that the second miscarried fetus was deformed, a circumstance that convinced Henry the child's loss was due to Anne's sexual depravity, most historians reject that notion. By 1536, Henry had become infatuated with another woman of the court, Jane Seymour, and supporters of Catherine and other opponents of the Boleyns were exploiting that attraction to promote Jane as an alternative queen. Having fallen out with Anne over various political issues, Cromwell, by interpreting flirtatious dalliance as evidence of actual **adultery**, convinced Henry that his wife was unfaithful. In May 1536, Anne and five alleged lovers, including her brother, George Boleyn, who was accused of **incest**, were arrested and executed for treason.

Less than two weeks later, Henry married Jane Seymour, who in October 1537 gave birth to Henry's longed-for son, the future Edward VI. Because Jane died of puerperal fever twelve days later, little can said about the nature of her brief marriage. She succeeded in reconciling the king with Princess Mary, but had little political influence and her demure personality is hard to recover from the surviving record. Henry was devastated by her loss and later ordered that he be buried next to her at Windsor, but the search for a new wife began within days of her death and much of Henry's grief over Jane may have stemmed from the selfish realization that, after two outspoken wives of dubious fertility, he had lost a submissive wife who could bear sons.

In 1540, Henry married Anne, the daughter of the duke of Cleves. In keeping with German practice, Anne had not been trained in the courtly arts; she did not sing or play an instrument, wore dowdy clothes, and had neither the wit nor the English to amuse her husband. She was also apparently without any sexual knowledge and thus unable to arouse a king, who, it appears, was now impotent. Although Henry slept with her for months, he did not, according to the later testimony of both parties, consummate the union, a fact that provided a basis for dissolving the match after only six months. Intriguingly, Henry adopted Anne as his sister, and she lived her life out in England, quietly.

Henry's fifth marriage, contracted only weeks after the end of the Cleves union, was to Katherine Howard, who came to Henry's attention through her politically ambitious uncle, the duke of Norfolk. Young (about nineteen or twenty), attractive, and witty, Katherine made her aging husband feel young again by apparently reviving his sexual powers. However, unlike Anne of Cleves, Katherine was not sexually naïve, and her uncle's rivals at court soon uncovered evidence that she had not come to her Henry as a virgin. Further investigation revealed that she had also behaved improperly after her marriage, having formed at least the intent to commit adultery with a young courtier named Thomas Culpeper. Devastated, Henry sent Katherine to the Tower, where she was executed in February 1542.

In July 1543, Henry married Katherine Parr, a childless, twice-widowed woman in her early thirties who offered pleasant companionship rather than sexual excitement. Intelligent, kind, and well-educated, Katherine knew how to divert a king made increasingly irascible by his deteriorating health. Although her zeal for reformed belief caused some marital friction, Henry's sixth marriage lasted until his death. Katherine brought comfort to Henry's last years and helped bring his three children closer to their father and to each other.

Henry's death in January 1547 is often ascribed to advanced syphilis, which is blamed for some of his earlier sexual and reproductive problems and for his mental and physical deterioration in the 1540s, when he grew increasingly suspicious of plots and intolerant of opposition. However, little can be said with certainty about Henry's medical history. He is known to have suffered for years with ulcers on his legs, but these may have been the result of diabetes, poor circulation, or any number of other conditions. Beyond the fact that his doctors, in treating the ulcers, gave him medicines sometimes prescribed for syphilis, there is little evidence to support the supposition that Henry had the disease. *See also* Impotence.

Further Reading: Erickson, Carolly. *Great Harry: The Extravagant Life of Henry VIII*. New York: Summit Books, 1980; Pollard, A. F. *Henry VIII*. New York: Harper and Row, 1966; Ridley, Jasper. *Henry VIII: The Politics of Tyranny*. New York: Viking, 1985; Scarisbrick, J. J. *Henry VIII*. New Haven, CT: Yale University Press, 1997; Smith, Lacey Baldwin. *Henry VIII: The Mask of Royalty*. Chicago: Academy Chicago Publishers, 1982; Warnicke, Retha M. *The Rise and Fall of Anne Boleyn*. Cambridge: Cambridge University Press, 1989; Wagner, John A. *Bosworth Field to Bloody Mary: An Encyclopedia of the Early Tudors*. Westport, CT: Greenwood Press, 2003.

John A. Wagner

HERMAPHRODITES. In Renaissance Europe, persons with ambiguous genitals were referred to as "hermaphrodites," a term derived from a myth recounted in the Roman poet Ovid's *Metamorphoses*.

Hermaphrodites played varied cultural roles. They appeared in alchemical symbology to represent the perfection attained by the balanced union of opposites, but deformed monsters, appearing as omens of ill, were also frequently described as hermaphrodites. Hermaphroditism was often rhetorically associated with male and female **homosexuality** and transvestism. Effeminate monarchs suspected of sodomy, such as **Henry III** of France, were libeled as hermaphrodites. Henry and his court were the subject of a satire entitled *The Isle of Hermaphrodites* (1605) by the classical scholar Thomas Artus.

There was a marked increase in European medical interest in hermaphrodites in the late sixteenth century. Sex between females was often conceptualized in medical writings in terms of one partner being a hermaphrodite and using an organ resembling the penis, rather than an artificial dildo, to penetrate the other. The recently discovered clitoris offered a way to explain hermaphrodites without having to admit the possibility of indeterminate gender—many hermaphrodites could now be described as women with enlarged clitorises. Some medical writers of the mid-sixteenth century, including the great anatomist Andreas Vesalius, believed that normal women did not have clitorises, which were thought to be exclusive to a small group of "women hermaphrodites."

In addition to physicians and surgeons, European judges were also concerned with hermaphroditism because individuals with ambiguous genitals were not permitted to live in intermediate genders but needed to be assigned as either males or females. The tendency in the sixteenth century was to move away from the medieval reliance on the hermaphrodite's own testimony as to his/her gender identity toward an increased role for medical experts, including physicians, surgeons, and **midwives**. Experts were not always restricted to examining the genitals and chest (the French surgeon Ambroise Pare recommended examining the vagina to see if it was capable of receiving a penis and if it produced menstrual discharges, and the penis to see if it was capable of erection and ejaculation), but sometimes extended their role to evaluating the **masculinity** or femininity of the overall personality and bearing, including voice and carriage. *See also* Medicine.

Further Reading: Daston, Lorraine, and Katherine Park. "The Hermaphrodite and the Orders of Nature: Sexual Ambiguity in Early Modern France." In *Premodern Sexualities*, edited by Louis Fradenburg and Carla Freccero, 117–36. New York and London: Routledge, 1996.

William E. Burns

HINDUISM. Hinduism is one of the great world religions. It began 3,500 years ago with the Aryan invasion of the Indus River Valley region. Hinduism by the early modern period held to its core beliefs of devotion to the Vedas as the source of all truth and to the **caste** system.

The vast multitudes of India had come to worship millions of gods and goddesses with a rich variety of cultic practices, some of which were more widespread than others. However, the Hindus, under the influence first of Muslim invaders and later of Christians during this era, began to move in the direction of monotheism. Their numerous male gods came to be a Trimurti of Brahma, Vishnu, and Shiva. Only a few people were devotees of Brahma, and there are only a few temples dedicated to him. However, great numbers became devotees of Vishnu or Shiva. Hindu gods were believed to come to earth in the forms of different avatars, and the avatar Krishna became one of the most popular.

The story of Krishna was told in the *Bhagavata-Purana* ("ancient stories of the Lord"), which begins when a king of Mathura's wife became the victim of a demon's lust. The demon assumed the form of her husband and seduced her while she was walking in the woods. From their union was born a son named Kansa, who was extremely cruel from the day of his birth. Upon reaching manhood he dethroned his father and began a terrible reign of tyranny. The people and the gods appealed to Vishnu for help. Vishnu took a white hair and a dark hair from his head. The white hair was incarnated as Balarama and the black hair was incarnated as Krishna. Then a voice prophesied that Krishna would be born to Devaki, the wife of Vasudeva, to accomplish the divinely appointed mission of killing Kansa. In time, Devaki gave birth to Krishna as her eighth child; however, another infant, the new-born son of Yasoda, the wife of a herdsman name Nanda was substituted for Krishna. Kansa, hearing of the birth of Devaki's eighth child killed the substituted son of Yasoda.

Krishna grew to manhood as the son of Nanda and Yasoda. As a young child Krishna performed heroic deeds and also endeared himself

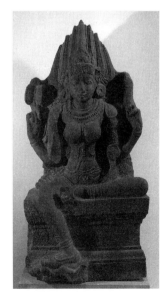

Kali, goddess of destruction, basalt, fourteenth to fifteenth century. © The Art Archive/Musée Guimet Paris/Dagli Orti.

to women as a mischievous child. As a teenager he played a trick on the *gopis* (wives of the cow herders). They were all madly in love with Krishna, although they were all married. Once, he discovered where they had left their clothing while bathing in the river and hid their clothes. He then climbed a tree and made each naked *gopi* come before him as a suppliant to claim her clothes. On another occasion he danced with the *gopis*, but he was able to multiply his hands so that he appeared to be dancing with each individual *gopi*. This made each one believe that she alone had the true hand of Krishna. He also played the flute and was popular with musicians.

Radha was Krishna's favorite *gopi*. Her husband was jealous and once sought to find them together, but what he found was Radha worshipping Kali, which was really Krishna in the form of Kali. The deception calmed her husband. Eventually Krishna fulfilled his destiny by killing the evil Kansa in a terrible battle. He then went on to fall in love with Rukmini, but had to fight several battles to win her. In one battle, he killed a king who had a **harem** of 16,100 damsels. Krishna wed all of them in a ceremony and then multiplied himself so that they each enjoyed their wedding night with him simultaneously.

The stories of Krishna produced a Krishna cult that promoted a *bhakti* movement in which the channeling of **love** to Krishna became a way of salvation. The love for Krishna was celebrated in romantic poetry, music, paintings, and sculptures. The poems, songs, and art gave expression to Krishna's love life with Radha, Rukmini (his first wife), and the *gopis* as expressions of the strong passions of women who are longing for an absent lover. Stories of Krishna were also told in the *Mahabharata*, which is the great Hindu poem that reached its modern form in the early modern period. It is the longest poem in the world.

By the early modern period, the stories of Krishna no longer emphasize him as the prince who liberates people from evil as they had done in the medieval era. Rather he was portrayed as the symbol of the passionate union of the believer with the god through romantic love. Radha becomes the object of his attention and his passionate lover. Her willingness to commit **adultery** is a symbol of her spiritual devotion to her god before all.

Poets celebrated the love of Krishna and Radha. Krishna Das Kaviraj (c. 1575), Sur Das (1483–1573), Parmanand Das, and Kumbhan Das all wrote Hindi poems about the two lovers. That of Sur Das used the thirty-six traditional modes of Indian music, the Ragas and Raginis, as the vehicle for holding thirty-six love poems. He was followed by Keshav Das of Orchha (fl. 1580), Govind Das (fl. 1590), Bihari Lal (fl. 1650), and Kali Das (fl. 1700). Bihari Lal's poem, the *Sat Sai*, celebrated the love of Krishna and Radna in seven hundred verses.

Paintings of Krishna and Radha depicted many scenes for both of their stories. In an illustration in the *Bhagawata Purana* (1790), the naked *gopis* are seeking their clothes from Krishna. In an illustration to the *Gita Govinda* (1610), Krishna dances with the *gopis*. In the closing scene of the work, Krishna and Radha are shown in an embrace. In an illustration to the *Rasamanjari* of Bhanu Datta (c. 1690), Radha is shown extinguishing the lamp in preparation to making love to Krishna. In an illustration to the *Sursagar* by Sur Das (1650), Krishna and Radha are shown engaged in sexual intercourse.

Shiva was often worshiped in temples using two sexual symbols, the lingam and the yoni. The lingam symbolizes Shiva's phallus, while the yoni represents either a vagina or a vulva. Both sex symbols represent energy. Shiva is a re-creator god, whose expenditure of energy is used to re-create life. Shiva is often depicted with his consort,

Sati, who is usually depicted as a voluptuous woman. However, she can take several forms that reflect different aspects of Shiva's attributes. Sati may be Parvati, reflecting gentleness; Durga, representing mystery; or Kali, representing ferocity.

In Hinduism there have been three major paths to karmic deliverance. The ways of asceticism and meditation have not attracted as many devotees as has the way of emotional devotion, or *bhakti*. During the early modern period Shiva *bhakti* flourished.

Hinduism promoted worship of goddesses more than most other religions. Devotees were Saktas, who often followed tantric practices. Some of the devotional practices were centered on the consorts of the gods, such as Parvati, the consort of Shiva. Among the widespread practices was devotion to the Great Mother Goddess, who was called by many names, including Devi. Intense loving emotions were devoted to her. She could be represented as loving, cruel, or deadly.

The divine feminine was represented by many goddesses. The most popular representations were Durga and Kali. The story of Durga ("awe-inspiring") was told in the *Markandeya Purana*. She was created as a pure woman warrior to destroy a demon, and was presented in the statues and paintings of the early modern era with ten arms, which she used to destroy evil, a serene face with a halo above, and as riding on a tiger, destroying dangerous obstacles.

Kali ("dark") was depicted wearing a necklace of human skulls with a hideous face and teeth dripping with blood. The hands of her many arms all held weapons. Cruel and deadly to her enemies, she was usually kind to her children. When a plague of demons could not be controlled by the Hindu gods and goddesses they called upon Kali to destroy the demons. The Thuggee cult worshipped Kali by killing people, most often travelers. They were responsible for at least 50,000 murders, and possibly as many as 2,000,000, between 1600 and 1700. They frequently would join a party of travelers and then strangle them as the opportunity arose. The loot they stole was devoted to Kali.

Some of the dances of India are derived from the goddesses. Others were of the gods, and from Shiva in particular, as is displayed in the famous bronze Shiva cast by Nataraja in 1600. The god was depicted as a dancer whose dance brought life, but when he tired of dancing the world ended. The dance of Kali is one of the feminine dances.

In Kerala, a state at the southwestern tip of the Indian subcontinent, many forms of dance developed. One of these, called Kathakali, began in the 1600s as a form of story-play. Several schools of this form of dance developed, and some were performed by men only.

Devi as Bahuchara Mata was worshipped by she-men (*hijra*), who dressed and lived as women. They were often employed at birth rituals. Some *hijra* were homosexuals. When discussed in classical Hindu literature, being a *hijra* was not viewed favorably, likely because *dharma* required marriage and the producing of children.

During the early modern period, India was dominated in the northern part of the subcontinent by the Islamic Mogul Empire. At times Muslim rulers controlled much of India, but never all of it. Hindu resistance was often fierce and successful, and in addition the Hindu population was always much larger than that of the Muslim conquerors. The Moguls often destroyed Hindu temples and looted their treasures, in obedience to the Koranic injunction to destroy idolatry, which abounded in the iconic worship practices of the Hindus. Many of their temples were filled with voluptuous statutes depicting Hindu myths.

Hindus resisted Muslim attacks on their religion by intensifying their Hinduism. They increased to fanaticism their devotion to cows, nonviolence in some cases, and to vegetarianism. Some Hindus formed naked groups of militants trained in yoga and carrying a trident. In south India devotional *bhakti* movements dedicated to Vishnu or Shiva arose. Some devotes of Shiva became Lingayats, who wore around their necks a replica of Shiva's phallus.

Some Hindu cultural practices were copied by the Muslim invaders, while they tried to suppress others. One practice they found offensive was **sati** or *sutee*, meaning "virtuous woman," which was the practice of a widow immolating herself in her husband's funeral pyre. In some cases widows were forcibly cast into the funeral pyre if she refused to do so voluntarily.

The practice of *sati* came from the story of the goddess Gaurī or Dākshāyani, who goes by a thousand other names. The goddess was a consort of Shiva's and became a symbol of marital devotion. Her father despised his son-in-law, which so insulted Sati that she used her yoga powers to self-immolate herself with the prayer that in a future rebirth she would be born to a father who would appreciate her marital devotion. She was later reborn as a new avatar, Parvati, daughter of a good king, and again the wife of Shiva. The story was celebrated in the Tantra literature of the time. *See also* Asia; Christianity; Islam; *Kama Sutra*.

Further Reading: Archer, W. C. *The Loves of Krishna in Indian Painting and Poetry*. Mineola, NY: Dover Publications, [1957] 2004; Dallapiccola, A. L. *Hindu Visions of the Sacred*. London: The British Museum Press, 2004; Fuerstein, Georg. *Tantra: The Path of Ecstasy*. Boston: Shambhala, 1997; Hawley, John S., ed. *Sati, the Blessing and the Curse: The Burning of Wives in India*. New York: Oxford University, 1994; Kulke, Herman, and Dietmar Rothermund. *A History of India*. New York: Barnes & Noble, 1986; McGilvray, Dennis. *Symbolic Heat: Gender, Health and Worship among the Tamils of South India and Sri Lanka*. Ahmedabad: Mapin Publishing Pvt. Limited, 2008; Payne, Ernest A. *The Saktas: An Introductory and Comparative Study*. Mineola, NY: Dover Publications, [1933] 1997; Warshaw, Steven. *India Emerges: A Concise History of India from Its Origin to the Present*. Berkeley, CA: Diablo Press, 1992.

Andrew J. Waskey

HOMOEROTICISM. Homoeroticism is sexual attraction between men. It is not a term that is ordinarily applied to attraction between women. For some researchers, the term "homoeroticism" is to be distinguished from "homosociality" because the former includes an element of sexual attraction that the latter does not. "Homosociality" may best be considered today as a continuation of "male bonding" that has typified male social behavior for as long as history has been recorded. Hunters out on a three-day hunt without the presence of females were to our ancestors as likely an example of male bonding as an all-male poker game or fishing trip is today.

With the addition of sexual attraction, homosociality tips into homoeroticism, the prelude to intimate sexual activity. At various times in history, homoeroticism took a prominent place in art and literature. In ancient Greece, vase painting often included graphic scenes of homoerotic art. In the Italian Renaissance, painters like Caravaggio and sculptors like Michelangelo used homoeroticism to empower some of their finest pieces. No one today who looks at Caravaggio's "Boy with a Basket" or his "Amor Vincit Omnia" would dispute the homoeroticism in those paintings. Likewise, for all the talk of its "idealized male form," Michelangelo's grand David statue in Florence relies for much of its power on a naked male body designed to appeal to the libido.

In the English Renaissance, homoeroticism came of age in English poetry. Of the 154 sonnets William **Shakespeare** penned, 126 were written to a young man with whom he was smitten, and some of these sonnets are vividly homoerotic, particularly the earliest ones. Richard Barnfield, a Shakespeare contemporary, openly published verses proffering love of one young man for another. There is some evidence that Barnfield was punished for his love poetry. He was twice disinherited by his father, perhaps because his gentle homoerotic pastoral lyrics embarrassed his family. We do not know who the actual personae were in Barnfield's poems, but in literature homoeroticism was sometimes masked as a tribute to a friend, often dead. Thus, later in the Renaissance, John Milton's poem to his friend Charles Diodati carries sentiments of male love that could not be perceived then as overtly "homosexual."

Although critics have accepted the homoerotic verses of Shakespeare and Barnfield for many years, there is yet reluctance to accept homoerotic readings of various Renaissance writers considered paragons of heterosexuality. John Donne, for example, has generally been revered as a "lady's man," and most of his love lyrics are read quite rightly as quintessentially man-woman poems. But Donne wrote a series of private poems that were published after his death as "verse letters," and some of these, particularly those written to young Thomas Woodward, are highly charged with homoeroticism. Similarly, the Renaissance lyrics of Sir Philip Sidney's friend Fulke Greville contain strains of homoeroticism. *See also* Homosexuality.

Further Reading: Crompton, Louis. *Homosexuality and Civilization*. Cambridge, MA: Belknap Press, 2003; Goldberg, Jonathan, ed. *Queering the Renaissance*. Durham, NC: Duke University Press, 1994; Klawitter, George. *The Enigmatic Narrator: The Voicing of Same-Sex Love in the Poetry of John Donne*. New York: Peter Lang, 1994; Turner, James Grantham, ed. *Sexuality and Gender in Early Modern Europe*. Cambridge: Cambridge University Press, 1993.

George Klawitter

HOMOSEXUALITY. "Homosexuality" as a term is not an old one, as it was coined only at the end of the nineteenth century by the Austrian writer Karl-Maria Kertbeny. What it denotes, of course, is ancient. Sexual attraction between members of the same sex is found in the oldest literature and in some traditions it was, and continues to be, honored. Of course, many homosexuals have been vilfied by various cultures and churches, persecuted, and often murdered or executed. The Renaissance was no exception in this respect, although persecutions in the Western world were not generally organized by governments or religious institutions, and executions were rare. The prevailing attitude in England and on the continent was very much "don't ask, don't tell."

In Europe, the use of medieval ecclesiastical penitentials (lists of sexual sins with suggested penances used by priests in administering the sacrament of Confession) died out during the Renaissance because Reformation Protestantism did not practice the sacrament of Confession. For Catholic penitents, of course, the questions asked in examination continued to prove as much an occasion for sin as the sin itself, and undoubtedly gave naïve penitents new ideas for sexual variations. Italy was largely tolerant of homosexuality, although legal strictures against it existed on the books. In Florence, "The Office of the Night" became a kind of vigilante group sanctioned by the city's fathers to rout homosexuals out of hiding, but the pogrom was short lived. Italy, in fact, by the time of Shakespeare had such a notoriously relaxed attitude about homosexual practice that English fathers routinely warned their sons about travel in Italy.

Renaissance England also experienced a similar, unofficial softening of attitudes, while not relaxing its official laws against homosexual acts. In England the Reformation brought new power to the state over the church under **Henry VIII** (r. 1509–1547), and secular courts took over responsibility for punishing what they considered various moral abominations, including sodomy. By 1540, Henry had grouped penalties for sodomy together with other penalties in a move designed to wrest power and social control away from the clergy. The punishment on the books was harsh: the convicted sodomite would not only be executed, but all his lands and revenues would be confiscated to the state. The law was repealed under Henry's daughter Mary I, but reinstated under the first parliament of her sister, **Elizabeth I** (r. 1558–1603). The new sodomy law of 1559 was, however, more a moral weapon than the political weapon it had been under Henry. For this reason, perhaps, it came to be rarely invoked throughout the English Renaissance, and by the time of King James I (r. 1603–1625), who was a homosexual himself, it was roundly ignored. Very few men were actually hanged for homosexual behavior in England during this period.

In some cultures, the matter of partner hierarchy is important in homosexual relationships. In ancient Greece, many homosexual pairings consisted of an older man mentoring a younger one, who would be ushered into Greek life by a sexual liaison with someone who was already established in society. Similarly in the Renaissance, the practice of both fellatio and **anal sex** was common enough (as is witnessed by various references in drama and lyric poetry), with the young man usually serving as passive partner, denoting his secondary position in the relationship. Literary references to **Ganymede**, the darling cupbearer boy of Jupiter, can be found in playwrights like **Shakespeare**, Ben Jonson, and Christopher **Marlowe**.

In recent years, much attention has been paid to Shakespeare's use of **cross-dressing**. One example is that of Viola in *Twelfth Night*, who undergoes a kind of sexual transformation when she changes her clothes to disguise herself as the young man Cesario. Since all roles on the Renaissance stage were played by men and boys, such cross-dressing is all the more convoluted, as onstage there is a boy playing a girl who cross-dresses as a boy. Although there are no fully overt homosexual characters in any of Shakespeare's plays, critical attention has been paid to the love between Antonio and Bassanio in *The Merchant of Venice* and the possible attraction of Iago for Othello. The most blatant use of homosexuality in Renaissance drama, however, was by Christopher Marlowe, who wrote an entire play, *Edward II*, based on the love of an English king for his minion, Piers Gaveston.

Amongst Renaissance lyrics, the most famous instances of homosexual love occur in Shakespeare's sonnets. Although critics continue to disagree on Shakespeare's own sexual orientation, no readers can miss the homosexual overtones of the sonnets, particularly numbers 1 through 17. Shakespeare was apparently not ashamed to air his love for a young man, and the bulk of the sonnets (1 through 126) concern male-male love. Only in the final sonnets of his sequence does Shakespeare turn his attention to a woman. Of other poets in the English Renaissance, Richard Barnfield stands out as a person who was not afraid to publish poems about male-male love. In fact, after the success of his lengthy "Affectionate Shepherd" poem in 1594, he published a second volume with twenty sonnets expressing love for the same "Ganymede" he had idealized in the early book.

As the sixteenth century turned into the seventeenth, English anti-sodomy laws remained unaltered. The most notorious application of the anti-sodomy laws came with the prosecution of Lord Castlehaven for sodomy, amongst other crimes; he was executed in 1631. However, as with most such cases, Castlehaven had been prosecuted for a large collection of sundry crimes, such as treason, rape, and blasphemy, and sodomy was often lumped together with similar charges in court cases where the number and salacious nature of the accusations might make up for the lack of a solid case for any of them.

See also: Americas; Anal Sex; Henry III; 'Ishq; Lesbianism; *Zinā*

Further Reading: Bray, Alan. *Homosexuality in Renaissance England*. London: Gay Men's Press, 1982; Crompton, Louis. *Homosexuality and Civilization*. Cambridge, MA: Belknap Press, 2003; Pequigney, Joseph. *Such Is My Love*. Chicago: University of Chicago Press, 1985; Smith, Bruce R. *Homosexual Desire in Shakespeare's England*. Chicago: University of Chicago Press, 1991; Summers, Claude, ed. *Homosexuality in Renaissance and Enlightenment England*. New York: Haworth Press, 1992.

George Klawitter

IL CORTEGIANO. See The Book of the Courtier

ILLEGITIMACY. See Bastardy

IMPOTENCE. Impotence is understood as either an erectile dysfunction or the obstruction of male seminal emission in a regular or permanent way. For the early modern period, the temporary detraction of male potency is frequently mentioned along with other maledictions of alleged **witches** and is prominently depicted in ***The Malleus Maleficarum*** by Jakob Sprenger and Heinrich Kramer. In his *Démonomanie des sorciers*, Jean Bodin believed that the spell of impotence (*nouer l'aiguillette*) was cast fairly often at wedding ceremonies, which aggravated the deed by harming the administration of a God-given sacrament. According to Martin del Rio's *Disquisitionum magicarum libri sex* (1599), the fear of such spells at weddings was so common that in some places hardly anyone would dare to get married in broad daylight.

Another influential work was Reginal Scot's *Discoverie of Witchcraft* (1584), which ascribed the inability to achieve seminal emission to magical disturbance, while permanent erectile problems were regarded as a sign of natural frigidity. Scot drew strongly on the studies of the German physician Jan Weyer, whose *De praestigiis daemonum* was first published in 1563 and many times reprinted and translated. Weyer, though not doubting the general existence of witchcraft, believed that most cases of impotence were due to the illness of melancholy rather than a matter of magic spells. According to scholar Winfried Schleiner, it also seems possible that the great French writer Michel de Montaigne was familiar with a case reported by Weyer in a later dispute. In one of his *Essais*, Montaigne argues that temporary impotence was primarily a psychological matter (*imaginatio*); he supports this with evidence from the case of a French nobleman (probably the Comte de Gurson), whom he himself healed using a placebo.

Still, psychological as well as physical reasons for impotence remained relatively obscure. Not until the early eighteenth century, did medical debate on the condition markedly increase. Apart from the intellectual discourses on impotence, sexual strength has constantly played a role in the premodern imagination, especially for the construction of manhood. According to the German Rietberg land law of 1697, any man willing to settle had to prove his manliness by "being able to draw a bow, please his wife in bed, and follow his master to the battle field." Many similar examples are known.

Until modern times, the inability to achieve penile erection (*impotentia coeundi*) was regarded as an impediment to **marriage** in canon law, and throughout the early modern era **divorce** processes based on that issue can be traced in the records of most European marital courts. Several sources on the forensic examination of such cases were published by Karl Sudhoff in his *Archiv für Geschichte der Medizin*. Female impotence received much less attention. *See also* Magic, Love, and Sex; Witches.

Further Reading: Bajada, Joseph. *Sexual Impotence. The Contribution of Paolo Zacchia, 1584–1659*. Rome: Editrice Pontifica Università Gregoriana, 1988; Behrend-Martínez, Edward. "Female Sexual Potency in a Spanish Church Court, 1673–1735." *Law and History Review* 24, no. 2 (2006): 297–330; Entin-Bates, Lee R. "Montaigne's Remarks on Impotence." *Modern Language Notes* 91 (1976): 540–54; Gelin, Henri "Les noueries d'aiguilette en Poitou." *Revue des Etudes Rabelaisiennes* 8 (1910): 122–33; Schleiner, Winfried. *Melancholy, Genius, and Utopia in the Renaissance*. Wolfenbütteler Abhandlungen zur Renaissanceforschung X. Wiesbaden: Harrasowitz, 1991.

Hiram Kümper

INCEST. Incest is a difficult concept to explain for many reasons, not the least of which is the fact that it is neither universally defined nor understood. It also does not help us to understand the concept when scholars cannot trace its origins. What we do know is that the concept of incest is socially constructed, which means that each society decides for itself what constitutes it. Commonly, incest prohibits individuals who are related either by blood (consanguinity) or by marriage (affinity) from marrying or from having sexual relations with one another. Incest prohibitions vary from culture to culture and have even changed over time within a particular culture. Not all human societies ban incestuous relationships. There are cultures that do not even have a word for incest and, hence, where it cannot by definition occur. Other societies allow certain groups of relatives to intermarry while barring others from so doing. Ancient Egyptian, Incan, and Thai societies, for example, permitted sibling **marriages**, and even required them among royalty, but no one outside of this elite group could intermarry with a family member. During the Hellenistic era some nation-states permitted marriages between half brothers and half sisters, but only if they were of the same father. Half siblings of the same mother could not wed. Further, it is important to distinguish between sex and marriage when considering the concept of incest. Some preliterate warring tribes encouraged siblings to engage in sexual intercourse before battle because they thought it made the warriors braver. While sibling sex was permissible in that specific circumstance, those same siblings could not wed.

Prohibitions against sexual or marital relationships may establish a bar between consanguinal or blood relatives or affinal or marital relatives or both. Some of the oldest known prohibitions against incest come from ancient Near Eastern societies such as the Hammurabi Code of Mesopotamia, the Hittites of Asia Minor, and the ancient Hebrews of Syria and Palestine, whose incest rules can be found in the Old Testament texts of Leviticus and Deuteronomy. The ancient Greeks also had rules barring sexual relationships between family members. In medieval and early modern Europe, the religious and political rulers of Christendom helped to define incest for Western culture. The Emperor Justinian (527–565), for example, banned marriages within five degrees of kinship and, five hundred years later, Pope Gregory VII (1073–1085), extended the ban to seven degrees of kinship. Interestingly, though authorities and scholars seem most concerned about incestuous relationships between a father and his daughter, this is the one coupling that is not banned in the Old Testament texts that the Church uses as its authority. Incest prosecutions, however, were conducted in Church courts and, therefore, Church leaders determined what constituted an incestuous relationship in territories under their control.

According to marriage doctrine in early modern Europe, both consanguinity and affinity posed a bar to marriage and before a couple announced their intentions, they had to make sure they were not related within the prohibited degrees of kinship. For instance, **Henry VIII**, while still heir to the throne in 1503, required a dispensation from the pope to marry Catherine of Aragon, the widow of his elder brother, Prince Arthur. If a couple wed and then later discovered they were related within the prohibited degrees, the Church would grant them a **divorce**. On the scale of sexual sin, Western theologians determined that incest was a more serious offense than **adultery** but not as serious as sodomy, while Eastern Christians viewed incest on par with all other sexual sins.

In Indian cultures of Southeast Asia, Hindus required men who had sexual relations with their wives' sisters to do penance, but some Hindu cults actually praised men who had incestuous sex as more spiritual than those who did not. Chinese Buddhists frowned upon incestuous unions. While incest with a sister was not so serious, Buddhists asserted that men who had relations with their own mothers had to suffer punishment in nine different hells and lost their families up to three generations. Chinese law also prohibited marriages within certain degrees of kinship. Historically speaking, it should be noted that incest rules are not intended to protect children from sexual abuse, but rather to control sexual relations and to regulate marriage. *See also* Anal Sex; Buddhism; Christianity; Hinduism.

Further Reading: Arens, W. *The Original Sin: Incest and Its Meaning*. New York: Oxford University Press, 1986; Bullough, Vern L. *Sexual Variance in Society and History*. New York: John Wiley & Sons, 1976.

Mary Block

INCUBI/SUCCUBI. The concept of human-demon sex characteristic of the European witch hunt created the theological problem of how a material human body could have sex with an immaterial spirit. Christian theologians in the Middle Ages, elaborating on the natures of angels and devils, claimed that devils, while ultimately spirits, could create a "body" out of compacted air. Sexually male demonic bodies were called incubi and sexually female ones succubi. The "sons of God" in the Biblical book of Genesis who copulated with the "daughters of men" were frequently identified as incubi, although not all demonologists accepted this identification. Incubi and succubi were frequently discussed in the context of demonstrating the physical reality of demons, since if demons could engage in sex they could not be denied to be real.

The artificial nature of the demonic body was particularly useful in explaining how women could conceive children by demons. (Male demonologists were usually far more interested in the question of intercourse between female humans and incubi than the reverse.) The standard explanation of interfertility between human women and demons (the question of whether a human male could father a child with a demoness was not often discussed) went back to the Scholastic theologian Thomas Aquinas (c. 1224–1274). Aquinas claimed that the demon first formed and inhabited a female body as a succubus, had intercourse with a human male, and preserved the semen. (It was also widely believed that demons collected semen emitted in wet dreams.) It then formed and inhabited a male body as an incubus, ejaculating the preserved semen into a human woman's vagina. The actual father of the woman's child was not a demon, but a human male. Despite this fact, many argued that the children conceived by demonic intercourse were more likely to become **witches** themselves, and to be powerful ones. Toward the end of the witch-hunt period, Franciscan philosopher and consultant to the Roman Inquisition Lodovico Maria Sinstrari (1622–1701) tried to distinguish between incubi/succubi and demons proper in his unpublished *Demoniality*, but his ideas had little influence. The intellectual problem of human-demon sex was mostly on the academic level. For ordinary people, the relationship of spiritual devils to carnal intercourse was not a problem because devils were thought of as material. *See also* Christianity.

Further Reading: Stephens, Walter. *Demon Lovers: Witchcraft, Sex, and the Crisis of Belief.* Chicago and London: University of Chicago Press, 2002.

William E. Burns

INDEX OF PROHIBITED BOOKS. Established by Pope Paul IV in 1557 during the interval between the second and third sessions of the Council of **Trent**, the *Index of Prohibited Books* (*Index Librorum Prohibitorum*) was a list of publications censored by the Roman Catholic Church because, through their immorality or doctrinal error, they posed a serious danger to the Church and to all faithful Catholics. In an effort to mitigate the severity of the Church's earliest lists, the Council of Trent in the 1560s revised Church laws on book censorship, which prompted Pope Pius IV to issue a new list of banned publications, the so-called Tridentine Index, in 1564. In 1571, maintenance of the list became the responsibility of the Sacred Congregation of the Index, which regularly updated the list with new writings that had been denounced in Rome for error or immorality. Catholic authors could defend their writings and books could be removed from the list if the authors published new editions with the corrections called for by the Sacred Congregation in the *Index Expurgatorius*. Publications considered correctable appeared on the list with the mitigating clauses *donec corrigatur* ("forbidden if not corrected") and *donce expurgetur* ("forbidden if not purged").

The *Index* was designed by the Church to prevent unwary Christians from falling into sin because of the growth of literacy and the increasing access afforded to all classes of people to publications of all kinds. In the Church's eyes, the development of the printing press by Johannes Gutenberg in the fifteenth century and the emergence of an increasingly affluent and educated middle class in the sixteenth century only seemed to heighten the danger presented to the faithful by the harmful doctrines of the Protestant reformers. As books, pamphlets, and tracts on many topics became readily available, the Catholic Church believed that the power of the printed word could do great damage if it promoted false teaching that contradicted Church doctrine and led people to embrace Protestant ideas. If not closely monitored, the printed word could also promote moral decay by addressing topics that were lustful and improper.

Many of the authors and publications banned during the **Reformation** period were condemned for heresy, such as the works of the reformers John **Calvin**, Martin **Luther**, and Huldrych Zwingli. Other authors were condemned for challenging the Church's worldview or for in some way questioning the Christian faith as taught by the Church. For instance, Galileo Galilei (1564–1642) was condemned for his lectures and correspondence, most notably for his *Dialogue Concerning the Two Chief*

World Systems (1632). His defense of Nicolaus Copernicus's (1473–1543) heliocentric theory of the solar system—Copernicus's *De Revolutionibus* was placed on the *Index* in 1616—caused the *Dialogue* to be condemned only five months after its publication. Placed on trial in 1633, Galileo rejected his scientific theories and survived. Giordano Bruno (1548–1600), a speculative Aristotelian philosopher and a Dominican friar for most of his life, failed to recant the errors detected in his *On the Infinite Universe and Worlds* (1584) and other works, and was burned at the stake.

In later centuries, more works and authors were condemned for writing works of fiction that were considered immoral and too sexually explicit. Among the publications that appeared on the *Index* for sexual content were Samuel Richardson's *Pamela* (1744), Gustave Flaubert's *Madame Bovary* (1864), and all the love stories of such nineteenth-century writers as Stendhal, George Sand, Honore de Balzac, Alexandre Dumas, and Eugene Sue. Although the *Index* was abolished by Pope Paul VI in 1966, the Church reaffirmed the moral obligation of Catholics to refrain from reading or circulating works that endangered faith and morals. *See also* Christianity.

Further Reading: "Galileo and the Inquisition." The Galileo Project. Rice University. http://galileo.rice.edu/bio/narrative_7.html; Galilei, Galileo. *Dialogue Concerning the Two Chief World Systems*. Translated by Stillman Drake. Berkeley and Los Angeles: University of California Press, 1953; Gilmour, Peter. "Don't read this!" *U.S. Catholic* 68, no. 9 (2003): 6; Godman, Peter. "Inside the archives of the Inquisition." *TLS* (1998): 15; Halsall, Paul, ed. *Modern History Sourcebook*. http://www.fordham.edu/halsall/mod/indexlibrorum.html; "Index librorum prohibitorum, 1557–1966. [Index of prohibited books]"; Nesvig, Martin Austin. "'Heretical Plagues' and Censorship Cordons: Colonial Mexico and the Transatlantic Book Trade." *Church History* 75, no. 1 (2006): 1–37.

Nicolás Hernández, Jr.

INFANTICIDE. Infanticide is the killing of newborn infants. During the sixteenth and seventeenth centuries, infanticide emerged throughout western Europe as a particular capital offence, differentiated from murder and manslaughter. Murder was the most sacrilegious and heinous crime of all and the murder of children was regarded with particular horror. In all European countries, the new legislation replaced the presumption of innocence with the presumption of guilt: a woman who concealed the birth of an illegitimate baby that subsequently died was presumed to have murdered it. The prosecution rates for infanticide increased (more women were executed for infanticide than witchcraft) and those accused were often young, unmarried (single or widowed), and poor (Ruff, 150–51). **Midwives** were at risk of accusations of both infanticide and witchcraft because their knowledge of agents to control fertility was increasingly regarded with suspicion (Bicks, 137).

A complex mix of religious, moral, economic, and social forces brought about this pan-European shift. Illegitimacy was regarded as morally repugnant and spiritually damaging because it was evidence of illicit sexual activity. It also placed a financial burden on parishes and local communities, which had to support illegitimate children left in their care. The new laws defined infanticide as an exclusively female crime and strengthened the association between illegitimacy and female guilt (moral as well as legal). However, the legislation was not always popular and was being ignored by some judges and jurors in England as early as the mid-seventeenth century (Walker, 153). In the eighteenth century, infanticide laws were increasingly criticized and the English statute of 1624 was repealed in 1803 (Jackson, 32). Court records show that reasons for committing infanticide included shame, mental derangement, economic hardship, and neglect (Wrightson). The assize reports from the Old Bailey in London record eighteen indictments for infanticide between 1674 and 1700. All the women accused were sentenced to death, but responses to them ranged from condemnation of their unnatural and cruel behavior to compassion for one young woman, whose baby died in October 1679 after her landlady turned the woman out into the street while she was in labor (www.oldbaileyonline.org).

Evidence from court records is only one way of understanding attitudes toward infanticide in the early modern period. Popular and sensational narratives of infanticides and filicides (i.e., the murder of older children) were printed throughout Europe. The writers of *occasionels* in France, *flugschriften* in Germany, and pamphlets in England all fashioned accounts of actual crimes into quasi-fictional narratives with identifiable generic conventions in response to reader expectation, social mores, and the politico-religious tensions of the period. These publications were small (quarto and octavo), short (four to fifty pages), and cheap, putting them within reach of all levels of early modern readers. From a surviving corpus of approximately 400 English prose murder narratives printed between 1573 and 1700, around thirty deal with child-murder (Robson, 304–37).

Although the "barbarity" of child-murder is one of the main selling points of these accounts, the narratives are typically constructed around the central figure of the murderer with the reader's attention only temporarily deflected to the victim(s). The generic conventions of English murder pamphlets demanded an emphasis on sinning and repentance, Protestant proselytizing, and equal measures of admonition and exhortation. The child-murderers represented are mostly women—single, married, and professional (midwives, baby-minders, and wet-nurses)—but a significant number of men are there as well, such as disgraced clergymen, errant Jesuit priests, and enraged fathers.

In German *flugschriften*, female child-murderers are portrayed as vicious and promiscuous, themselves the daughters of careless parents, and are subjected to violent, tormented executions (Wiltenburg, 235–37). In France, the story of Anne Belthumier's survival of her hanging in 1589 for infanticide is represented as a miracle, showing that faith can save and God will correct earthly judicial error (Chartier, 63–68). English pamphlets demonstrate a range of responses to child-murder. There are overtly misogynistic accounts that emphasize the immorality and cruelty of the women who murder their infants. Others have salacious and sensational titles to attract potential readers but the narratives aim to arouse compassion. *Blood for Blood* (1670) narrates how Mary Cook—"melancholy" and suicidal—murdered her two-year-old daughter; the writer describes the crime as cruel but the circumstances as "tragical." The story of widowed Mary Goodenough (*Fair Warning to Murderers of Infants* [1691/1692]) is even more pathetic. Driven by poverty into an adulterous affair with a baker in an attempt to feed her children, Goodenough became pregnant, concealed the birth of the baby, and left it to die. Undeniably guilty under the terms of the 1624 Act, she was condemned to hang. The writer admonishes anyone tempted to adultery, but rather than berating Goodenough for lewdness, suggests that it was the adulterous baker who was most to blame.

German, French, and English pamphlets all used stories of child-murder as propaganda in the religious conflicts of the period, giving the crime a significant political dimension. Catholic French theologians published stories of the Protestant ritual murder of babies during the Wars of Religion (1562–1599) (Rucaut, 18–20); Protestant German writers showed the most violent child-murders being committed by Catholic nuns (Wiltenburg, 237), and English pamphleteers used male and female child-murderers to warn of the potential dangers of Catholic rule throughout the seventeenth century (Robson, 151–55, 167–72).

In Europe, court records and cheap print show child-murder as a crime that was mostly committed by women. In early modern China (late Ming [1368–1644] and early Qing [1644–1911] dynasties), the *victims* of child-murder were overwhelmingly female. Although newborn infants of both sexes were drowned to limit family size, girls were the most vulnerable (Brook, 163). Factors contributing to this were a patrilineal inheritance system that favored male children, a rise in the price of dowries, poverty, and local custom (Waltner, 197–205). In China (as in Europe), economic, religious, and social factors combined to inspire infanticide and also to try and proscribe it. Infanticide was illegal throughout China, although it was not a capital crime, and legal texts, magistrates' manuals, and moral texts all represent child-murder as a threat to social order (Waltner, 195). Confucian doctrine taught that the killing of female children had cosmic significance, leading to an imbalance between yin and yang (Kinney, 101). Mirroring developments in early modern Europe, a rise in population and prosperity in China, combined with improving distribution networks and an expanding readership, also saw a rise in the popularity of colloquial fiction (Furth, 9; Roberts, 183–84). The appetite for printed stories was used by government authorities to propagate the idea that female infanticide was wrong. Morally uplifting songs with a similar message were circulated in an attempt to reach the illiterate (Waltner, 203). There are records and stories of women (mothers and midwives) killing newborns but a father killing his daughter was represented as particularly damaging because the deliberate and violent dissolution of the father/child bond was regarded as morally damaging and politically reprehensible (Waltner, 201 5), once again giving the crime of child-murder a significant public and political dimension. *See also* Abortion and Contraception; Confucianism.

Further Reading: Bicks, Caroline. *Midwiving Subjects in Shakespeare's England*. Aldershot: Ashgate, 2003; Brook, Timothy. *The Confusions of Pleasure Commerce and Culture in Ming China*. Berkeley and Los Angeles: University of California Press, 1998; Chartier, Roger. "The Hanged Woman Miraculously Saved: An *occasionel*." In *The Culture of Print Power and the Uses of Print in Early Modern Europe*, edited by Roger Chartier, 59–91. Translated by Lydia G. Cochrane. Cambridge: Polity Press, 1989; Dolan, Frances E. *Dangerous Familiars Representations of Domestic Crime in England 1550–1700*. Ithaca, NY: Cornell University Press, 1994; Furth, Charlotte. "Concepts of Pregnanacy, Childbirth and Infancy in Ch'ing Dynasty China." *Journal of Asian Studies* 46 (1987): 7–35; Hoffer, Peter C., and N.E.H. Hull. *Murdering Mothers: Infanticide in England and New England 1558–1803*. New York: New York University Press, 1984; Jackson, Mark. *New-Born Child Murder: Women, Illegitimacy and the Courts in Eighteenth-Century England*. Manchester: Manchester University Press, 1996; Kinney, Ann Behnke. *Representations of Childhood and Youth in Early China*. Stanford, CA: Stanford University Press, 2004; The Proceedings of the Old Bailey, London 1764–1834. www.oldbaileyonline.org; Roberts, J.A.G. *The Complete History of China*. Stroud: Sutton, 2003; Robson, Lynn. *"No Nine Days' Wonder": Embedded Protestant Narratives in Early Modern Prose Murder Pamphlets 1573–1700*. PhD dissertation, University of Warwick, 2003; Rucaut, Luc. "Accusations of Infanticide on the Eve of the French Wars of Religion." In *Infanticide: Historical Perspectives on Child Murder and Concealment 1550–2000*, edited by Mark Jackson. Aldershot: Ashgate, 2002; Ruff, Julius R. *Violence in Early Modern Europe 1500–1800*. Cambridge: Cambridge University Press, 2001; Walker, Garthine. *Crime, Gender and Social Order in Early Modern England*. Cambridge: Cambridge University Press, 2003; Waltner, Ann. "Infanticide and Dowry in Ming and Early Qing China." In *Chinese Views of Childhood*, edited by Ann Behnke Kinney. Honolulu: University of Hawai'i Press, 1995; Wiltenburg, Joy. *Disorderly Women and Female Power in the Street Literature of Early Modern England and Germany*. Charlottesville: University of Virginia

Press, 1992; Wrightson, Keith. "Infanticide in Earlier Seventeenth-Century England." *Local Population Studies* 15 (1975): 10–22.

Lynn Robson

'ISHQ. The word *'ishq* is Arabic in origin but has been borrowed by the Persians and Turks as well as numerous other Muslim societies. It is often defined as **love** but this definition must be expanded and explained. *'Ishq* refers specifically to passionate love driven by an overpowering desire to obtain its object. Love (*ùubb, maùabbat, hawä*) is usually characterized as three types: natural, intellectual, and divine. The compelling physical desires of the body are recognized as natural and are expressed as profane heterosexual or homosexual love. The intellect and soul manifest themselves as an intellectual love and divine mystical love of God respectively. However, the Sufi mystics of **Islam** typically abandoned reason and intellect in their quest of divine love.

'Ishq, as secular earthly passionate love, permeated Arabic, Persian, Turkish, and other literatures. Attached to this persistent theme were the sadness, longing, and suffering of the lover for his or her beloved. This theme immortalized the tortures of love endured by famous lovers in Middle Eastern literature such as Majnun and Layla, Khusraw and Shirin, Salämän and Absäl, and Mahmud and Ayaz. Secular love poetry proliferated in the lyric form of the *ghazal*, which was typically between five and fifteen couplets long. While heterosexual love was the norm, a strong current of homosexual love is found especially in classical Persian poetry. However, in Persian, the lack of a third person gender-specific pronoun allowed this to remain ambiguous. Within the courts and more elite classes, it was not an uncommon practice to sleep with prepubescent and adolescent boys. Once they reached puberty and were able to grow beards, new boys were found. In the *Qäbüs-näma*, a work of the Mirror-for-Princes genre, the prince is advised to sleep with boys in the winter and girls in the summer.

'Ishq as manifested as divine, sacred love also became a major theme of poetry. In many cases in popular poetry, the language of the mystics was adopted so that it is extremely difficult, if not impossible, to differentiate between the longing of the body or the soul, although all expressions are primarily physical. The stories of famous lovers became very popular subjects for mystical narrative and didactic poems (*see* **Sufi Romances**). The expression of *'ishq* within Islamic mysticism is very involved and complicated. It becomes an obsession and quest for the eternal, the transcendent and the sacred. The lover is constantly in pursuit of the beloved.

The ultimate goal of the Sufi path was to obtain unity with God, which culminated with the annihilation of self. This journey took the seeker through a long series of stages and states. This was depicted in many ways. The seeker or lover in literature took on many forms besides the typical lover/beloved image. Sometimes the lover was depicted as a beggar before the king. Sometimes the lover was likened unto a moth that enamored of the flame of a candle, flew into the fire and was consumed by it. *See also* Homosexuality; Middle East.

Further Reading: Arkoun, M. "'Ishk." In *Encyclopaedia of Islam*, edited by P. Bearman, Th. Bianquis, C. E. Bosworth, E. van Donzel, and W. P. Heinrichs. Leiden: Brill, 2007; Schimmel, Anne Marie. *As Through a Veil, Mystical Poetry in Islam*. New York: Columbia University Press, 1982.

Mark David Luce

ISLAM. In 632, Mohammed, the founder of Islam, died unexpectedly at Medina, leaving behind a religious community centered there, about 180 miles north of Mecca.

ISLAM

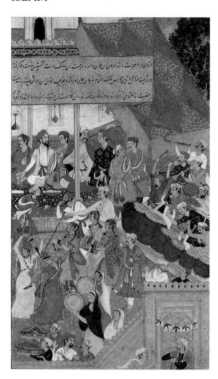

The marriage entertainment of Akbar's brother, from "Akbar Namar, Story of Akbar," c. 1561. © The Art Archive/ Victoria and Albert Museum London/Sally Chappell.

The revelations he had received as a prophet were collected from pieces of bone, parchment, palm leaves, and the hearts of his followers into the Koran, along with the *hadiths*, Mohammed's sayings and deeds. The Koran and the *hadiths* became the sources of *shari'a* (shariah), or Islamic law, that developed in the next several centuries.

Mohammed taught that the basic spiritual problem for humans was ignorance. The Koran (and eventually the *hadiths*) formed the law that would guide people on the path (*sunna*) to paradise. Humans were not viewed as corrupted radically by sin but, rather, as afflicted with problems caused by ignorance. Consequently, in the area of human sexual life, there was a general acceptance of sexual drives as natural, rather than inherently sinful. However, adultery or fornication were prohibited and severely punished as matters that were evil ("*shirk*").

Mohammed, as the warrior leader of his religious community, had approximately a dozen wives, as well as some concubines. Later scholars have claimed that many of these marriages were made for political reasons, or to bring widows under his protection. The slave girl Maria al-Qibtiyya, a Coptic Christian, was given to Mohammed by the ruler of Egypt. She may have been freed and married by Mohammed; she bore him a son, Ibrahim, who died young.

Mohammed's example was imitated to a degree by his followers. Mohammed had decreed that Muslim men may have only four wives, and, importantly, that they must be all treated equally. Later Sunni schools of *shari'a* allowed up to four wives, four concubines, and four slave girls at one time, and stipulated that they must all be treated equally. Mohammed's limitation that men could have only four wives at one time was actually not an endorsement of polygamy, but a limitation on it.

Divorce was also easy for Sunni Muslim men, but virtually impossible for Muslim women. All that was necessary for a man was to say to a wife, in the presence of witnesses, "I divorce you" three times. Provisions for her maintenance would have to be made, but otherwise the man was free to move on to a new woman immediately.

Islam, in the early modern period, was a religion that shaped three great empires; the Mogul Empire in India, the Safavid Empire in Persia, and the Ottoman Empire, based in Turkey and the Balkans; and a number of smaller kingdoms in central **Asia**, Egypt, and North **Africa**. Each of these three empires was extremely wealthy during this period due to trade and the booty of conquests. Enormous sums were available to be spent on artistic activities such as architecture, jewelry, and furnishings.

While traditional Islamic art has always been limited to calligraphy (especially of sayings from the Koran), geometric designs, and designs developed from plants, the art of this period included an enormous number of paintings of people. The Persian tradition of painting was very rich and influenced the Moguls as well as the Ottomans, who commissioned portraits of the Sultans.

The Mogul (Persian, Mughal) empire had begun when Babur—a descendant of Tamburlaine and through him a descendant of Genghis Khan—conquered northern

India in the 1520s. His descendants were to remain as the rulers of much of India for several centuries, but were to achieve their greatest cultural attainments during the early modern period.

The Mogul court promoted a refined culture while often expressing Islamic opposition to the sexual expressions of the religions of India as, for example, when Babur had the faces and genitals of naked Jain statures carved in living rock at Gwalior knocked off. As Muslim warriors, the Moguls were often chivalrous in their treatment of the women of the families of other Muslim princes who were defeated by them. It was the custom to return the harem of another unmolested. In contrast the captured young sons of non-Muslim princes were often castrated, while their daughters were prostituted or sexually abused.

In the practices of the times it was common for the harem to number many more young women than the traditional maximum of twelve. In the early modern period it flourished under Akbar and other emperors. The number of women in Akbar's **harem** was probably 5,000. Some women of harems were older women who simply lived there. Some were Slavic or Abyssinian "Amazons" who guarded the harem. Some were servant girls, and others were presentation princesses. The latter were lovely young women who were presented to the Emperor as wives by royal or noble families that sought an alliance with the Moguls. For example, in 1562 the Raja of Jaisalmer presented a daughter to Akbar, whom he graciously accepted for political reasons. Despite the size of their harems, siring heirs was to prove more difficult for the Mogul dynasty than the opportunities available should have allowed.

To maintain sexual vigor at the court, physicians were kept on call who could tend to the health of the emperor and that of his harem. The physician might have to examine a woman of the harem who was semi-clothed and behind a screen. In some cases harem women faked an illness to have the hand of the physician examine the woman's breast or privates, which was recorded by several European physicians.

Having many wives—the Mogul emperor's often numbered in the hundreds—was justified by the Koranic distinction between wives who were in a lower form of **marriage**, *muta*, which was considered to be temporary, versus those who were *nikah* because their marital status was the result of an orthodox Muslim ceremony, which could only be between a free Muslim woman and a Muslim man. In contrast, *muta* was considered to be a private act between a man and a woman and the religious issue was not relevant.

Akbar rejected the interpretations of the orthodox Muslim legal scholars. He was far more tolerant of non-Muslims, and he also engaged in practices contrary to Mohammed. For example, he washed his privates before sex rather than afterward, as Mohammed had done. To protect women in general, Akbar and others sought to end the Hindu practice of **sati**. In this practice, Hindu wives were expected to throw themselves onto their husband's funeral pyre. He also sought to end child marriages.

An extensive harem also flourished under Shah Jahan but he particularly loved Arjumand Banu. Her title, Mumtaz Mahal, meant "favorite of the palace." She bore him thirteen children before dying in **childbirth**, delivering the fourteenth while on a military campaign. Deeply grieved, Shah Jahan ordered the building of an enormous tomb for her, the famous Taj Mahal. It was planned on the basis of a garden. However, Shah Jahan's Shalimar Bagh built at Lahore is considered to be the most beautiful of all Mogul gardens outside of the Shalimar Bagh on Lake Dal in Kashmir. The Taj Mahal was built as an imitation of a garden in the Muslim paradise. Inlaid with fine stones and gemstones, it was covered with carvings of sayings from the Koran in Arabic.

The wealth of the Moguls was enormous. Much of it had been looted from Buddhist and Hindu temples. However, many new gemstones came from the alluvial diamond fields of India near Golconda, which would be exhausted during the reign of the Moguls. Many of the diamonds and other jewels were use to encrust the Mogul Peacock Throne, an extravagant work that would be broken up and carted back to Persia by Nadir Shah in 1739.

The Persians eventually created their own Peacock Throne with some of their spoils from India. The Persian Empire had arisen from one of the Sufi orders of the Mongol period, the Safavids. Sheikh Safi al-Din (1252–1334), its founder, inspired a legacy of charismatic warrior leaders who converted many Turkomen tribes in eastern Turkey and Azerbaijan to their Shi'ite teaching. As mystical Sufis, the Safavids were able to use poetry to inspire their followers. They also used it to spread their ideology. About the beginning of the early modern period, the Safavid Empire was centered in Tabriz. However, the threat of Ottoman military power forced its transfer to several locations, including Isfahan, which became an architectural and artistic triumph. The Safavids promoted the revival of Persian traditions of art and architecture. Persian miniature portraits of love scenes and of other scenes became an important part of the legacy. During the period of Safavid consolidation of power, Turkic was replaced by Persian and Shi'ite Islam was imposed or widely accepted.

Among peculiar Shi'ite practices are temporary marriages (*mut'a*), often between a young man and an older widow. It is also called *nikah al-muwaqqat*, and is based on the Koran 4:24. It is called *sigha* in Persian. *Mut'a* allowed sexual intercourse and it provided monetary support for the woman. Persian managers of caravansaries offered *mut'a* wives to travelers staying the night.

Shi'ite legal scholars (*ulama*) developed a more conservative approach to **divorce** ("*talaq*"). A Shi'ite man could not divorce by repeating the divorce formula three times on one occasion. "I divorce you" had to be repeated on different occasions before two witnesses while sober and calm, which delay allowed opportunity for reconciliation. Shi'ite Shari'a also provided more generously for women in inheritance than Sunni practice. Scholars have claimed that this is due to the role that Fatima, the daughter of Mohammed and wife of Ali, plays in Shi'ite piety.

The Ottoman Empire was ruled by the Turkish sultan. Upon ascending to the throne, it was the practice of the sultan to have all his competing brothers executed to eliminate any rival claimants to the throne. In contrast, the Safavids would simply imprison their siblings, while the Moguls originally sent them off to remote frontiers to fight before finally also adopting the practice of killing all rival siblings.

In the Ottoman Empire, the harem was the sultan's. The Topkapi was the pleasure place built for the sultan in Constantinople, where the sultan and his harem resided. It was common for the sultans to keep company with a different woman each night. Those who became favorites of the sultan were often in danger from their rivals. Murders were not unknown as a way of eliminating a rival or the son of a rival. **Eunuch** slaves guarded the women of the Sultan's harem. Any male caught attempting to invade the harem was severely punished.

As an Islamic empire all Ottoman men who could afford more than one wife were allowed to have them. Slaves were also purchased for sexual reasons. While forbidden by Islamic law, **homosexuality** and pedophilia were quietly practiced by the rich and powerful in some cases.

The Ottomans were ruling a vast mosaic of conquered peoples. They organized them into Milets, which were ethnic groups headed by a man appointed for the purpose of being the liaison between the sultan and the people of the Milet. For example, the Patriarch of Constantinople was the head of the Christian Milet.

Among the responsibilities for the head of the Milet was the delivery of the tax (*jizya*) on the non-Muslims (*dhimmi*). Akabar had eliminated this tax in India, but the Ottomans often had it paid by the taking of children in the *devshirme* system. Pretty young girls were often prepared for the harem while boys might be castrated and put into various forms of service. Other boys would be put into the fearsome slave army of the sultan, the Janissaries. *See also* Buddhism; Castration; Christianity; Hinduism; Middle East; Polygamy/Polyandry; Slavery.

Further Reading: Daniel, Elton L. *The History of Iran*. Westport, CT: Greenwood Press, 2001; Gascoinge, Bamber. *A Brief History of The Great Moguls*: New York: Carroll & Graf Publishers, 2002; Hodgson, Marshall G. S. *The Venture of Islam: Conscience and History in a World Civilization*. 3 vols. Chicago: The University of Chicago Press, 1974; Kinross, Lord. *The Ottoman Centuries: The Rise and Fall of the Turkish Empire*. New York: Morrow Quill Paperbacks, 1977; Kissling, Hans J. *The Last Great Muslim Empires: History of the Muslim World*. Princeton, NJ: Markus Wiener Publishers, 1996; Kulke, Herman, and Dietmar Rothermund. *A History of India*. New York: Barnes & Noble, 1986; Wiebke, Walther. *Women in Islam: From Medieval to Modern Times*. Princeton, NJ: Markus Wiener Publishers, 1999.

Andrew J. Waskey

JEANNE D'ARC. *See* Joan of Arc

JOAN OF ARC (c. 1412–1431). Joan of Arc (in French Jeanne d'Arc), a French peasant girl whose improbable military leadership raised the English siege of Orléans and revived the cause of the French royal House of Valois, is the most enigmatic and compelling figure of the Hundred Years War and perhaps in all of French history. Shrouded in myth, declared a Catholic saint in 1920, and endlessly analyzed or glorified by artists, politicians, and historians, Joan and her brief public career have over the centuries become emblematic of a wide variety of causes and hopes. As a result, it is difficult to say much with certainty about Joan in terms of her appearance, personality, or sexuality.

Born about 1412 into a prosperous peasant family from the Lorraine village of Domrémy, Joan, at about age thirteen, began hearing the voices of Saint Margaret, Saint Catherine, and the archangel Michael, who exhorted her to go to the aid of the Dauphin Charles, the uncrowned king of France. Because of civil war and English invasion, Charles's assumption of his late father's crown and the continuance of his dynasty were in jeopardy. In February 1429, Joan, who was now perhaps seventeen or eighteen, persuaded the dauphinist commander at Vaucouleurs to provide her with an escort to Charles. Advised by her voices to cut her hair and assume male attire, Joan traveled for eleven days through enemy territory to reach the dauphin's court. After being kept waiting for several days while the dauphin's councilors debated the advisability of receiving her, Joan was summoned to court, where she made a sensation by immediately picking Charles, whom she had never seen, out of a crowd. Joan and the dauphin then held an intense private conversation during which Joan, by unknown means, convinced him that she had been sent by God to defeat the English and see him crowned.

However, before dispatching her to Orléans with an army, Charles sent her to Poitiers to be interrogated by a panel of theologians charged with ensuring her religious orthodoxy, and then to Tours for a physical examination conducted by his mother-in-law to ensure that Joan was a virgin. Having passed these tests, Joan, riding at the head of her men, entered Orléans on April 29. Although she wore armor like any soldier, Joan's only weapon was her special standard, which had been designed on instructions from her voices. Driven by Joan's sense of urgency and her confidence in her mission and inspired by her courage—she refused to leave the field after being wounded by an arrow—the French attacked fiercely, forcing the English to lift the siege on May 8. In June, Joan led

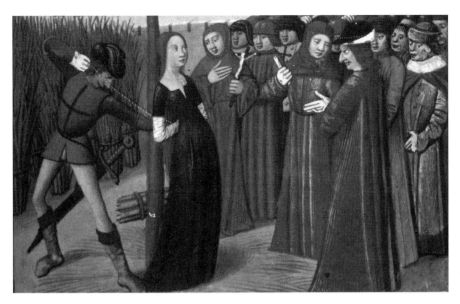

Execution of Joan of Arc, from "Les Vigils de Charles VII," by Martial de Paris. © Giraudon/Art Resource, NY.

another campaign that cleared the Loire Valley of English garrisons and concluded with a major victory at Patay, thereby clearing the way for the dauphin to travel to Rheims, the traditional French coronation site, and be crowned king on July 17.

Military success now made Joan a political force at court, where she urged vigorous prosecution of the war. However, the failure of her ill-considered assault on Paris in September caused her influence to decline, leading her to depart the court secretly in May 1430 to help repel an enemy attack on Compiègne. On May 23, Joan was captured by the Burgundians, who sold her to their English allies. Anxious to discredit the Valois cause by associating it with witchcraft and heresy, the English put Joan on trial for both in February 1431. Examined by bishops and theologians who were appalled by her use of male attire, Joan was condemned to death. Before sentence could be read, Joan recanted, denying her voices, confessing to blasphemy and sorcery, and promising to wear women's clothes. Sentenced to life imprisonment, Joan asked to be sent to an ecclesiastical prison, where she could have female attendants. However, she was returned to the English military prison, where, four days later, she overthrew her recantation by resuming male attire. Although Joan said that it was more suitable to dress like a man while in the keeping of men, historians have surmised that the English, angry that she had escaped the flames, sent soldiers to gang-rape her or ordered her jailers to hide her women's clothes. In any event, her subsequent admission that her voices had returned sealed her fate. Joan was burned at the stake in Rouen on May 30, 1431.

In the 1450s, the French king ordered a new trial to reverse the verdict of 1431 and clear Joan's name. Comprised largely of the recollections of men who had fought with her, the records of this trial provide most of what is known about Joan as a person. Joan's squire, Jean d'Aulon, testified that he often saw Joan in various states of undress as he tended her wounds and helped her in and out of her armor. Having on several occasions seen her naked legs and breasts, he described her as "a young girl, beautiful and well-formed" (Richey, p. 141). Her close companion, Jean, duke of Alençon, also found her naked breasts "beautiful," which, since the contemporary ideal of beauty called for small, firm, and high breasts, means they may have been of such description. A doctor who examined her while she was imprisoned declared her to be "*stricta*" (e.g., narrow in the hips), but did not confirm d'Aulon's statement that Joan was never known to menstruate, an assertion that has over the years generated many otherwise unsupported claims regarding Joan's femininity or her mental or physical condition. A courtier who had seen Joan at the French court said she had black hair cut short like a man's, a claim that was seemingly verified when a historian later found a short strand of black hair embedded in the wax used to seal one of Joan's letters.

At the rehabilitation trial, most of Joan's military comrades swore that they had never felt any sexual arousal around her, being inspired instead by her words and strength of purpose. However, the squire Gobert Thibault testified that men did feel sexual desire for her but did not dare act upon it because of her chaste demeanor and the aura of saintliness that, in the men's minds, surrounded her. Whether or not Joan was raped in prison is uncertain, but we do know that Joan had earlier violently resisted the attempts of an English guard to fondle her breasts. All indications are that, while of pleasant appearance, Joan was completely absorbed by what she considered her divine mission and showed no interest in attracting men sexually.

Further Reading: Pernoud, Régine. *Joan of Arc: By Herself and Her Witnesses*. London: Scarborough House, 1982; Pernoud, Régine, and Marie-Véronique Clin. *Joan of Arc*. Translated by Jeremy Duquesnay Adams. New York: St. Martin's Press, 1999; Richey, Stephen W. *Joan of Arc: The Warrior Saint*. Westport, CT: Praeger, 2003; Warner, Marina. *Joan of Arc: The Image of Female Heroism*. New York: Knopf, 1981; Wheeler, Bonnie, and Charles T. Woods, eds. *Fresh Verdicts on Joan of Arc*. London: Garland, 1996; Wood, Charles T. *Joan of Arc and Richard III: Sex, Saints, and Government in the Middle Ages*. Oxford: Oxford University Press, 1991.

John A. Wagner

JUDAISM. Judaism is the religion of the Jewish people, who characterized a small but widespread minority in early modern Europe. While Judaism originated with the religion and culture of ancient Israel in the first millennium BCE, the rabbinic Judaism that became normative for Jewish communities of the medieval and modern periods was formulated in late antiquity, concurrent with the growth and articulation of Christianity.

Jews settled throughout the Christian and Muslim worlds. Generally, Jews living in Muslim lands are called Sephardim, while Jews living in Christian lands are called Ashkenazim. More specifically, Sephardim refers to those Jews expelled from Spain in 1492, and who settled throughout the Mediterranean. The Jewish communities of the eastern Islamic world are sometimes called *Edot haMizrah* (communities of the East). Ashkenazim properly refers to Jews from central Europe. Jewish communities that were predominately Ashkenazic or Sephardic would often have a minority community of Sephardim or Ashkenazim, much like a Protestant community in a Catholic majority or vice versa.

Jews did not gain citizenship in Christian countries until after the French Revolution. Generally excluded from guilds and burgher (town) rights, and not possessing large areas of land, Jews were granted "privileges" to live in various jurisdictions, and were protected by the authorities that granted those privileges. Authorities often looked to Jewish moneylenders for financing because Church law restricted Christian money lending. High debts, as well as the Jews' alien status within society, encouraged anti-Jewish feeling from the populace. Anti-Judaism, the precursor to modern anti-Semitism, occasionally materialized in "blood-libels," where Jews were accused of desecrating the Host. Sometimes real violence erupted, most famously in the Rhineland during the First Crusade, when mobs, inspired and helped by Crusaders on their way to the Holy Land, killed thousands of Jews in a fit of apocalyptic fervor. At other times Jews were expelled from the countries they were living in, giving rise to the image of the Wandering Jew. And yet, some Jews became successful merchants on an international scale, making use not only of liquid capital but also of a network of Jewish merchants reaching into the Far East. A number of these successful merchants came into the employ of local leaders and became known as "Court Jews." Most Jews lived in restricted areas, often in town ghettoes, or as was the case in the Russian Empire, in the "Pale of Settlement," a large area in Poland and Ukraine where Jewish settlement was permitted.

Jewish culture was remarkably literary. Universal primary education was an ideal in Jewish communities, centuries before the European nations began to do so. Jews spoke the languages surrounding them, and often spoke Jewish dialects like the Ladino of Spanish-origin Jews, and the Judaeo-German, or Yiddish, of the Ashkenazic Jews. Hebrew, though, was the language of Jewish literary culture and was also used to communicate by letter with Jews of other lands. The greatest evidence of Jewish culture is literary. There are few artistic or architectural examples of Jewish life. A few synagogues survive, and material culture was best preserved through ritual items. Cemeteries provide rich testimony to the values of Jewish culture, telling the story of communities and identifying family structures. Jewish cemeteries reveal the honor bestowed upon scholars, rabbis who served as teachers and as authorities of Jewish law.

While the Jews were spread through innumerable jurisdictions, Jewish law, or *halakhah*, governed Jewish life. There was no central legal authority, and rabbis were ultimately granted authority through community acceptance. The surrounding authorities considered the Jewish communities as corporate bodies, and as such, the Jewish communal authorities had governing power. The rabbis, as the scholars of Jewish law, communicated with their rabbinic colleagues in a vast network of study of the legal texts, traditions, and precedent.

Rabbinic law, based on the Bible and disseminated in the Talmud, was interpreted through the ages in responsa written by major authorities. Jewish law was systematically codified only a few times in history. The code of Maimonides (d. 1204), called the *Mishneh Torah*, continues to be influential among Jewish legal scholars to this day. The reigning authoritative code, first published in Venice in 1565, is the *Shulhan Arukh* (literally, the Ordered Table). This code of law has been the standard authority throughout the Jewish world ever since. It was written by the Sephardic authority Joseph Caro of Safed (Palestine). At the same time, the Ashkenazic authority Moses Isserles of Prague was working on a comprehensive code. Isserles appended his rulings when they differed with Caro's, as glosses to the code, so that the combined work covered both Sephardic and Ashkenazic practice. The *Shulhan Arukh* covers all areas of Jewish life, and governed Jewish communal life in the early modern period. The *Shulhan Arukh*, as a product of the sixteenth century, offers excellent evidence of Jewish life, including sex, love, and marriage.

The *Shulhan Arukh* is divided into four sections, one of which (the *Even HaEzer*) is devoted entirely to the laws of marriage and divorce. Marriage was considered a *mitzvah*, or commandment, an expectation of all Jews. Marriages were arranged, which was particularly important since Jewish law does not recognize marriage to non-Jews.

Eligible marriage partners were often quite restricted (due to the laws against incest and other legal restrictions), so Jews had to rely on arrangements with other Jewish communities. Jewish law does permit a woman to own property, and there are examples of single women, usually widows, who engaged in trade. The most famous example is Glueckl of Hamelin, in Germany, who left behind rich memoirs. However, once married, the wife was expected to work to support the household. Any income she earned while married, or earnings from her separate property, was given over to her husband. Women only inherited property when there were no male children.

Jewish law provides for what we would call no-fault divorce. A man could choose to divorce his wife and draw up the writ of divorce, called a *get*. He did not have to demonstrate cause. However, only the man could initiate the divorce. A woman could appeal to the rabbinic court for help in procuring a divorce for cause. Grounds for that appeal were a husband's negligence in providing food, raiment, or regular conjugal relations. When a man and woman were divorced the woman received an economic settlement that was always agreed to in advance of the wedding in a document called a *ketubbah*. The *ketubbah* is still used today in Jewish marriages, but its economic substance is no longer employed in the distribution of property. In the early modern period, as in earlier times, the *ketubbah* governed the settlement that the husband owed his wife in case of divorce. The same settlement was owed to the wife by the husband's children after the husband died.

Ancient Jewish law permitted a husband to have more than one wife, but this was proscribed for Ashkenazic communities in the eleventh century. Polygamy continued in Sephardic communities through the middle of the twentieth century. Adultery and incest were strictly forbidden by ancient law. Nonmarital relations that were not incestuous or adulterous (i.e., premarital or postmarital sex) were not treated with the same severity, but were still generally frowned upon by Jewish law and tradition. Marriage was considered the proper context for sexual relations. Within marriage, sex was consecrated and became a holy act.

Regular conjugal relations were, as mentioned above, one of the principal marital obligations of a husband toward his wife. The frequency of sexual relations (*onah* in Hebrew) was determined by the husband's occupation at the time of marriage. If he were a merchant who traveled for long periods, then he would only be required to have conjugal relations with his wife a few times a year. But if he worked locally, or was a man of leisure, then the requirement was at least once weekly. That the sexual relationship was framed as a legal obligation of the husband toward his wife indicates that sex was independent of procreation. The Jewish legal requirement to have children is incumbent only upon men. That is, a woman was not considered a "sinner" if she was not married with children, while a man was. Additionally, the requirement of regular conjugal relations applied whether or not the wife was fertile. That is, during pregnancy, nursing, after menopause, and if a woman was known to be generally infertile, the marital obligation of conjugal relations still applied. While ancient Jewish law provided that a man should divorce his wife if they are married for ten years and have not had children, Moses Isserles wrote in his gloss to the *Shulhan Arukh* that "in our time," that is, sixteenth-century Europe, "we do not compel him to divorce his wife because there are no children." Rather, if the couple wished to remain married then they remained married, and their conjugal relationship remained a Jewish legal obligation, even though it was deemed non-procreative.

The marital sexual relationship, while required by Jewish law, was regulated with periods of abstinence. Based on ancient biblical law, a woman, during her menstrual period and a week afterward, was considered ritually impure and did not engage in sexual contact with her husband. At the end of her period of impurity (*niddah* in Hebrew), she immersed in a **mikveh** (ritual bath). Jewish law required that construction of a *mikveh* be the top priority of any Jewish community, to insure that marital relations could always resume after the periods of impurity. The observance of the laws of ritual impurity, sometimes called "family purity," tended to insure that husbands and wives engaged in marital relations when the woman returned from the *mikveh*, thus institutionalizing regulated sex in marriage.

The *Shulhan Arukh* does provide specific guidelines on sex. Couples should engage in sexual relations only in private, not in the daytime, and not in the light. A man should not kiss a woman on the genitals or even look at her genitalia. However, elsewhere in the *Shulhan Arukh* and other Jewish legal literature the law is stated clearly that "all is permitted" within a marital relationship, including **anal sex**. Most authorities understood the strictures of the *Shulhan Arukh* to be sagely advice rather than legal prohibitions. Since the law permitted all forms of sexual intimacy between a husband and wife (as long as the wife was not ritually impure), the sociological implication is that the rabbis recognized that while the times and contexts of sex could be regulated, its forms and expression could not.

Jewish tradition often speaks of the relationship between God and the people of Israel as analogous to the love between a husband and wife. The intensity of love and erotic passion is seen as a metaphor for the mutual attraction between God and Israel. In mystical circles, this was used as an explanation of the holiness inherent in the sex act between husband and wife. While there is some literary evidence for love and erotica, and quite ample remains of "secular love poetry" from the Spanish Jewish community, the more overwhelming examples of love between God and Israel testify that there was real love between husbands and wives. Were there not, then the widespread metaphor of the love-relationship between God and Israel would be ineffective. Jewish culture saw the relationship between a husband and wife as one of deep love, of provision and protection, of intimate sexual expression, and as a covenanted arrangement of mutual obligations. *See also* Menstruation.

Further Reading: Feldman, David M. *Marital Relations, Birth Control and Abortion in Jewish Law.* New York: New York University, 1968.

David J. Fine

JULIAN OF NORWICH (1342–c.1416). Julian of Norwich was born in 1342 to a nobleman's family in Norwich, England. Her books, *Showings of Divine Love* and *Revelations of Divine Love* are well-known contributions to medieval theology. Sometime in her early adulthood, she became an anchoress at St. Julian's church, choosing the patron saint of the church as her namesake. Julian lived in an anchorhold for approximately forty-three years; she gave advice to the visitors who came to her window, and wrote two versions of her book of visions. The author Margery Kempe, one of the few other extant female Middle English writers, visited Julian sometime in 1413 to obtain spiritual advice. Obeying the *Ancrene Wisse*, the thirteenth-century rulebook for these women who were "buried" in a cell, she seems to have remained in her anchorhold until her death in about 1416.

In her influential visions, Julian writes that she prayed for three gifts from the hand of her God: to understand Jesus Christ's Passion in a more palpable manner, to receive a deathly illness, and to receive three wounds. These wounds would consist of contrition, compassion for her fellow man, and a greater longing for God. At the age of thirty, she did experience an almost fatal illlness which led to a temporary paralysis. In the midst of the illness she had a series of visions. Upon reflection and meditation, Julian wrote *A Vision Showed to a Devout Woman*, sometimes more commonly referred to as *Showings*. The first version, which seems to be written soon after her experience, later gave way to the expanded second version of her text, *A Revelation of Divine Love*. Instead of choosing Latin, the language of the medieval Church, Julian instead wrote in her vernacular, English. Her texts are some of the few that can still be studied as examples of Middle English female authorship.

According to her own account, *Revelation* is not merely an expansion of the first book but an actual rephrasing of her first vision; the book also contains the addition of later visions to amount to a book much larger than the first. It shows the influence of theologians and other writers, including the English mystic Richard Rolle.

As indicated by the title of her second book, one of Julian's major discourses is Divine Love, not only between Christ and humans but also within the Trinitarian godhead. She envisioned a moving image of the Passion, focusing on Christ's sacrifice for humans. At one point, in a particularly inspirational and forward-looking moment, she even pictured God as a Mother comforting the hurting sinner as a broken child, instead of the traditional view of God as Father. From her sweeping vision of all of creation as a hazelnut in God's hand to her most famous quote, "Sin is necessary, but all will be well, and all will be well, and every kind of things will be well," this Middle English writer tried to comfort her fellow Christians. *See also* Christianity; Mystics.

Further Reading: Bradley, Ritamary. *Julian's Way: A Practical Commentary on Julian of Norwich*. London: HarperCollins Religious, 1992; Dinshaw, Carolyn, and David Wallace, eds. *The Cambridge Companion to Medieval Women's Writing*. New York: Cambridge University Press, 2003; Julian of Norwich. *Revelations of Divine Love*. Edited and translated by John Skinner. New York: Doubleday, 1997; Underhill, Evelyn. *Mystics of the Church*. Eugene, OR: Wipf and Stock Publishers, 2002.

Katherine R. Cooper

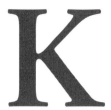

KAMA SUTRA. Composed by Mallanaga Vatsyana, some time between the second and fifth centuries CE in Vedic **India**, the *Kama Sutra* is commonly known as a guide to sensual pleasure or as a salacious book of anecdotes. The book, however, is much more. Only one book in seven deals with techniques of physical lovemaking. The rest of the *Kama Sutra* offers a completely philosophical, matter-of-fact treatise on men and women, covering subjects as diverse as how to furnish and decorate a house, how to woo a bride, how husband and wives are to behave to one another, how religious festivals are to be celebrated, how the kitchen is to be provisioned, and how a garden should be planted. The *Kama Sutra* is an attempt to define the relationship between a man and a woman; the sexual act stands at the heart of the relationship, but the book addresses questions and circumstances in which the act is performed. The approach is that of a *Shastra*, or scientific text, composed in *sutras*, or aphorisms.

Philosophically, the *Kama Sutra* emphasizes the balance in life between *Kama*, *Dharma*, and *Artha*, the three great goals of Hindu life. *Kama* is the name of the Hindu god of love, and it means pleasure of all senses, not just sexual. As the text explains, *Kama* is the delight of the body, mind, and soul: "awaken eyes, nose, tongue, ears and skin, and between sense and sensed, the essence of *Kama* will flower" (Sinha, 1997). *Dharma*, from Sanskrit *dhru*, "to hold," is religious, moral, and social duty; it means acting in accordance with religious teachings, the laws of society, and one's own conscience and nature. *Artha* defines the duty to amass wealth and possessions for the benefit of one's family; it includes learning and craft-skills. *Kama*, *Dharma*, and *Artha* are to be pursued in harmony; bound together and practiced properly, each one must benefit from the other two. Like a dance, the *Kama Sutra* offers sensation-provoking techniques that flow perfectly from one figure to the next, improvised but effortless. The work describes then a scientific and logical attempt at teaching the ways to fully appreciate the beauty and essence of life, be it spiritual or physical, private or public.

Considered fundamental in the education of the women of royal families, the original *Kama Sutra* listed the womanly skills required to serve and entertain husbands and lovers (Indian movie director, Mira Nair explored this historical aspect in her 1997 film *Kama Sutra*). The text describes the general arts necessary to a good wife—singing, dancing, playing instruments, speaking foreign languages, painting, calligraphy, making garlands and floral bouquets, cooking delicious foods, the ability to distinguish between true and false gems, sewing, color-making and dying, treating birds and animals, keeping the body neat and clean, and braiding hair and dying it with henna.

The *Kama Sutra* also emphasizes the intimate arts necessary to a good lover—reading a lover's thoughts, expressing love, showing acceptance through bodily postures and unfastening of clothes, allowing slow intimate touching, scratching lovingly with nails and biting, exposing the private parts, participating artfully in intercourse, encouraging and pleasing the partner, feeling full satisfaction and satisfying the partner, role playing (i.e., pretending anger and reconciliation), pleasing the angry partner, concluding the sexual act, and leaving the sleeping partner. Although patriarchal and male-dominated, Vedic India viewed women's needs and desires in matters of sexual pleasure and satisfaction as equal to those of men. The *Kama Sutra*, therefore, is in some ways a remarkably modern and progressive text; it presents women as active sexual agents, fully entitled to erotic pleasure. However, in some other ways, the *Kama Sutra* comes across as a testimony of an archaic sensibility for it proposes the acceptance of **adultery** (for men) as a way of life, endorses the Machiavellian exploitation of women for men's economic and political advancement; and justifies the **rape** of reluctant women.

In this absence of absolute morality, characteristic of early **Hinduism**, the *Kama Sutra* explains the concept of **love** with no conditional right and wrong. It recommends that the lover spurn classifications, but at the same time it describes four types of love: (1) simple love of intercourse—a habit, a drug; (2) the separate addiction to specific aspects of sex—kissing, embracing, or oral intercourse; (3) the mutual attraction between two people—instinctive, spontaneous, and possessive; and (4) the one-sided love springing from the lover's admiration for the beauty of the beloved. Satisfaction of the first two types depends on physical proficiency, whereas satisfaction of the second two types depends on the harmony and instinct between the partners above all rules. The *Kama Sutra* recognizes the difference between love and sex, and discusses the subject without subtlety and romantic-spiritual language.

Further Reading: Sinha, Indra, trans. *The Love Teaching of Kama Sutra with Extracts from Koka, Shastra, Ananga Ranga and Other Famous Indian Works on Love*. New York: Marlowe & Company, 1997.

Lucia Bortoli

KNOX, JOHN. See *The First Blast of the Trumpet Against the Monstrous Regiment of Women*

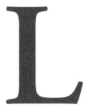

LA MALINCHE (c. 1502–c. 1529 or 1551–1552). La Malinche, also known as Dona Marina and Malinal, was born between 1502 and 1505 in what is now the eastern Mexican state of Veracruz. She was the slave, interpreter, strategist, and sexual partner of the Spanish conquistador Hernán Cortés; the mother of the first Mexican mestizo, or mixed-race child; and has been mythologized as the mother of her country, its first and greatest betrayer, and a passive symbol of the conquest of Mexico.

Very little is actually known about La Malinche, and what few facts exist often contradict each other. She is referred to by word and image in the indigenous Nahuatl account of the conquest, the Florentine Codex, and in accounts by a few contemporaries of Cortés, most notably Bernal **Díaz del Castillo.** They all agree that La Malinche was born into a noble family, but was sold into slavery as a child. She was eventually given as a gift, along with gold, jewels, and twenty other female slaves, to Cortés soon after his arrival in Tabasco in 1519. Cortés needed a translator who could speak both Nahuatl (the language of the Aztec Empire) and Chontal Mayan, and La Malinche was fluent in both languages, possibly because of her previous owners. La Malinche quickly learned Spanish and, by the time the Spanish reached Tenochtitlan, the Aztec capital, in late 1519, she had become Cortés' secretary, sole translator, and strategist. She also taught the Spanish about local customs and religion, and helped them to find local foods and shelter.

La Malinche showed exceptional bravery at numerous points during the Spanish campaign. She, along with other indigenous people, helped Cortés avoid a number of ambushes, especially when the Spanish were in Tenochtitlan. She is also credited with ensuring that diplomacy often took place instead of slaughter. In 1522, she gave birth to Don Martin Cortés, who is the first recorded mestizo, or mixed-race child, in Mexico. She is recorded again during Cortés' Honduras campaign, acting once again as strategist, translator, and secretary. She married another conquistador, Juan Jaramillo, in 1524, and had a daughter with him; then she vanishes from the historical record. Some letters from her children indicate that she died around 1551 or 1552, but some historians put her death in about 1529.

La Malinche was highly regarded during her lifetime. Her **marriage** to a Spaniard indicates that she was accorded status and value by the Spanish, and she was addressed, both by the Mexica and by the Spaniards, with honorifics. Cortés himself said that, after God, Malinche was the greatest reason for his success in Mexico. In succeeding centuries, however, she became mythologized by Mexican nationalists as the betrayer of her nation; seen as the "Mexican Eve," she was the Bad Woman, who betrayed her

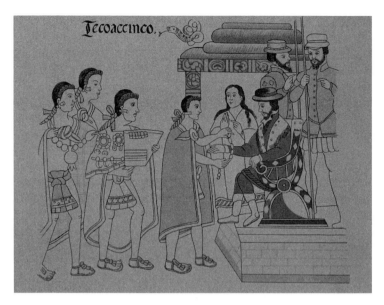

Ambassadors of Aztec emperor Montezuma bring presents to Hernán Cortés and Dona Marina, from the Lienzo de Tlaxcala codex, from original paintings by Tlaxcala artists in the 1560s. © The Art Archive/Mireille Vautier.

blood and her nation for sex, and embodied a negative and irrational national identity and sexuality. Her name has even given rise to a modern Mexican term, "malinchismo," which means to betray one's country and race by mixing with European or outside influences.

Her sexual relationship with Cortés has also been used as a symbol of Mexican submission to outside influence in modern Mexican literature. More recently, her denigration and defamation for patriarchal purposes have moved Chicana and Mexican women writers to see in her a symbol of their own racial, cultural, and ethnic tensions, contradictions, and oppression. Undoubtedly clever, quick-witted, and brave, her gender and her sexual relationship with Cortés make La Malinche a highly problematic symbol for modern Mexicans. *See also*: Americas; Concubines; Explorers.

Further Reading: Cypess, Sandra Messinger. *La Malinche in Mexican Literature: From History to Myth*. Austin: University of Texas Press, 1991; Esquivel, Laura. *Malinche: A Novel*. New York: Atria, 2006 (see for useful bibliography); Romero, Rolando, and Amanda Nolacea Harris, eds. *Feminism, Nation and Myth: La Malinche*. Houston: Arte Publico Press, 2005; Taylor, John. "Reinterpreting Malinche." *Ex Post Facto* 9 (2000): http://userwww.sfsu.edu/epf/2000/jt.html.

Kristen Pederson Chew

LESBIANISM. The full extent of sexual and romantic love between women in the Renaissance will remain unknown, due to the scattered nature of documentation, but the idea was not unknown. The common, documented habit among women of all social classes of sharing a bed may have facilitated sexual relations, when they were desired. A description of an erotic interaction between two women, with implied mutual **masturbation**, appears in Fernando de Rojas's novel *Celestina* (1499), and may have reflected a common reality among prostitutes. There are also several cases in legal records of women covertly adopting male clothing and social identity to live with other women as their "husbands." Not all descriptions of love between women imply sexuality, however. Some Renaissance Neoplatonic circles also endorsed a spiritual love between two women, a love compatible with physical **chastity.** Like other Neoplatonic activities, this form of love was reserved for persons of high social status.

The rare references to lesbianism found in Renaissance writings generally reflect male understandings rather than actual female practices. Much of the discourse on sex between women in Renaissance Europe drew on the classical tradition, particularly the works of the Roman poets Ovid and Martial, the Greek satirist Lucian of Samosata, and, above all, the lyric poet Sappho of Lesbos. Sex between women was also exoticized by being located in other contemporary cultures. Many European traveler accounts found lesbianism relatively common in the Islamic world, while fostering it was one of the litany of charges that Protestant polemicists made against Catholic convents. Pierre Brantome, who recounted the scandals of late sixteenth-century French courtiers, ascribed an allegedly widespread fashion for sex between women to Italian influence. (Brantome's work also contains one of the rare Renaissance uses of the word "lesbian" to refer to sexuality between women.) Brantome, like other male writers, did not conceive of lesbianism as an equal alternative to heterosexuality, but as a way for women to avoid **pregnancy** or enjoy sex in the absence of a man. He insisted that women themselves recognized the superiority of heterosexual sex.

Religious condemnation of lesbianism drew on St. Paul's Letter to the Romans in the Bible, but, like other forms of sex in the period, lesbianism was increasingly identified throughout much of Europe as a crime as well as a sin. Although lesbianism was never persecuted with the intensity of male **homosexuality**, an increased legal hostility that had begun in the High Middle Ages continued and intensified with the overall emphasis on purifying the community characteristic of Protestant and Catholic reformations. The 1532 *Constituo Criminalis Carolina* incorporated the death penalty for lesbian sexual activity into the law of the Holy Roman Empire, but its inclusion was not followed by a wave of persecutions. Legally prohibiting sex between women was characteristic of the Roman legal tradition that dominated most of Continental Europe. The common-law tradition of England did not prescribe a legal penalty for lesbianism, while Orthodox Russia continued to treat it as a sin rather than a crime. Some legal commentators distinguished between different acts, suggesting that women who used instruments to penetrate each other, counterfeiting the penis, deserved far harsher penalties than *tribades* or *fricatrices,* Greek and Latin terms with the literal meaning of "rubbers," referring to women who rubbed their pubic areas together. The few documented executions for female same-sex activities usually involved aggravating circumstances of gender transgression such as the use of a device for penetration or female-to-male transvestism.

Legal persecutions of lesbians were more common in northern Europe than in the Mediterranean area—no executions of lesbians are known from Italy in the Renaissance. One case of persecution of a cross-dressing lesbian occurred in the Bavarian city of Speyer in 1477, when Katherina Heltzeldorfer was executed by drowning. The case reveals the importance of Heltzeldorfer's ambiguous gender in conceptualizing her sexuality. The testimony of women who had contact with Heltzeldorfer identified her sexual aggressiveness as characteristically male, and analogized their relations with her to those with men.

Medical, legal, and clerical understanding of lesbianism in the West was transformed in the late sixteenth century by the discovery of the clitoris as an object of male knowledge. Particularly in France, women who had sex with women were increasingly defined as possessing freakishly enlarged clitorises. *See also* Cross-Dressing; Platonic Love; Prostitution.

Further Reading: Crompton, Louis. "The Myth of Lesbian Impunity: Capital Laws from 1270–1791." *Journal of Homosexuality* 6 (1980–1981): 11–25; Puff, Helmut. "Female Sodomy: The Trial of Katherina Heltzeldorfer (1477)." *Journal of Medieval and Early Modern Studies* 30 (2000): 41–61; Traub, Valerie. *The Renaissance of Lesbianism in Early Modern England.* Cambridge and New York: Cambridge University Press, 2002.

William E. Burns

LITERACY. The early modern period witnessed an increase in the amount of people who could read, write, and have access to schooling in western Europe and its colonies. It is difficult to provide concrete numbers for this growth, since the only direct means of measuring early modern literacy is the perusal of legal documents to determine how many persons were or were not able to write their signatures. Nevertheless, literacy scholars agree that factors such as the advent of the printing press, the **Reformation** and Counter-Reformation movements, and the processes of national unification and imperial expansion created the need for mass literacy and the conditions that made it possible.

Johann Gutenberg's printing technique enabled the reproduction of books on an unprecedented scale, creating the possibility for individuals outside the upper classes and the professional elites to access books and to publish their own writings. In addition, the formation of a wider literate public was stimulated by the growing administrative demands of the emerging nation-states. Both Reformation and Counter-Reformation advocates took advantage of the wider audience that **printing** made possible, and in turn, the continued struggle between Protestants and Catholics worked also as an incentive to provide education and extend literacy throughout western Europe. Furthermore, according to Kenneth A. Lockridge, Protestantism was the main force behind the development of a system of formal schooling in New England (186), and in the Spanish and Portuguese colonies, the Catholic Church organized a solid system of elementary education and catechism instruction.

Literacy (in the Western conceptualization of the term as *alphabetic* literacy) was a central instrument in the colonization of the New World. Amerindian cultures possessed technologies for recording and transmitting information, such as the Aztec *amoxtli* (elaborate pictographic records made on tree bark) and the Inca *quipu* (a system of strings of different lengths and colors, in which knots were used as marks). However, as Walter D. Mignolo explains, because such methods were non-alphabetic, Europeans defined these cultures as illiterate and developed an extensive educational system to establish European legal, economic, political, and religious institutions on the American continent.

These cultural changes brought about a multiplication of educational centers on both sides of the Atlantic, and thus made a fundamental contribution to the spread of literacy. The expansion, however, was not evenly distributed across lines of class, gender, and race. For instance, while elementary instruction and training in practical skills were provided to the indigenous people in the colonies, royal universities and Jesuit colleges were established for male Europeans and their male descendants only. In Europe, the level of education that a person could obtain was also determined by his or her place in society. The upper levels of education were the exclusive realm of men of the upper and middling social ranks, and, in general, schools were more widely available in urban centers than in rural areas. Women's education, when women received one at all, was in most cases limited to the basic reading and writing skills that would be useful in their roles as wives, mothers, and supervisors of the household.

Ideologies of female sexuality intersected with ideologies of female literacy in the limitation of women's education. The mastery of languages, and the knowledge of Latin in particular, were associated with a lack of **chastity** in women, both at a metaphorical level (a woman who desired to learn, and was eloquent, was seen as a woman who harbored sexual desires and would not contain her sexuality) and at a more practical level, since regular interaction with a tutor was seen as a circumstance propitious for seduction. Along these lines of concern, conduct books, such as Juan Luis Vives' 1523 *De institutione feminae chrisitanae* (*On the Instruction of a Christian Woman*), which was written to guide the education of **Henry VIII**'s daughter Princess Mary, warned women against speaking in public as well as against reading literary works; they were warned not only against works that dealt with **love** (from Greek and Roman amatory elegy to chivalric romances and sentimental novels), but also those that dealt with war, since they could lead girls to vividly imagine the male body.

In turn, literary works of the period often built on the associations between female education and sexuality. For instance, in his famous play *El caballero de Olmedo* (*The Gentleman from Olmedo*), the Spanish dramatist Lope de Vega presents an old *alcahueta* (go-between) who passes herself as a Latin teacher for young Inés, and who uses this opportunity to pass letters between Inés and her lover. A scene in William **Shakespeare**'s *The Taming of the Shrew* revolves around a similar situation. To woo Bianca, two of her suitors disguise themselves as Latin and music tutors, respectively, and the girl engages in flirtatious conversations with them while she "translates" a passage of Ovid's *Heroides* and learns musical notes. What is more, early modern women writers, such as Lady Margaret Cavendish, explored these equivalences in their own texts. In the preface to *The Description of a New World, Called the Blazing World* (1669), Cavendish playfully suggests that she has become the "mistress" (or "authoress") of her fictional work, because she could not be the "mistress" of a powerful ruler such as Alexander or Caesar. In the words of Margaret W. Ferguson, "statements about one's own or someone else's literacy seem[ed] often to work like statements about one's own or someone else's sexual experience" (10).

Further Reading: Ferguson, Margaret W. *Dido's Daughters: Literacy, Gender, and Empire in Early Modern England and France*. Chicago: University of Chicago Press, 2003; Houston, R. A. *Literacy in Early Modern Europe: Culture and Education 1500–1800*. New York: Longman, 1988; Lockridge, Kenneth A. "Literacy in Early America 1650–1800." In *Literacy and Social Development in the West: A Reader*, edited by Harvey J. Graff, 183–200. New York: Cambridge University Press, 1982. Mignolo, Walter D. *The Darker Side of the Renaissance: Literacy, Territoriality, and Colonization*. Ann Arbor: University of Michigan Press, 1995.

Belén Bistué

LITERATURE, EUROPEAN. The period in Europe spanning the late thirteenth century to about the middle of the seventeenth century, which we have come to call the Renaissance, or, more recently, the early modern period, has long been characterized in relation to the advent of perspective and proportion in art, the use of the vernacular in literature, and the philosophy of Humanism, or the impulse to see man, rather than God, as the center of the universe. In this way, the revival of Protagoras' anthropocentric fifth century BCE claim that "man is the measure of all things" underscores the mode of thought predominant in the early modern period. Scholars associate the Renaissance with the nineteenth-century Swiss historian Jacob

Burckhardt, who uses the term in his book *The Civilization of the Renaissance in Italy* (1860). Though many aspects of his analysis have now been discredited, Burckhardt posits that the emergence of Italian Renaissance aesthetics, political thought, and philosophy significantly and consciously broke with the ideas of the Middle Ages, and modeled itself instead on those of ancient Greece and Rome. It would be misleading, however, to say that the Renaissance signifies merely a revival of classical aesthetics and beliefs, just as it would be misleading to believe that the term "early modern" signals some teleological path to our own day. That the European Renaissance was, at its core, an original and innovative era across artistic genres and philosophical ideals lies at the heart of Burckhardt's theory as well as our own understanding of the period today.

Literary innovation and diversification was particularly strong during the Renaissance. Poetic forms borrowed from classical antiquity, such as epics (like those of Dante Alighieri (1265–1321), Ludovico Ariosto (1474–1533), Edmund Spenser (1552–1599), and John Milton (1608–1674)) and eclogues, or pastorals, evidenced in the work of Jacopo Sannazaro (c. 1457–1530), Garcilaso de la Vega (1501–1536), Pierre de Ronsard (1524–1585), and Spenser again, became reinvigorated through, among other things, an increased use of both religious and secular allegory. At the same time, medieval forms, like the courtly Romance by writers straddling the medieval and Renaissance periods, like Sir Thomas Malory (1405–1471) and the author of the anonymous Spanish *Amadis of Gaul* (1508), remained quite popular through the early modern period, despite a growing number lampoons of the genre, notably Miguel de Cervantes Saavedra's (1547–1616) satire of the chivalric romance, *Don Quixote* (Part I 1605; Part II 1616). Satire, also a classical genre, underwent a modernization during the Renaissance. An excellent example is Desiderius Erasmus' (1466–1536) *Praise of Folly* (1511), which tied together the traditional antique encomium with the satire form, or François Rabelais' (1494–1553) grotesque and carnivalesque *Pantagruel* (c. 1532).

New literary forms emerged as well. For example, the frame tales of Giovanni Boccaccio (1313–1375), Geoffrey Chaucer (1342–1400), and Marguerite de Navarre (1492–1549) contrasted high and low styles by juxtaposing bawdy tales filled with religious corruption and all sorts of sexual indiscretion with tales of courtly romance and moral parables. The new fourteen-line sonnet form, innovated by Francesco Petrarca (Petrarch) (1304–1374) and later developed by Sir Phillip Sidney (1554–1586), Garcilaso de la Vega, Lope de Vega (1562–1635), and, of course, William **Shakespeare** (1564–1616), among countless others, revolutionized love poetry. Playwrights were also increasingly prolific during the Renaissance, often transgressing the traditional boundaries of comedy and tragedy. Shakespeare, Christopher **Marlowe** (1564–1593), Lope de Vega, Pedro Calderón de la Barca (1600–1681), and Pierre Corneille (1606–1684) revolutionized dramatic forms across Europe. More traditional tragedies and comedies, like those written by the so-called neoclassicists in France (Jean Racine (1639–1699) and Molière (1622–1673)), as well as by Shakespeare and his Elizabethan contemporaries, conformed not only to classical Aristotelian dramatic rules but, perhaps more importantly, corresponded to the aesthetic demands of their day and appealed to both courtly and popular audiences.

The role of women has sparked heated debate among scholars over the last thirty years, initiated by Joan Kelly in her seminal 1977 essay "Did Women Have a Renaissance?" Until recently, a handful of women writers, such as Christine de Pizan (1365–1429), de Navarre, and Madame de La Fayette (1634–1693) in France, and Aphra Behn (1640–1689) in England, were considered exceptions in the male-dominated early modern period. Since the 1970s, scholars have uncovered a huge number of texts written by noblewomen, nuns, and even professional writers, consisting of literary, sociopolitical, philosophical, and epistolary works, with the aim of better defining and interpreting women's role in the Renaissance. Heralded as "new voices" of the Renaissance, these women include Italians Tullia **d'Aragona** (1510–1556), Moderata Fonte (1555–1592), Isabella Andreini (1562–1604), and Arcangela Tarabotti (1604–1652), British writers Isabella Whitney (c. 1540–c. 1580), Elizabeth Cary (1585–1639), and Margaret Cavendish (1623–1673), and the French poet Louise Labé (c. 1520–1566). Moreover, what are now considered misogynistic gender roles espoused in social treatises by male Italian Renaissance writers like Leon Battista Alberti (1404–1472) and Baldesar **Castiglione** (1478–1529), have come under additional scrutiny.

What is particularly significant about a number of these women authors is the way in which they diverge from stereotypical poetic conceits first developed by Petrarch in *Il Canzoniere* (started c. 1327), a collection of love poems addressed to the fabled Laura. For example, Labé became famous for inverting Petrarchan sonnet conventions with a male love object and a female poet-lover, as well as for further problematizing the trope of unrequited love by finding fault with the man. Poets like Labé paved the way for other deviations from the Petrarchan sonnet, which praises love as a neo-Platonic virtue and idolizes physical attributes such as golden hair, coral-red lips, and white breasts. Shakespeare's Sonnet 130 ("My mistress' eyes are nothing like the sun," published 1609) and Lope de Vega's Folk Song VII (published posthumously) are both love poems that negate Petrarchan conventions and, like Labé's sonnets, infuse the poems with a sense of realism.

Another realist motif in Renaissance poetry, the *"carpe diem"* theme, is evidenced in the works of the Metaphysical and Cavalier poets. The most famous examples include Andrew Marvell's (1621–1678) "To his Coy Mistress" (1681) and Robert Herrick's (1591–1674) "To the Virgins, to Make Much of Time" (1648), which begins "Gather ye rosebuds while ye may." These overtly sexual verses (though succumbing to sexual desire was not always the theme of *carpe diem* poems) remind us that what we see of time is all we have and once youth and strength are gone, old age, weakness, and death are all that follow. These realist motifs in poetry also serve to underscore the Humanist vein of the Renaissance.

Further Reading: Boccaccio, Giovanni. *The Decameron*. Translated by G. H. McWilliam. London and New York: Penguin Books, 1995; Braden, Gordon. *Petrarchan Love and the Continental Renaissance*. New Haven, CT: Yale University Press, 1999; Burckhardt, Jacob. *The Civilization of the Renaissance in Italy*. Translated by S.G.C. Middlemore. London and New York: Penguin Classics, 2004; Castiglione, Baldessar. *The Book of the Courtier*. Translated by George Bull. London and New York: Penguin Classics, 2003; Chaucer, Geoffrey. *The Canterbury Tales*. Translated by Nevill Coghill. London and New York: Penguin Books, 2003; Clarke, Danielle, ed. *Renaissance Women Poets*. London and New York: Penguin Classics, 2001; de Navarre, Marguerite. *The Heptameron*. Translated by P. A. Chilton. London and New York: Penguin Books, 1984; Gardner, Helen, ed. *The Metaphysical Poets*. London and New York: Penguin Classics: 1985; Greenblatt, Stephen. *Renaissance Self-Fashioning: From More to Shakespeare*. Chicago: University of Chicago Press, 2005; Grossman, Edith, ed. *The Golden Age: Poems of the Spanish Renaissance*. New York and London: W. W. Norton & Company, 2006; Labé, Louise. *Complete Poetry and Prose: A Bilingual Edition*. Translated by Deborah Lesko Baker and Annie Finch. Chicago: University of Chicago Press, 2006; Petrarch, Francesco. *Selections from the Canzoniere and Other Works*. Translated by Mark Musa. New York: Oxford University Press, 1999; Salzman, Paul, ed. *Early Modern Women's Writing: An Anthology 1560–1700*.

New York: Oxford University Press, 2000; Stortoni, Laura Anna, ed. *Women Poets of the Italian Renaissance: Courtly Ladies and Courtesans*. New York: Italica Press, 1997; Woudhuysen, H. R., ed. *The Penguin Book of Renaissance Verse*. London and New York: Penguin Books, 1993.

Adele Kudish

LOVE. Most of modern culture urges us to think of love, from the outset, as a private matter, personal, inward, profoundly ours, and, where other persons enter, as the bond that firms the most intimate of ties with lovers, children, or parents. This idea reflects the deep-set individualism of our whole culture, which is introspective, liberal, and focused on consumption. The premodern European attitude was sharply different in regards to love. Although premodern Europeans loved as intensely as do we and others elsewhere, love, as they conceived it, was as public as it was private, as collective as individual, as objective as subjective. Moreover, love, for the premodern era, was not only feeling but action; it was a behavior, thoroughly encoded. It was also an ideal and a principle: social, political, divine, and cosmic. So, although also intimate and private, love was meat for social ethics and social action, for political theory and praxis, and for religion and philosophy. Love, therefore, figured in the several moral codes that glossed and shaped premodern collective life and, in short, played out very differently from love today.

At the same time, premodern love, at its core, sprang from universal feelings, deeply rooted in humans as animals. Neuroscience suggests that, in humans as beasts, love has two strands: infatuation and attachment. In human brains, both of these strands are based on certain neurotransmitters and shaped by certain organs inside our skulls that house and handle feelings. These same transmitters and, to a degree, these same brain parts, do the same job for other mammals, for birds, and for all creatures prone to spells of intense sociability. Love, or a feeling like it, serves procreation in several ways, by luring mates to one another, overcoming habitual caution and aversion, or, in raccoons for instance, sheer orneriness, and then rewarding the cooperation that helps rear young. Attachment, in some species, including humans, also serves non-procreative bonds, such as those that bind a foraging troop or pack, or, perhaps, even a mere herd or flock. Dogs, whose genes still remember their prehistoric careers as genes of wolves, illustrate brilliantly the sociable, non-procreative capacities of love-like feelings. Such social love was also often salient to premodern humans.

To root premodern love in premodern culture, it pays to start with social principles and habits. An historian of Florence, Richard Trexler, makes a profound and telling distinction. Florentines, he said, had two social and political modes, which he labels "contract" and "sacrifice." This distinction, helpful for Florence, serves handily for all medieval and Renaissance Europeans. A contract, whether legal or social, whether formal or informal, is a witting exchange where terms are clear and fixed. In their purest form, contract exchanges, whether economic, social, or political, were not only precise; they were also finite and easily closed. Sacrifice, at first glance, was, and is, contract's inversion. In a sacrificial exchange, one party says, "Take this offering from me! I want nothing back!" However, a contract and sacrifice actually have much in common. Both, usually, are reciprocal. Although sacrificers neither want nor expect anything back, they await the reward, the counter-sacrifice. As anthropologists note, sacrifice, unlike contract, is not closed, but open. Lacking clear measure, its exchanges are hard to stop. A moment's reflection on Christmas cards, dinner invitations, blandishments and courtesies, and all those words and deeds that keep friends, couples, and families happy, will illustrate the open-ended nature of generous actions. Moreover, a moment's contemplation on the play of contracts in social relationships will illustrate their power to undermine them. **Prostitution**, for instance, awakens queasiness and scorn for its reduction of sex to contract; a loving couple should, we think, eschew bare bargains.

Premodern Europe knew and used contracts. Nevertheless, for practical and ideological reasons, it leaned on sacrifice far more than contemporary society does. Practically, European institutions were too weak to enforce contracts readily. States, police, and law courts lacked reach. Geographically, Europe was fragmented, opaque, and viscous. Where institutions faltered, personal relationships took up the slack. Sacrifice, employed across social networks, helped render folk reliable. Accordingly, Europeans wrapped themselves in vast skeins of mutual exchange, giving gifts and hospitality, lending services and money, imparting precious information, saying prayers and buying Masses for one another, and, sometimes, risking their necks helping friends in fights. This flurry of mutual help made good the weakness of the state, and of banks, insurance, medicine, communications, and information storage; in short, it helped Europeans confront the many dangers of their risky world. As for ideology, Europeans lived by several value systems that spurned contract and embraced sacrifice. Of these, the chief three were family ethics, honor, and faith. All three draped sacrifice in love's mantle.

Family, in 1500, had functions modern families often lack. The modern family is chiefly a foyer for residence, nurture, companionship, and consumption. Premodern families, as households (which might include wider kin, servants, apprentices, and other residents), had those same jobs but also engaged, far more than now, in production, education, worship, and, above all, politics and governance, for the family was a pillar of the polity, buttressing social control. Families, nuclear and extended, thus not only policed their members; they also might engage in petty warfare; feuds or vendettas; an aspect of that state-free governance the social sciences call self-help. With so many tasks and burdens, families needed the loyalty, or, to rephrase, the sacrifices of their members. It was not an ideal state of affairs; the more services a family performs, the more it harnesses those inside it. The stripped-down modern family, loose-jointed and fragile, is the half-happy fruit of physical and economic security and institutional competence. Old families relied on a familial ethic, a norm of love and loyalty that, when strong, would bind, trammel, and mobilize its members, and allay the inevitable tensions among its members over access to property or liberty from its head's commands.

Honor was another zone of love. Honor, once thought typically Mediterranean, in fact shaped lives everywhere, from Scotland to Russia to Portugal. As an ethic, honor praised a plethora of sacrifices: hospitality, largess, courageous actions, and virtues, especially truthfulness—often costlier than evasion or lies. At its heart, honor preached loyalty: to lords, vassals, patrons, kin, friends, associates, self, and city, and to all that was sacred. It was a particularist code, lauding a man for defending, regaling, and exalting all his allies. Female honor accrued to the chaste; **chastity**, a sacrifice curbing both sex and assertiveness, expressed loyalty to one's house's males—father, brothers, and husband. Manifold sacrificial acts, aligned with honor, cemented premodern solidarities, attaching clients to patron, kinsmen to clan, guildsmen to guild, neighbors to quarter, partisans to party, citizens to town, and soldiers, cops, and bandits to their captains. Honor's exchanges, of gifts, services, favors, obeisances, compliments, and oaths, as befitted sacrifice, used love's language.

Premodern political discourse melded the idioms of family, of honor, and of law. A monarch might use patriarchal language, admonishing subjects to love him like a father. Meanwhile, feudal language spoke of honor and loyal love to lords. Communal polities—cities, towns, and villages—also invoked both honor and law. Most political units, when they urged sacrificial actions, readily evoked love. Among soldiers and officials, very gradually, mere pay took over, but, to military and public officers, service long looked nobler when a mummery of blandishments and broadband exchange masked a relationship's mercenary core.

Meanwhile, law itself by nature generally eschewed love and cherished contract. Premodern legal systems, of state, church, and even town and village, often bore the stamp of ancient Roman law, where contract ruled supreme. At the same time, veins of customary and feudal law ran through the mass of precepts. Nevertheless, law, as an instrument of governance, was generally not inclined to love, but to compliance, seeking not the eager heart but the bent neck. Sixteenth-century Scotsmen distinguished between "love and law," sundering mediation and social settlement from judicial arbitration. Their distinction distilled the law's distance from control's more social processes.

Religion evoked love in countless ways. **Christianity**, the ascendant faith, built its ethics, theology of salvation, and vision of both history and the cosmos on a monumental sacrifice, Jesus' voluntary death, an act of love inviting imitation. Catholic and Orthodox practice brimmed with sacrificial actions of body, mind, and spirit. Many were ascetic: pilgrimage and crusading, fasting, vigils, bare feet, hairshirts, flagellation, sexual abstinence, prayer, and contemplation all helped the faithful repay God, Mary, and the saints for the double grace of providence in this world and salvation in the next. Other pious actions, less ascetic, verged on gift giving: spending for candles, masses, indulgences, and art in churches and other holy spaces, and for myriad works of charity. Medieval doctrine strove to banish any shade of contract; no such outlay should purchase providence or grace. To think or practice otherwise was the sin of simony, and a heresy. The Protestant **Reformation** demurred; to a Protestant eye, all such works aped the act of purchase. Christians of all denominations agreed that love should pervade any exchange between the faithful and God's realm. Grace, essential to salvation, was an act of love, a holy gift, and never a commodity. Christian love differed from the love that honor championed, for it was universal, and no respecter of persons. Love of neighbor should befall all Christians; honor's affections, by contrast, were trenchantly particularistic.

Because love entangled so variously with social and political relationships, in both language and in practice it engaged its opposites. At the other pole stood hatred. Premodern Europeans hated, socially and politically, in flagrant ways no longer current or legitimate. Hatred was a normal condition, both individual and collective. Like love, hatred eschewed contract's finite reciprocity. Rather, it too urged abandon. A hatred, then, like a love, engendered broadband exchanges, acts not amorous but odious, likewise open-ended; like love, hatred snaked through social networks. The most spectacular chains of malicious actions were the personal feuds and big vendettas that might mobilize an extended family or a clan of kinfolk and their dependents. Thus, alongside friendship stood its antonym, enmity; Romance languages oppose the terms neatly (*amici, inimici*, for instance, in Latin and Italian). Like love and friendship, hatred and hate-soaked violence served as yet one more form, also outside the law, of social control; fear of endless violence might stay an arm or quell a risky yen. Feud by nature was hard to stop; rivals seldom agreed that mutual harm had finally balanced. Accordingly, peacemakers stepped in to quash the mayhem. A formal peace, a mini-treaty, sometimes notarized, might stage fictions of mutual love: sacrificial words of pardon, tears, the exchange of kisses and embraces, shared cake and wine, and the shouldering of penalties against a breach. Peace-brokers were often clergy, who, ideally, stood outside the sanguinary ethic of honor. The state, with its law and paper records, might guarantee the truce.

Amidst so many social and political habits of loving, individual Europeans did still fall in love and bond to intimates. Love, especially infatuation and desire, was the theme of endless song and poetry. It shaped knightly romance, a medieval genre still thriving in the Renaissance, and often inspired dance, drama, and gala tournaments. Doctrines of love, some traceable back to Plato and Ovid, others imbued with Christian mystical strains and feudal notions of gracious service, posited that love ennobled the male lover, urging him to deeds of virtue to earn assorted tokens from his beloved's heart and body. Meanwhile, the short story, another genre, often treated love as the mischievous disturber of family life's good order. Since many, especially the elite, married for economic, social, and political strategy, infatuation was more likely outside marriage than in, especially if some restless female May lay in a December's boring bed. Such marriages did happen, as when a grizzled widower took a second or third wife. Short-story writers like Chaucer and Boccaccio treated their happily indignant readers to titillating stories of adulterous intrigues where a dodderer's well-merited loss of honor added moral sauce.

Premodern Europeans, eyeing romance, often stressed not love's pleasures but its pains. Love, said their writings, was like an illness. The lover suffered, lost appetite and sleep, and had an unsettled mind and body. Jealousy tormented him, and despair warred eternally with hope. Ovid and medical doctrines supported this idea of love as sickness and bodily affliction. Moreover, romantic love, in general, disturbed the social order. It subverted parental desires to manage their offsprings' marriages, upset the dominion of husbands over wives, and subverted the chaste good order of the church, especially at nunneries. Sometimes, as at the end of a William **Shakespeare** comedy, love, by priming a marriage, bolstered good order. But, in the eyes of folk magic, infatuated love was a darker force. **Witches** and wise women, for a fee, could call it up, as could any woman armed with the right prayers and paraphernalia. In Italy, women used spells to inflict the men they wanted with "the hammer" (*il martello*), a passion that would unman and bind them, bending them to a woman's will.

After 1650, as western Europe slid slowly toward the Enlightenment, the earlier love order disbanded. As states grew more robust, honor slowly abandoned violence and drifted into a mild civility. As this happened, vendetta receded and the costly demands of many social solidarities, family among them, became less urgent. Magic slowly lost its grip. In politics, theories of social contract, pragmatic and individualistic, swept away more patriarchal ideas that prized contract's opposite, sacrifice. Meanwhile, as families shed some tasks, parents gradually came to give offspring more liberty in choosing mates, and an ideal of companionate **marriage**, with love at its center, rather than interest and administration, spread across the upper and upper middle classes. Love therefore shifted its position, shedding old jobs and, ever more, retreating into the narrow modern corner where it now resides: romance and domestic affection. *See also* Eros; Love Sickness; Platonic Love.

Further Reading: d'Aragona, Tullia. *Dialogue on the Infinity of Love*. Edited and translated by Rinaldina Russel and Bruce Merry. Chicago and London: University of Chicago Press, 1997 (see pp. 27–42 for high doctrines of sexual love); Davis, Natalie Zemon, and Arlette Farge. *History of Women in the West*. Vol. 3: *Renaissance and Enlightenment Paradoxes*. London and Cambridge, MA: Belknap Press of Harvard University Press, 1993 (see pp. 64–84 for the roles of love and sexuality for women); Stone, Lawrence. *Family, Sex and Marriage in England 1500–1800*. New York: Harper and Row, 1979 (see for a social history in one country); Trexler, Richard. *Public Life in Renaissance Florence*. New York: Academic Press, 1980 (see pp. 19–33 for ideas of governance and sacrifice in public life).

Thomas Cohen

LOVE SICKNESS. Being sick with love is not just a poetic trope; today's medicine diagnoses love sickness as an illness characterized by a drop in the serotonin level of the brain resulting in such symptoms as anxiety; depression, including insomnia; loss of appetite; and various degrees of confusion. Similarly, being "madly in love" identifies a state of euphoria or an elevated mood and self-esteem. Brain scans of individuals passionately in **love** show great activity in the anterior cingulated cortex and caudate nucleus similar to those found in the neuroanatomy of obsessive-compulsive disorder (OCD).

Modern medical technology has only validated what physicians have suspected since antiquity—matters of the heart can cause troubling physiological conditions of varying severity and duration. Hippocrates (470–410 BCE) and Galen (129–201 CE) warned about the dangers of the disease because it was difficult to cure and could potentially lead to death. They explained its physiology within the theory of the Four Humors (a balance between blood, yellow bile, phlegm, and black bile), which determined the state of health and mind of the individual; love sickness would result from an excess of black bile residing in the infected liver. The symptoms of the disease included lack of appetite, sleeplessness, and sadness. Treatments consisted of purges and internal remedies. Among the Arabs, Avicenna (980–1037) confirmed love sickness as the "disease of sadness," a physical and mental affliction caused by obsession with the object of love. Ibn Al Nafis (1213–1218) further described its symptoms as change of color in the face and accelerated heartbeat. As treatment, Avicenna recommended baths and topicals, defamation of the desired object, and coitus. In medieval Europe, Bernard of Gordon (c. 1310) and Valesco de Taranta (1380–1418), among many others, followed their predecessors' humoral medical definition of love sickness and further differentiated between *amor heroes* (the obsessive preoccupation with a beloved), *melancholy* (excessive sadness and fear), and *mania* (excessive anger). Love sickness could develop into *mania* in severe cases. In terms of symptoms and remedies, they followed their predecessors' teachings. Throughout history, physicians concurred on the "genteel" nature of love sickness as "the lovers' malady of heroes": "the noblemen who, because of their wealth and the softness of their life suffer this passion" (Gerard of Berry, c. 1230).

During the Renaissance, the interpretation of the disease acquired a new perspective; philosophers and theologians became interested in the medical debate and transferred the attention from the patient's conditions onto the cause of his ailment: the lady, the object of his desire. In *The Anatomy of Melancholia*, the sixteenth-century British cleric Robert Burton re-proposed a thesis, stated earlier by the Italian Marsilio Ficino (1433–1499) and the Frenchman Francois Valleriola (1504–1580), that identified the cause of love sickness with the "evil" effects of the lady's beauty of proportions—face, eyebrows, cheeks, hair, and, above all, eyes, because they are the "seats of love" itself. The eyes of the lady would emit noxious vapors that in the lover's body would cause blood poisoning and a general infection.

The seventeenth-century Frenchman Jacques Ferrand, who wrote the Renaissance medical *summa* on the diseases of erotic love, shifted the discussion of the leading causes of love sickness to the reproductive organs and sexual hyper-excitation. Men and women alike were ruled by erotic instincts and amorous desires that would lead to different degrees of love sickness—mania, melancholy, or uterine fury. For Ferrand, sexual desires and passions generated heat that would burn the natural humors of the body and change them into noxious vapors; in the form of burnt blood, they would reach the brain causing obscured mental vision and distorted judgment and melancholy. Viewed as unbridled creatures who were prisoners of their sexual urges and therefore prone to promiscuity and deviance, women would develop melancholic conditions from the overheating of the uterus and the swelling of the clitoris.

Ferrand explained love sickness in social and psychological terms by focusing on the nature of the relationship between the lovers. He not only supported the thesis that the female body was responsible for the male patient's sickness, but also helped criminalize the female patient by linking the disease to the physiology of the female sexual organs. By the end of the seventeenth century, female anatomy became the fashionable site of morbid investigation and treatment of a multitude of emotional and physical symptoms treatable only through the physician's administration of purges and pharmaceuticals. *See also* Medicine.

Further Reading: Bartels, A., and S. Zeki. "The Neural Basis of Romantic Love." *Neuroreport*, 17 (2000): 3829–34; Haynes, Alan. *Sex in Elizabethan England*. Stroud, England: Sutton Publishing, 1999; Money, John. *Love and Love Sickness: The Science of Sex, Gender Difference, and Pair-Bonding*. Baltimore: Johns Hopkins University Press, 1980.

Lucia Bortoli

LOVE SONGS. In Renaissance Europe, musicians repeatedly turned to romantic love and sexual desire as subjects for their compositions, with a number of prominent genres and methods of engaging romantic themes.

During the late fourteenth and early fifteenth centuries, courts in Avignon, southern France, and northern Italy housed a chivalric culture in which *chansons* ("songs") of the *ars subtilior* ("more subtle art") flourished. Influenced by the medieval tradition of *fine amour* ("refined love"), this music addresses idealized romantic love, often in the form of admiration for an unattainable woman. *Ars subtilior* songs are organized in *formes fixes* ("fixed forms": polyphonic *ballades*, rondeaux, and virelais) and are characterized by complex melodies, rhythms and relationships among voices. This elevated, refined style is sometimes mirrored in the songs' musical notation, with elegant visual imagery reflecting their texts. *Belle, bonne sage* (c. 1400), a three-voice rondeau by Baude Cordier, exemplifies this; in the manuscript *Chantilly, Musée Condé 564*, this love song is inscribed in the shape of a heart.

Throughout the fifteenth and early sixteenth centuries, the polyphonic *chanson* retained an important role in European court life. Court chapels were instrumental in the development of the *chanson* during this period. Rulers like Philip the Good of Burgundy (r. 1419–1467) maintained particularly impressive chapels, employing the most talented performers and composers from across Europe to provide music for church services and secular entertainments. Such chapels provided musical training for promising young students and fostered an international musical style through increased interaction among musicians from France, England, Italy, and the Burgundian lands.

An approach to composition based on a preference for consonance, strictly controlled dissonance, and *contenance angloise* ("English quality") distinguishes this international style from music of the preceding centuries. This style is described by Johannes Tinctoris (c. 1435–1511) in *Liber de arte contrapuncti* (1477), a treatise defining principles of composition based on procedures used by musicians like

Gilles de Binchois (c. 1400–1460), John Dunstable (c. 1390–1453), Guillaume Du Fay (c. 1397–1474), Jean de Ockeghem (c. 1410–1497) and Antoine Busnoys (c. 1430–1492). Such composers wrote particularly refined chansons in the formes fixes. Their chansons feature tuneful melodies, rhythms that are intricate but less complex than those of the *ars subtilior* and the frequent use of syllabic text setting. By the beginning of the sixteenth century, composers had abandoned the *formes fixes*, and musicians like Josquin des Pres (c. 1450–1521) and Henricus Isaac (c. 1450–1517) were producing songs with structures defined solely by their texts. This practice is exemplified in *Mille regretz* (c. 1520), a four-voice chanson attributed to Josquin. This piece explores a speaker's regret at having abandoned his lover; each remorseful utterance receives a unique musical setting.

Love songs so deeply penetrated the fabric of fifteenth-century European court culture that they were often used as source material for sacred music. Du Fay's four-part *Missa se la face ay pale* (c. 1450s) is one such example. The tenor line of each movement in this setting of the Mass Ordinary is a variation on a single, secular *cantus firmus* ("fixed melody"): the tune from Du Fay's ballade of the same name.

In the sixteenth century, the Italian madrigal emerged as an important musical genre. After the publication of Pietro Bembo's edition of Francesco Petrarch's *Canzoniere* (1501), composers became interested in setting verse by major poets like Petrarch (1304–1374), Torquato Tasso (1544–1595) and Giovannni Battista Guarini (1538–1612). Such writers' work is centered on social play, with themes of love, sex, and wit interwoven in ways meant to surprise, delight and amuse readers.

Sixteenth-century Italian composers sought to create music that reflected the artfulness of poetic language. *Il bianco e dolce cigno* (1538), a four-voice madrigal by Jacques Arcadelt (c. 1507–1568), is an example of a composer's attempt to help music illuminate textual form and meaning. This poem's speaker contrasts the literal death of a swan with the figurative death of an orgasm; in turn, Arcadelt uses repeated descending melodic figures to illustrate the words "*mille mort' il di*" ("a thousand deaths a day"). Composers like Adrian Willaert (c. 1490–1562), Cipriano de Rore (1515/1516–1565), Maddalena Casulana (c. 1544–1590s), Orlando di Lasso (c. 1532–1594) and Carlo Gesualdo (c. 1561–1613) refined the madrigal over the course of the century, using chromaticism and increasingly literal madrigalisms to create expressive settings of poetic texts.

Madrigals were an extremely popular form of entertainment, with over 2000 collections published between 1530 and 1600. These collections inspired the development of the genre outside Italy. Thomas Morley (1557/1558–1602) and Thomas Weelkes (c. 1575–1623) used Italian madrigal techniques to create musical settings of English poetry. Mogens Pedersøn (c. 1583–1623) studied composition in Venice, eventually returning to Denmark to compose Italian-language madrigals for King Christian IV (r. 1588–1648).

Other genres of secular song flourished simultaneously with the madrigal. Beginning in the 1540s, the *villanesca*, a strophic, homophonic song for three or four voices, flourished in Naples. *Villanesche* are lighthearted, usually focusing on relationships between frustrated men and deceitful women. They often assume a rustic tone, using pastoral imagery and borrowing or imitating folk melodies. Under the reign of Francis I (r. 1515–1547), the Parisian *chanson* gained popularity. These *chansons* were simpler than those of the fifteenth century, and are characterized by brisk rhythms, syllabic text setting, and homophonic textures, which allowed amateurs to read and perform them easily. While some of these pieces are of a serious nature, most are settings of amorous, humorous texts. *Pilons l'orge*, by Claudin de Sermisy (c. 1490–1562), is a typical lighthearted *chanson*; this *malmariée* presents the thoughts of a beautiful young woman who despises her aging husband.

Despite their popularity, Renaissance love songs were sometimes greeted with resistance, especially among clergy members who viewed them as morally corrupt. In the dedication to his settings of the *Song of Songs* (1584), Roman Catholic composer Giovanni Pierluigi da Palestrina (1525/1526–1594) admitted that he was ashamed to have written love songs early in life. Protestant reformer Martin **Luther** (1483–1546) published collections of chorale settings in order to provide a wholesome alternative to lascivious secular musical entertainments. Purifying church music was a subject of debate at the Council of **Trent** (1545–1563), where some reformers suggested purging the liturgy of masses based on secular *chansons*. This policy was never adopted.

Further Reading: DeFord, Ruth I. "Musical Relationships Between the Italian Madrigal and Light Genres in the Sixteenth Century." *Musica Disciplina* XXXIX (1985): 107–68; Fallows, David. *Songs and Musicians in the Fifteenth Century*. Brookfield, VT: Variorum, 1996; Freedman, Richard. "Paris and the French Court under François I." In *The Renaissance from the 1470s to the End of the 16th Century*, edited by Iain Fenlon, 174–96. Englewood Cliffs, NJ: Prentice Hall, 1989; Haar, James. *Essays on Italian Poetry and Music in the Renaissance, 1350–1600*. Berkley and Los Angeles: University of California Press, 1986; Oettinger, Rebecca Wagner. *Music as Propaganda in the German Reformation*. Aldershot: Ashgate, 2001; Rees, Owen Lewis. "*Mille regretz* as a Model: Possible Allusions to 'The Emperor's Song' in the Chanson Repertory." *Journal of the Royal Musical Association* 120, no. 1 (1995): 44–76; Wegman, Rob C. "Johannes Tinctoris and the 'New Art.'" *Music & Letters* 84, no. 2 (2003): 171–88; Wegman, Rob C. "New Music for a World Grown Old: Martin Le Franc and the 'Contenance Angloise.'" *Acta Musicologica* 75, no. 2 (2003): 201–41; Wright, Craig. "Tappissier and Cordier: New Documents and Conjectures." *The Musical Quarterly* 59, no. 2 (1973): 177–89; Wright, Craig. *Music at the Court of Burgundy, 1364–1419: A Documentary History*. Henryville, PA: Institute of Medieval Music, 1979.

Brooke Bryant

LUTHER, MARTIN (1483–1546). Martin Luther is considered by many to be one of the most influential people in Western history. He was prolific and complicated, fiery and personal, intense and thoughtful; he was also the founder of the Christian Protestant movement. When he posted his 95 theses against the abuse of indulgences (the written forgiveness of sins) at the German city of Wittenberg in 1517, he began a protest that would change not only Christianity but the flow of human history.

Born to a peasant family in 1483 in Eisleben, Saxony, his father, Hans, wanted his son to become a lawyer. Martin Luther, after receiving his Bachelor of Arts and Masters of Arts, began to study for a law degree. His concern about the viability of confession and the sacraments, the relationship between God and man, and the destruction of sin was an almost daily anxiety. In July 1505, when caught in a storm and fearing for his life, he made a vow to enter a monastery if St. Anne would save him. Later, he entered an Augustinian order. In 1508 he traveled to Wittenberg to lecture and study while working on his doctorate in theology. After a later visit to Rome, he received his degree in 1512.

Around the same time another member of the clergy, the Dominican friar Johann Tetzel, was sent by Pope Leo X to gather money for St. Peter's Basilica. By selling papal indulgences, he was able to raise money. While there is some discussion as to whether Tetzel's selling tactics were sanctioned by the Pope, he certainly seems to have extended the doctrine of indulgences to a new level. He may have even offered forgiveness to those who had no remorse or to those planning to commit future sins.

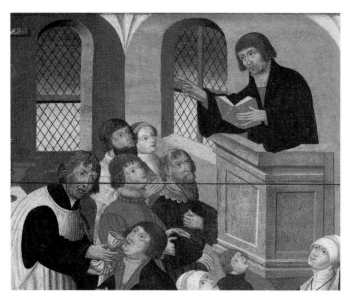

Martin Luther, 1561. © The Art Archive/Nationalmuseet Copenhagen Denmark/Dagli Orti (A).

Luther, and others in the Church, objected to this "empty" forgiveness. When asked by his students to validate the indulgences, Luther posted an invitation for an academic dialogue on the abuse of indulgences along with his *Disputation for Clarification of the Power of Indulgences*, now called the 95 Theses, on the church door at Wittenberg, October 13, 1517. Unwittingly, thus began the Protestant **Reformation.**

As a result of his criticisms of the Catholic Church, particularly his arguments for salvation by faith alone and not the sacraments of the church, Luther was summoned to Rome by Pope Leo X in 1521. To aid Luther and to impede the trip, which was a dangerous one, Fredric III, the Elector of Saxony, asked the Holy Roman Emperor Charles V to call an imperial Diet, or general assembly, at Worms, where Luther could defend his views. At the trial Luther was ordered to recant his recent writings; Luther refused. He was then formally excommunicated, and the sympathetic Elector Fredric then placed him in hiding. It was at this time that Luther was able translate the New Testament, which he finished in 1522, making the Bible available in German for the first time. Besides translation work, Luther also wrote prolifically on subjects such as marriage, government, and economics, while arguing for an active change within the Roman Catholic Church. He also corresponded with the famous humanist monk and writer Desiderius Erasmus of Rotterdam. In contrast to Luther, Erasmus argued that the Church should be reformed, but in a more internal and peaceful way.

Another of Luther's contributions was his articulation of the Christian doctrine of the priesthood of the believer. Instead of going to the priest to speak to God, a Christian could approach God in private without clerical assistance. This doctrine also emphasized literacy so that the individual could understand Scripture without the intervention of the clergy.

Luther also argued against the celibacy of monks and nuns, which was met with mixed feelings. As a result many willingly left their convents, while others were forced out. Of her own volition, the former nun Catherine von Bora became Luther's wife in 1525. He affectionately called her "my Lord Katie," and together they had six children and took in at least eleven other children. Luther put forth views of traditional marriage, which allowed his wife the management of their household and encouraged women to be active in education and raising children.

Martin Luther was a complex thinker and revolutionary; his writings reflect a variety of opinions on a range of topics. After a lifetime of writing, preaching, and teaching, the father of the Protestant Reformation died in 1546 of complications from a stroke. *See also* Calvin, John; Christianity; Henry VIII, King of England.

Further Reading: Althaus, Paul. *The Theology of Martin Luther*. Translated by Robert C. Schultz. Philadelphia: Fortress Press, 1966; Bainton, Roland Herbert. *Here I Stand: A Life of Martin Luther*. New York: Abingdon-Cokesbury Press, 1950; Brecht, Martin. *Martin Luther*. Translated by James L. Schaaf. 3 vols. Philadelphia: Fortress Press, 1985–1993; Luther, Martin. *Works*. Edited by Helmut T. Lehmann et al. 55 vols. St. Louis: Concordia Publishing House, 1955–1959.

Katherine R. Cooper

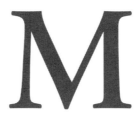

MAGIC, LOVE, AND SEX. The connection between magic, love, and sex has a long history in popular belief. Since ancient times, the symbolic objects that have been used in love magic are as varied as the cultures that employed them. Magic is concerned with acquiring power, which provides the ability to control humankind's most compelling interests and drives. Hence, the resultant importance and appeal of employing magic in obtaining love and sex.

In India, where human beings were believed to have sprung from trees, sap was considered to aid procreation. In early sixteenth-century Spain, the potato, which was brought to Europe by the Spanish conquistadors who conquered the Inca Empire in Peru, was believed to cure **impotence**. In certain Australian tribes, boys were not allowed to eat lizards because of the creature's physical resemblance to the shape of the penis; it was feared that consuming the lizard would leave a boy possessed with an uncontrollable desire to engage in sexual intercourse. In the British Isles, the Anglo-Saxons used the marigold in love charms, and the best-known aphrodisiac from the ancient world is the mandrake plant. Pliny the Elder maintained that a mandrake root that resembled the shape of a phallus would secure genital love. In **Asia**, the root of the ginseng plant was considered to be a true aphrodisiac. Aphrodisiacs were generally taken in the form of a love potion over which a magical spell had to be spoken as the philter was being prepared. Related to love magic is the anaphrodisiac, or lust-killer, which was supplied by magicians and was particularly popular during the early modern period. The early fifteenth-century Arabic/North African erotic book ***The Perfumed Garden for the Soul's Delectation***, contains a section on undoing spells and other charms.

There are two types of love magic. One is general and is effective on anyone. The other is individual, and often includes an object that has been infused with magic by a witch or wizard. The latter is much more effective, as it is personal and specially prepared. Due to its connection with **witches**, love magic was declared illegal in England, where the Witchcraft Statute of 1542 made it a crime to incite anyone to unlawful love. *Grimoires*, or early modern European textbooks of magic, such as the *Heptameron* or *Magical Elements*, include various instructions for making love amulets, as well as directions for magical procedures.

Magical power was believed to reside in the male and female sex organs, which played a major role in the Tantric cults that originated in India, and focused on magic and sex. Ritual sexual union is essential to Tantrism, a school both of **Hinduism** and **Buddhism** that became popular in many Asian countries. The most sacred mantra of tantric worship is that of the jewel (penis) in the lotus (vulva). The fourteenth-century manual *Hatha-Yoga-Pradipika* explains a technique whereby the practitioner of Buddhist Tantrism could learn to draw the ejaculated semen back through the penis, in an effort to avoid parting with this fluid, which was associated with the enlightened mind. *See also* Christianity; Europe; *The Malleus Maleficarum*.

Further Reading: Kieckhefer, Richard. "Mythologies of Witchcraft in the Fifteenth Century." *Magic, Ritual and Witchcraft* 1, no. 1 (2006): 79–107; Kramer, Heinrich, and James Sprenger. *Malleus Maleficarum*. Translated by Montague Summers. London: Pushkin Press, 1928. Reprint ed. New York: Dover, 1971; Thorndike, Lynn. *A History of Magic and Experimental Science*. 8 vols. New York: MacMillan, 1923–1958; Walker, Benjamin. *Sex and the Supernatural: Sexuality in Religion and Magic*. New York: Harper and Row, 1973.

Ronna S. Feit

MALINAL. *See* La Malinche

THE MALLEUS MALEFICARUM (Kramer, 1486). *The Malleus Maleficarum* (*The Witches' Hammer*) is a comprehensive and authoritative guide to the nature, powers, detection, and the prosecution of **witches**; it may also be one of the most infamous books ever written. The *Malleus* is the work of a German Dominican friar, Heinrich Kramer (Latinized Henricus Institoris), an inquisitor and a zealous defender of Catholic orthodoxy, who attempted to launch a sweeping persecution of witches in Germany during the 1480s. In 1484, in response to unexpected local resistance, Kramer obtained explicit papal sanction for his activities in the form of the notorious "Witch Bull," *Summis Desiderantes*, of Pope Innocent VIII. Kramer launched a witch hunt in Innsbruck the following year, an attempt that proved an unmitigated disaster. Kramer was obsessed with the sexual deviance of witches, which confused and irritated his hosts, as did the fact that his methods were both brutal and illegal. Eventually, the local authorities intervened to end the trials, free the accused women, and compel the unwilling inquisitor to leave town. The town's bishop declared Kramer both incompetent and senile. Insulted and humiliated, Kramer retired to Cologne, where he wrote the *Malleus* as a rebuttal of his critics and as a guide to future witch prosecutions.

Kramer worked hard to make the *Malleus* as authoritative as possible, adding the name of the widely respected Jacob Sprenger as co-author, although this was almost certainly done without Sprenger's consent. Published in 1486, the treatise is divided into three parts. The first part is a theologically informed demonstration that witchcraft and witches are real—so real in fact that not to believe in witches constituted heresy—although Kramer confronted his critics less with theology than with what passed in Kramer's mind for empirical evidence: the testimony of witnesses, the afflictions caused by black magic, and the confessions (coerced under torture) of the witches themselves. Kramer's most original contribution to the notion of witchcraft—the claim that, almost without exception, witches are women—is found in this part of the treatise. In the second part of the book, Kramer offers a highly idiosyncratic catalogue of witches' powers and behavior, derived in equal measure from coerced confessions and from folklore. The witches Sabbath, for example, while figuring

The title page of a late edition of *The Malleus Maleficarum*, 1669. Courtesy of the Dover Pictorial Archives.

prominently in other witch treatises of the day, is here almost completely absent, while sexual references abound, including everything from the conventional (the witch's power to cause impotence and infertility) to the bizarre (the witch's alleged predilection for stealing human penises). In the final section, Kramer provides a detailed guide to actual prosecution.

Despite its author's obsessions, the *Malleus* was a success; new editions appeared for over 200 years and the text was widely disseminated. To those predisposed to accept the reality of witches, the work was also persuasive. Within twenty years of the book's publication, scholars dealing with witchcraft accepted Kramer as an authority on the subject and the *Malleus* as a standard reference text.

Further Reading: Behringer, Wolfgang. *Witches and Witch-Hunts.* Malden, MA: Polity Press, 2004; Broedel, Hans Peter. *The* Malleus Maleficarum *and the Construction of Witchcraft.* Manchester: Manchester University Press, 2003; Kramer, Heinrich. *Malleus Maleficarum.* Edited by Christopher Mackay. 2 vols. Cambridge: Cambridge University Press, 2006.

Hans Peter Broedel

MANDEVILLE, SIR JOHN. See The Travels of Sir John Mandeville

MARGUERITE DE NAVARRE (1492–1549). Marguerite de Navarre, also known as Marguerite d'Angoulême, was born May 11, 1492, the oldest child of Louise of Savoy and Charles of Orléans, Count of Angoulême. Two years later her brother, François, was born and her father died, leaving Louise de Savoy to protect her children's royal interests. The three were virtually inseparable, with Louise de Savoy taking as her motto *Libris et Liberis*, "For my books and for my children." Raised first in Cognac, then Blois, Marguerite received the same education as her brother, whom Louise was grooming to be king, despite the unlikelihood of his succession. With access to her ancestor Jean d'Angoulême's fine library in Blois, Marguerite learned Latin, Greek, Italian, and Spanish and studied assiduously both the classical writers and Scripture. An accomplished horsewoman, she regularly joined François in jousts and military games. Both enjoyed exceptionally good health in their youth.

In 1509, at the age of seventeen, Marguerite married Duke Charles d'Alençon, as arranged by King Louis XII. The sixteen-year marriage resulted in no children. Marguerite had little in common with her uneducated husband and found the isolated château d'Alençon a stark contrast with the more convivial ones in which she had been raised. Her copious letters written at this time mention him only briefly. When Louis XII died in 1515 leaving no male heir, François, unexpectedly, gained the throne and married Louis XII's daughter, Claude. Marguerite, and Louise de Savoy then regularly traveled with the itinerant court. The king, his mother, and sister were popularly described as having one heart shared by three bodies. As Queen Claude became increasingly incapacitated by her multiple pregnancies, Marguerite often took her place in public functions. Her wit and beauty added to the already exuberant court atmosphere that prevailed with François's triumphant military campaign at Marignan at the beginning of his reign.

By 1521, however, the national mood had changed as the formidable armies of Charles V, Holy Roman Emperor, threatened all of France. Political uncertainty for Marguerite and her family paralleled religious doubts; in the early 1520s Marguerite took interest in the writings of Guillaume Briçonnet and Lefèvre d'Étaples that advocated formal reforms to the Church. Like many of the elite at this time, Marguerite became interested in the mystical elements of her faith and over a period of three years wrote a series of letters to Briçonnet that explored her spiritual doubts and concerns. These ideas she transformed into three long poems, *Dialogue en forme de vision nocturne*, the *Miroir de l'âme pécheresse* and the *Oraison de l'âme fidèle*. The first was a meditation on death and eternal life, inspired by the death of her favorite niece, Charlotte. With the death of Claude in 1524, François named his mother regent and Marguerite became his unofficial secretary of state, meeting with all visiting foreign dignitaries. After the king's 1525 defeat and capture in Pavia, Marguerite negotiated directly Francois's release with his captor, Charles V. In 1527, Marguerite married Henri d'Albret, King of Navarre, and became a queen in her own right. Her power was quite limited, however, given that Charles V controlled most of the kingdom's holdings, and she continued to spend most of her time with the French court. In 1528 her daughter, Jeanne, was born; two years later a son, Jean, died in infancy. Along with her mother and Margaret of Austria, Marguerite negotiated the landmark "Ladies' Peace," or Treaty of Cambrai of 1529, that put in abeyance the hostilities between France and the Holy Roman Empire. In 1533, amidst rising internal religious disputes, the Sorbonne condemned Marguerite's *Miroir de l'âme pécheresse* and she left the court to remain in Navarre. Clément Marot and Bonaventure Des Periers were among the multiple exiled writers whom she protected in her own kingdom. For the rest of her life she continued to travel extensively and to pursue political advantages for her brother and her own kingdom. She died December 21, 1549, two years after the death of François.

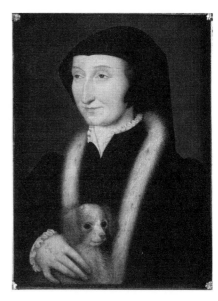

Marguerite of Angouleme, Queen of Navarre, 1544. © Réunion des Musées Nationaux/Art Resource, NY.

In the same period when she composed her mystical poetry, Marguerite also wrote four Biblical plays—*Comédie de la Nativité de Jésus-Christ, Comédie de l'Adoration des Trois Roys à Jésus-Christ, Comédie des Innocents* and *Comédie du Désert*, all of which belong to the tradition of the medieval mystery. Later, between 1535 and her death in 1549, Marguerite wrote seven secular plays. Three, *Le Malade, L'Inquisiteur*, and *Trop, Prou, Peu, Moins* are religious satires. *Comédie des quatre femmes* and *Comédie du parfait amant* have **love** as their motif while the two remaining, *Comédie sur le Trespas du Roy* and *Comédie jouée au Mont de Marsan* are more philosophical, offering meditations on death and conceptions of earthly life.

However, it is her collection of seventy stories patterned after Giovanni Boccaccio's *Décaméron*, the *Heptaméron*, for which Marguerite is best known. They address the many complexities inherent in male and female relationships, particularly in marriage, and reflect Marguerite's own brand of humor, ranging from the satirical to the ribald. Begun in 1542, they were not published until 1558, nine years after Marguerite's death. In her 1546 prologue, Marguerite acknowledges her debt to Boccaccio but underscores that her own stories are *veritable*, or true. As in the *Décaméron*, the *Heptaméron*'s characters tell tales to pass time as they await the repair of a bridge that has washed out during torrential floods in the Pyrenees. Her most notable innovation is the way in which the ten storytellers—five men and five women—discuss each others' stories, interpreting the actions and motivations of the subjects. She modeled her ten narrators after friends and family at the Navarre court, with Parlemente resembling Marguerite herself and Oisille, Louise de Savoy. **Love** is the main topic of the tales, with

Parlemente advocating a neo-Platonic view, claiming that perfect human love prepares one for divine love. The bawdy Hircan, with his disdain for courtly love, takes an opposite stance. The other storytellers take varying attitudes and not necessarily in defense of their own sex. With the *Heptaméron*, Marguerite creates complex and believable characters who tell tales of equally interesting acquaintances. Their intellectual and witty sparring reveals the oftentimes conflicting notions of honor, love, and friendship which dominated early modern French society. *See also* Diane de Poitiers.

Further Reading: Lyons, John D., and Mary B. McKinley. *Critical Tales: New Studies of the Heptaméron and Early Modern Culture.* Philadelphia: University of Pennsylvania Press, 1993.

Margaret Harp

MARLOWE, CHRISTOPHER (1564–1593). When **homoeroticism** is discussed in regard to English Renaissance literature, the name of Christopher Marlowe inevitably arises. Born in 1564 in Canterbury, he attended Cambridge on a scholarship because his father was a cobbler and unable to school his son. After receiving his BA in 1584, Marlowe stayed on at Cambridge for the master's degree, giving him three more years in which he could steep himself in the study of classics. Although many young university men at the time had their sights on law or church ministry, Marlowe himself seemed destined for a life devoted to poetry and the **theater**.

Among his poems, "Hero and Leander" is most notorious for its depiction of Neptune's fascination with Leander's body. Enamored of Hero, Leander swims the Hellespont to reach her, but en route Neptune laves the boy's body with water, and Marlowe delights in creating a blazon or anatomical description in poetry of Leander's muscles and limbs, stopping just short of the buttocks, which he playfully disdains to describe. Readers, however, are not fooled by the witty proximity to the seat of homoeroticism. "Hero and Leander" remains one of the finest epyllions—a brief narrative poem on a romantic or mythological theme—written during the English Renaissance.

A shorter lyric of homoerotic content is Marlowe's famous "Come Live with Me and Be My Love," a poem written in imitation of Virgil's second eclogue. With its pastoral setting, Marlowe places his homoerotic shepherd in a classic stance reminiscent of the Golden Age. The poem was soon answered by Sir Walter **Raleigh**'s "The Nymph's Reply to the Shepherd," which washed all traces of homoeroticism from its lyric tradition for hundreds of years. There is some evidence that Richard Barnfield's "The Affectionate Shepherd" influenced the writing of Marlowe's poem.

Of Marlowe's plays, *Edward II* has the most homoerotic content. In it, King Edward neglects his regal responsibilities as he dallies with his favorite Piers Gaveston. Eventually the English nobles rise up and depose the king in favor of his son. In a supreme act of sexual and poetic justice, Edward is executed by having a red hot poker inserted into his anus. In most productions of the play, however, this detail of the play is omitted. The king is simply crushed by a table. The homoerotic content of the play has never been denied, and the play remains the single most homoerotic piece of Renaissance theater to survive.

Although Marlowe's play *Dido, Queen of Carthage* begins with a whimsical homoerotic scene, the play does not sustain that tone. In the first scene, Jove plays with his boy lover **Ganymede**, and sets up an atmosphere that is in contrast to the ensuring treatment of Dido by Aeneas that follows in the play.

In his life, Marlowe made enemies not only among the theater crowd. There is some evidence that he served as an undercover agent for Sir Francis Walsingham, Queen **Elizabeth I**'s director of spying operations. In 1593, Marlowe was accused of heresy and blasphemy, possibly as a ruse to get him into protective custody. Among other things, accusations surfaced that Marlowe had said that Christ and John were lovers and that "all they that love not Tobacco and Boys were fools." Before Marlowe could face trial, however, he was stabbed in a tavern brawl at Deptford on May 31, 1593, and died. *See also* Anal Sex; Homosexuality; Shakespeare, William.

Further Reading: Bredbeck, Gregory. *Sodomy and Interpretation: Marlowe to Milton.* Ithaca, NY: Cornell University Press, 1991; Henderson, Philip. *Christopher Marlowe.* 2nd ed. New York: Barnes and Noble Books, 1974; Rowse, A. L. *Christopher Marlowe: His Life and Work.* New York: Grosset and Dunlap, 1966; Smith, Bruce R. *Homosexual Desire in Shakespeare's England: A Cultural Poetics.* Chicago: University of Chicago Press, 1991; Wraight, A. D. *Christopher Marlowe and Edward Alleyn.* Chichester, England: Adam Hart, 1993.

George Klawitter

MARRIAGE. There were few changes in the rules regarding marriage or in marriage behavior in the non-European world in the fifteenth and sixteenth centuries, but there were significant developments in the ideology and law of marriage in **Europe** during this time. At the beginning of the period, marriage formation and dissolution in many parts of Europe (especially on the geographical margins) were governed by custom rather than formal law. Marriage did not involve a priest or other intermediary, and often required no more than a statement by each partner that they married each other ("I marry you"), along with an exchange of rings or other tokens or, sometimes, a symbolic act such as drinking wine from the same cup. Communities recognized couples as married when they acted as married couples did, by living, eating, and sleeping together. Many customary systems also allowed for couples to separate. Among the Basques of France and Spain, for example, a couple could separate and remarry if they failed to have children after several years' cohabitation.

During the early modern period, however, the Church sought to bring more and more of these marginal regions more firmly under the jurisdiction of canon law, which regulated such matters as sexuality and marriage. For example, the earliest attempt to enforce the canon law of marriage in Iceland dates from 1429. From this time, it began to replace a customary system in which the consent of the woman was not required for marriage and which allowed for **divorce**.

Yet, in the sixteenth century, just as the Catholic Church began to use canon law, instead of local custom, as a method to standardize approaches to marriage throughout non-Orthodox Europe, it was challenged by the Protestant **Reformation**. The ensuing clash of Protestant and Catholic ideals forced a shift in the ideology and doctrines of marriage that

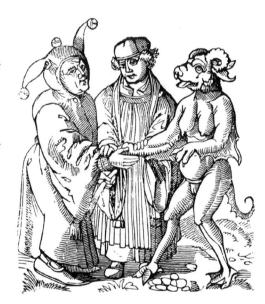

A reform minister officiating at the marriage of a fool and a she-devil. From Thomas Merner's anti-Lutheran pamphlet "Von dem grossen Lutherischen Narren," 1518. Courtesy of the Dover Pictorial Archives.

led in turn to changes in marriage laws and practices in many countries. The more general result was a secularization of marriage, and the creation of two broad approaches to marriage in central and western Europe—one Catholic and one Protestant. Over the longer term, the more secular approach to the ideology that was implanted in the sixteenth century became the dominant European model, making this period a turning-point in the history of marriage in Europe and later, by imperial extension, in many other parts of the world.

The ideology of marriage expressed in canon law had evolved during the thousand years prior to 1400. Laws regarding such issues as **celibacy**, obstacles to marriage (such as relationship by blood or marriage), definitions of consent, the role of priests, and divorce, varied over time and, depending upon the strength of the authority of the Church in particular parts of Europe, regionally. By the thirteenth century, the ideology of marriage and the body of canon law attached to it, had stabilized and provided for a system that valued celibacy higher than marriage, made marriage a sacrament, included a ban on marriages between individuals who were third cousins or more closely related, and prohibited divorce.

The reformers Martin **Luther** and John **Calvin** were only the most prominent theologians who eventually broke with the Catholic Church and laid the groundwork for the formation of Protestant churches in many European countries, states, and city-states. They and other reformers challenged Church doctrines and set in motion the trend toward more liberal and secular doctrines of marriage in Europe.

One fundamental shift was away from valuing celibacy higher than marriage, a medieval Church position expressed by the rule that clergy had to be unmarried. The reformers, for their part, argued for recognition of marriage as an institution ordained by God and available to all. Calvin criticized the Church's praise of **virginity**, while Martin Bucer (who led the Reformation in Strasbourg) condemned its admiration of the celibate life. They and others rejected such Catholic doctrines as offensive to what they regarded as God's gift of sexuality. Reformers held the doctrine of celibacy responsible for widespread illicit sexual activity, especially by priests and monks. Luther wrote that only one in several thousand people had the ability to stay a life-long virgin. He encouraged the clergy to marry, and led by his own example.

While revaluing marriage, the reformers also challenged the Church doctrine that it was designed primarily for procreation. They gave more emphasis to emotional ties within marriage and to the function of marriage in providing women and men with a stable sexual relationship that made fornication (sex between unmarried people) unnecessary.

Such reformulations of the character of marriage led to a rejection of the ways in which the Church dealt with marital breakdown. By 1400, Church courts could annul marriages, effectively declaring they had never existed because of a legal shortcoming in their formation, or grant separations, which allowed spouses to live separately but not to enter new marriages. But, following an interpretation of the New Testament, canon law did not permit divorce, or the dissolution of marriage such that former husbands and wives were able to remarry.

Most reformers argued that New Testament references to divorce ought to be read as permitting divorce for **adultery**, and most added desertion as a divorce-worthy offence. Over time, other grounds were added. Depending on jurisdiction, they included witchcraft, violence, and madness. At the same time, the Reformed Churches removed marriage from the list of sacraments and many reformers argued that its regulation was essentially a civil matter. In some regions, civil or mixed civil-ecclesiastical courts took jurisdiction of marriage and divorce law, while in others matrimonial litigation remained in the hands of ecclesiastical judges.

Reformed marriage doctrines also reduced the impediments to marriage, conditions such as relationship by blood or marriage that prevented two individuals from marrying. Church law banned marriage by third cousins or more closely related individuals, and also by individuals linked by a certain status or by a sexual relationship. For example, a man could not marry a woman with whom his bother had had a sexual relationship, a rule that bedeviled the marital status of **Henry VIII** of England when he sought an **annulment** of his marriage to his brother's widow, Catherine of Aragon, and a new marriage with Anne Boleyn, the sister of one of the king's former sexual partners. Such impediments were rejected by reformers as attempts to make marriage difficult. Certainly, in small communities such as most Europeans lived in during this period, it was increasingly difficult for men and women to find partners they could marry. The reduction of impediments facilitated marriage and, in the eyes of reformers, contributed to the stability of society.

The overall effect of changes in marriage ideologies and law in many parts of Europe in the sixteenth century was to shift the emphasis on marriage from its form to its content. More attention was paid to its emotional and sexual dimension, and the law began to embrace a more secular and contractual view of marriage. *See also* Bastardy; Christianity; Remarriage/Widows; Witches.

Further Reading: Phillips, Roderick. *Putting Asunder: A History of Divorce in Western Society*. New York: Cambridge University Press, 1988; Watt, Jeffrey R. *The Making of Modern Marriage: Matrimonial Control and the Rise of Sentiment in Neuchatel, 1550–1800*. Ithaca, NY: Cornell University Press, 1992.

Roderick Phillips

MASCULINITY. The study of masculinity considers the specific details of how boys and men are raised, how they relate with other people, and how they express their identities. Scholars focus on what cultural groups say boys and men are expected to do as well as on what kinds of objects (a Mustang convertible rather than a Volkswagen Beetle), animals (dog rather than a cat), and activities (football rather than ballet) cultures imprint with a male, rather than a female, subtext. Scholars also consider the ways understandings of masculinity flavor cultural and artistic productions.

Numerous scholars in ancient, medieval, and modern history have considered issues of masculinity in considerable depth, but the body of work for the early modern era remains small. With respect to men's private lives, ideas about the body and sexuality in Renaissance Europe have received the most attention. There are also important studies of changing expectations of **fatherhood** and husbands' rights and responsibilities, often embedded in works primarily devoted to women's history. Understandings of positive (or at least culturally approved) adult male roles have received much more attention than understandings of masculinity among boys, poor men, old men, or criminals. Tensions between generations have not yet received much attention. Gender expectations played an important role in attitudes toward Native Americans and the motivations of conquistadors, but most of the work on the effects of the European presence on Native Americans focuses on the seventeenth century and later.

It appears that the early modern era was one of rapid change for understandings of masculinity in many parts of the world. Western and central European ideology began to put a much greater emphasis on male responsibility, sexual restraint, and loving fatherhood than they had previously. This is evidenced not only by legislation but also by images and literature portraying good fathers and husbands as possessing self-control, personal authority, and vigor. In China, the Ming era placed a new emphasis on individualism, encouraging (elite) men to express themselves through poetry, to interact with (some) women as creative equals, and to cultivate their appreciation of the natural world through solitary retreats. The expanding Aztec empire in Mexico ranked men according to the number of war captives they had captured and offered for sacrifice, and encouraged boys to cultivate stoicism, obedience, truthfulness, and eloquence. The Maya seem to have emphasized a man's responsibility to farm, hunt, and fish, while the Inca treated the sexes as complementary and assigned male and female roles for public and ritual life. The sixteenth century arrival of western Europeans in the New World, bringing not only Christian ideology but also changes in social and economic organization, caused profound changes in the ways Native American men worked, parented, and acted as husbands, as did the increasingly large-scale importation of Africans as slaves in the Atlantic. The history of masculinity in the early Ottoman Empire and West African polities such as Benin and Ghana is yet in its infancy, but the rapid expansion of states in these regions must have had an impact on male identity development. Indeed, one of the hallmarks of the early modern period is the very large numbers of men put under arms throughout much of the world, but the implications of this have not yet received much attention with respect to gender.

Governments, heads of state, and politicians sometimes attempt to define themselves in terms of a particular kind of masculinity. Chinese emperors sought to present themselves as models of male Confucian orthodoxy, kowtowing to their mothers, offering the proper ritual sacrifices to their ancestors, studying the Confucian Classics, making and collecting fine art, and issuing land reform legislation intended to ensure family inheritances were equitable. Thus they demonstrated a good son's filial piety (obedience to and respect for their living and deceased ancestors), a man's intellectual prowess, and a mystic's appropriately channeled and controlled sense of the good, the true, and the beautiful. Fifteenth- and sixteenth-century European rulers, on the other hand, so strongly equated effective rule with military prowess that kings felt compelled not only to train in arms and lead troops into battle, but also to compete in tournaments. Courtiers, meanwhile, struggled to find ways to petition and companion rulers that their (potential or actual) employers would find personable but which would not compromise their honor or sense of self-worth. Early Ottoman emperors, whose state was built by *ghazi* warriors (initially bands of warriors held together by religious practice), particularly emphasized the role of the *ghazi* spirit of expanding and protecting the borders of Islam. *See also* Africa; Americas (North and South); Christianity; Confucianism; Cross-Dressing; Daoism; Eunuchs; Homoeroticism; Homosexuality; Hinduism; Islam; Judaism; Mistresses; Platonic Love.

Further Reading: Carrasco, Davíd, with Scott Sessions. *Daily Life of the Aztecs: People of the Sun and Earth*. Westport, CT: Greenwood Press, 1998; Cass, Victoria. *Dangerous Women: Warriors, Grannies, and Geishas of the Ming*. Lanham, MD: Rowman and Littlefield, 1999; Clendinnen, Olga. *Aztecs: An Interpretation*. Cambridge and New York: Cambridge University Press, 1991; Huang, Martin W. *Negotiating Masculinities in Late Imperial China*. Honolulu: University of Hawai'i Press, 2006; Ozment, Steven E. *When Fathers Ruled: Family Life in Reformation Europe*. Cambridge, MA: Harvard University Press, 1983; Reeser, Todd. *Moderating Masculinity in Early Modern Culture*. Chapel Hill: University of North Carolina Department of Romance Languages, 2006; Rocke, Michael. *Forbidden Friendships: Homosexuality and Male Culture in Renaissance Florence*. New York: Oxford University Press, 1996; Ruggerio, Guido. *The Boundaries of Eros: Sex Crime and Sexuality in Renaissance Venice*. New York and Oxford:

Oxford University Press, 1985; Sharer, Robert J. *Daily Life in Maya Civilization*. Westport, CT: Greenwood Press, 1996; Silverblatt, Irene. *Moon, Sun, and Witches: Gender Ideologies and Class in Inca and Colonial Peru*. Princeton, NJ: Princeton University Press, 1987.

Pamela McVay

MASTURBATION. In the Renaissance masturbation, or "self-pollution," was recognized as a sexual sin (and for Catholics a mortal sin), but it provoked little concern on the part of either clergy or physicians. Both Catholic and Protestant interpreters of the Biblical story of God condemning Onan for "spilling his seed upon the ground" usually described his sin as *coitus interruptus* and focused on the refusal to procreate (or, in Martin **Luther**'s case, the denial of sexual satisfaction to the woman) rather than masturbation. Although masturbation was often lumped with sexual intercourse between males and anal and oral intercourse between men and women in the larger category of sodomy, it attracted far less condemnation and concern than these practices. Nor was masturbation subject to the harsh legal penalties that other forms of sexual sin received, particularly with the religious reformations of the sixteenth century. Physicians too had little specific concern with masturbation, often not distinguishing between it and other methods of sexual climax. Jewish authorities also generally ignored masturbation, and the *shari'a* law of **Islam** had little concern with the practice except in the context of ritual purification.

One exception to the general Christian indifference to masturbation (the word itself, although derived from classical Latin, was not used in the Renaissance) was a short work of the early fifteenth century, commonly attributed to the French church reformer and chancellor of the University of Paris, Jean Gerson (1363–1429). Gerson discussed masturbation in the context of the confessional. The work takes the form of a description of a talk given by an experienced and diligent Paris theology master to a group of students. Gerson describes how a confessor must draw out an admission of the sin, which he saw as virtually universal among young males as well as adult men and women. Getting an admission of sin from the penitent was particularly difficult when dealing with masturbation, both because of the secret nature of the sin and the fact that many people saw nothing wrong with it. Gerson suggests that parents warn their children away from this sin at an early age. There is little evidence that Gerson's tract circulated widely or influenced clerical thought or practice.

Like most previous discussions of masturbation in the Western tradition, Gerson focused on men. Female masturbation was of less interest because women were not seen as fully responsible moral beings. Female masturbation was often treated in connection with **lesbianism**, as both were seen by male writers as ways for women to amuse themselves when lacking a man. As was the case with lesbianism, female masturbation was considered a much more serious sin if the masturbator used an instrument for penetration, "counterfeiting" the penis. The induction of orgasm through masturbation with the hands, solo or partnered, was sometimes considered an appropriate treatment for "female complaints." There was a revival of medical and clerical interest in female masturbation in the late sixteenth century, following the rediscovery of the clitoris as an object of authoritative male knowledge. *See also* Anal Sex; Christianity; Judaism; Oral Sex.

Further Reading: Laqueur, Thomas W. *Solitary Sex: A Cultural History of Masturbation*. New York: Zone Books, 2003.

William E. Burns

MEDICINE. Early modern medicine held firmly to the physiological models of health developed by classical authorities, especially the ancient physicians Galen and Hippocrates, which emphasized the fundamental importance of the four humors. These four fluids themselves had specific qualities, and health, both physical and psychological, depended on keeping the humors and their attendant qualities in balance. This balance, in turn, was maintained through healthy habits, such as a moderate diet, and sometimes through medical interventions. In matters of sex, differences between men and women could be explained by basic differences in the qualities of male and female bodies. Women's sex organs, for example, were sometimes said to be analogous to men's except that they remained internal, since the female body lacked the masculine heat needed to push them out. At the same time, however, the humoral model resulted in difficult puzzles. If, for instance women's bodies were cooler than those of men why did women have a stronger sex drive than their hotter male counterparts?

Since the Middle Ages, religious authorities had condemned contraception and, with particular vehemence, the **abortion** of a fetus that had quickened; that is, had begun to move in the womb. For this reason, and because of the prevalence of **midwives** who dealt with most issues surrounding **childbirth**, the physicians and scholars of the period paid relatively little attention to these matters. Nevertheless, contraception, which was very difficult to monitor in any case, was certainly practiced by individuals, though it is impossible to know for certain its relative effectiveness. Those experts who did write on the issue drew on ancient authorities such as Dioscorides and cited numerous plants such as rue—an herb still used in India for contraception—and various parts of the white willow, the so-called "chaste tree," in particular. Additionally, and perhaps even more importantly, folk tradition undoubtedly supplied suggestions for avoiding or eliminating **pregnancy**.

The moral implications of abortion were further complicated by concerns over medical ethics. The Hippocratic oath, for instance, forbids the use of medicine as a means to allow a pregnant woman to destroy her child. On the other hand, some authorities recognized that there were cases that justified abortions; a very young woman who became pregnant before her skeleton had fully developed was suggested as a candidate for abortion by the great medieval physician and philosopher Avicenna. In any case, several abortifacients were identified by contemporary experts.

The early modern moral position on sex itself was deeply affected by the emergence of syphilis at the end of the fifteenth century. The precise origins of the disease were unclear and it was commonly linked to foreigners in various European nations. In England, for example, syphilis was frequently termed *Morbus Gallicus*, the French disease. Though physicians of the period lacked a clear understanding of the transmission of the disease, it quickly became apparent that sexual contact was deeply implicated. Moreover since **prostitution** and other forms of sexual license were already frowned upon by authorities, and since disease was widely understood as one of the many punishments that God could bring down upon the wicked, medical explanations for the illness existed side by side with theological and moral accounts.

Numerous treatments for syphilis emerged in the sixteenth century, including hot baths and mercury unctions. A few suggested that since syphilis was contracted by sex with an unclean woman—that women could catch the illness from unclean men was rarely mentioned—that sex with a pure woman—a virgin—could serve as a cure.

Emotions in general were understood as both functions of humoral balance and possible sources of humoral imbalance. One extremely potent form of melancholia, described as an excess of black bile, was thought to both proceed from and contribute to overly strong feelings of love. As with other early modern ailments, it was often difficult to distinguish a **love sickness** that originated with physiological causes from one whose source was magical or demonic in nature, as it was believed that excessive passion could either proceed from bodily causes or be the work of the Devil. As the Devil could not afflict the soul directly, and since love emanated from the soul, he could only inflame love indirectly by manipulating the body through deceiving the senses or inflaming the brain with lustful fantasies. Drugs and philters could have a similar effect, though medical authorities stressed that, as with magic, they could inflame desires but could not absolutely compromise the free will of the individual. In the case of love melancholy, matters were particularly muddy since the Devil was thought to be especially capable in manipulating that humor. By contrast, physicians in the period sought increasingly to define madness, including melancholy, as a physiological condition, and not necessarily arising from spiritual torment.

Numerous treatments for love sickness were available. Renaissance physicians could, for instance, return to Avicenna, whose views on the issue were pragmatic, for several courses of treatment. These included directing the eye of the afflicted to some other object of affection, distracting the patient with other activities, and requiring the patient to listen to disparaging remarks about the beloved—preferably from old women. Reflections on the corruption of the flesh and on death were also cited as efficacious; one story of the time recounted how the philosopher Hypatia dissuaded an ardent suitor by showing him linens that had been stained with her menstrual blood. By contrast, some authorities suggested the opposite course, contending that vigorous sexual intercourse—not necessarily with the beloved—would help exhaust the violent passions and effect a cure. *See also* Love Sickness.

Further Reading: Beecher, Donald A., and Massimo Ciavolella. *Eros and Anteros: The Medical Traditions of Love in the Renaissance*. University of Toronto Italian Studies 9. Ottawa: Dovehouse Editions, 1992; Boehrer, Bruce Thomas. "Early Modern Syphilis." *Journal of the History of Sexuality* 1, no. 2 (1990): 197–214; Lawrence, Conrad I., et al. *The Western Medical Tradition, 800 BC to AD 1800*. Cambridge: Cambridge University Press, 1995; Riddle, John M. *Contraception and Abortion from the Ancient World to the Renaissance*. Cambridge, MA: Harvard University Press, 1994; Schleiner, Winfried. "Early Modern Controversies about the One-Sex Model." *Renaissance Quarterly* 53, no. 1 (Spring 2000): 180–91; Wiesner-Hanks, Merry E. *Christianity and Sexuality in the Early Modern World: Regulating Desire, Reforming Practice*. London: Routledge, 2000.

Todd H. J. Pettigrew

MENSTRUATION.   Early modern ideas on menstruation were heavily influenced by classical philosophers and physicians, like Hippocrates and Galen, who had established the basis of Western medical thought. These thinkers believed that all the body's fluids were interrelated and concluded that they were all forms of the same fundamental substance; therefore, each fluid could be transformed into one another. Consequently, although menstrual blood was thought to nurture the fetus in the womb, it was also understood that it changed to milk during lactation. These philosophers also examined the process of menstruation and deduced that periodic bleeding was not harmful to women; Hippocrates agreed that menstruation acted as a cleansing mechanism for the body, and therefore "menstruation had the function of purifying women of bad humors," which caused illnesses or diseases (Coutinho, 5). It was believed that if this bloodletting did not occur for women, wastes would build up within the body and cause illness. Galen, a respected follower of Hippocrates, concluded in turn that if menstruation cured the body of illness by natural bloodletting, then a physician-assisted bloodletting must also rid the body of diseases for women and for men. Therefore, menstruation was not only linked to blood flow, reproduction, and fertility, but also to purification and the term *purgation*. As menstruation was not clearly classified as being different from other types of bleeding/bloodletting and emissions from the body, it was certainly not uncommon to believe that women and men could alternatively experience a type of pseudomenstruation via other means or types of bleedings, such as nosebleeds, hemorrhoids, sputum, lactation, sweating, and the emission of semen.

An early modern viewpoint inherited from Aristotle was that women were moister and colder than men and were, therefore, sensually insatiable. Consequently, men were considered "more perfect," and early physicians developed a "hierarchy in which [men and women] differed by degree of heat" (Martin, 30–31). This hierarchal view cast a different light on women, and more so menstruating women, who were even colder and moister than usual, and "though all bodily fluids were seen as related, menstrual blood was still generally viewed as somehow different and dangerous" (Wiesner, 44–45). Peggy McCracken demonstrates that the significance of blood is gender-biased, and whereas women's blood via menstruation and parturition is regarded as inferior or suitable to certain social situations, men's blood via heroic gestures of war was of utmost consequence and importance. Therefore, she notes, "women's blood—menstruation and the blood of parturition—have long been associated with pollution in the Judeo-Christian tradition" (3). The negativity of this attitude toward menstrual blood in early modern thought was reinforced by classical thinkers such as Pliny the Elder (77 CE), who wrote that menstrual blood was so toxic that it destroyed crops and fruit, blunted knives, and even had the power to blight trees, kill bees, and make dogs mad. Also, Pliny claimed, sexual intercourse with a menstruating women during a full lunar eclipse could be harmful or even fatal to a man.

Beliefs surrounding particular menstrual practices were not only discussed and debated in medical and social circles, but were heavily imbued with religious taboos as well. Religious ideas from Old Testament Levitical blood laws considered menstruating women as tainted and impure, and although early modern Jewish communities had stricter rules, Christian penitentials and manuals of confession and pastoral care based their ideas upon the religious belief that women were unclean during menstruation. Because of this impurity, men were instructed to abstain from sexual relations with menstruating wives/women. In fact, during the sixteenth century, there was a belief that engaging in intercourse with menstruating women would "result in deformed or leprous children" (Wiesner, 45). Other Christian manuals and penitentials warned that "intercourse with an unpurified woman can cause bad things to happen . . . including infertility and weakness," and that "menstruating women are to do penance if they should enter a Church or receive communion" (Lee, 46, 44).

However, even though menstruating women might have been somewhat limited in social or religious circles because of their menstruating flesh, which experienced physical bodily suffering, this setback only caused them to excel in other religious situations. In effect, early modern piety drew from medieval devotion and beliefs, which "linked flesh, especially Christ's flesh, with woman" (Bynum 1991, 100), and Christ's bleeding body with woman's bleeding body, which caused "female spirituality to be "especially somatic" and which caused "not so much as a rejection of physicality as the elevation of it—a horrible yet delicious elevation—into a means of access to the divine" (Bynum 1989, 162). *See also* Christianity; Judaism; Medicine; Penitential Practices.

Further Reading: Amt, Emilie, ed. *Women's Lives in Medieval Europe: A Sourcebook.* New York: Routledge, 1993; Bynum, Caroline Walker. *Fragmentation and Redemption: Essays on Gender and Human Body in Medieval Religion.* New York: Zone Books, 1991; Bynum, Caroline Walker. "The Female Body and Religious Practice in the Later Middle Ages." In *Fragments for the History of the Human Body Part One,* edited by Michel Feher et al. New York: Zone Books, 1989; Coutinho, Elsimar M., and Sheldon J. Segal. *Is Menstruation Obsolete?* New York: Oxford University Press, 1999; Elliott, Dyan. *Pollution, Sexuality, and Demonology in the Middle Ages.* Philadelphia: University of Pennsylvania Press, 1999; Lee, Becky. "The Purification of Women After Childbirth: A Window onto Medieval Perceptions of Women." *Florilegium* 14 (1995–1996): 43–55; Martin, Emily. *The Woman in the Body: A Cultural Analysis of Reproduction.* Boston: Beacon Press, 1992; Mason-Hoyl, Elizabeth. *The Diseases of Women by Trotula of Salerno: A Translation of Passionibus Mulierum Curandorum.* Los Angeles: The Ward Richie Press, 1940; McCracken, Peggy. *The Curse of Eve, the Wound of the Hero: Blood, Gender, and Medieval Literature.* Philadelphia: University of Pennsylvania Press, 2003; Turner, Paul, ed. *Selections from The History of The World: Commonly Called The Natural History of C. Plinius Secundus.* Translated by Philemon Holland. Edited by J. M. Cohen. Centaur Classics Series. Carbondale: Southern Illinois University Press, 1962; Wiesner, Mary. *Women and Gender in Early Modern Europe: New Approaches to European History.* Cambridge: Cambridge University Press, 1993.

Sharmain van Blommestein

MIDDLE EAST. The empires of the Middle East in the early modern period were divided along ethnic, linguistic, and sectarian lines. The Ottoman Turks rose to power during this period, and their empire encompassed the Balkans, Anatolia, the Levant, most of the Arabian peninsula, and present-day Iraq and North Africa, but the political power of the Arabs was in eclipse. Ottoman society and administration were governed by Islamic institutions and legal systems, while the Ottomans guarded the holy shrines in Mecca and Medina and promoted Sunni orthodoxy. From early times, the Turks had adopted Persian as their courtly and literary language but, during this period, Ottoman Turkish emerged as a literary language replacing Persian and Arabic.

Centuries of conflict, invasion, and conquest had thoroughly mixed the peoples of the Middle East. The slave trade had brought slaves from all corners of the world and, with time, they had converted to **Islam** and been integrated into society. As a result, major cities, such as Istanbul, Damascus, Cairo, and Baghdad were truly cosmopolitan and multicultural. Within Ottoman administration, individual religious groups, such as the Christians and Jews, were allowed to maintain and control their communities.

As Ottoman power expanded out from its base in Anatolia, it conquered Muslim lands and simultaneously expanded into Europe; most notably, into the Balkans. At the beginning of this major period of conquest and expansion, there was a major shortage of trained religious leaders and judges, and it became common practice for Turks to study in Damascus and Cairo.

During the early modern period, a large number of Sufi sects and heterodox movements such as the Hurufis and Bektashis proliferated and manifested themselves as medicants who wandered throughout the lands, becoming known as dervishes. As part of their religious practices, they committed outrageous acts aimed at bringing blame upon themselves. These unorthodox acts included drug use, drunkness, illicit sexual relations, and all manner of unacceptable social behavior. They were condemned by orthodox Muslims, but it was within this atmosphere that many of the Christian and Muslim populations in Anatolia and the Balkans began to integrate.

MIDDLE EAST

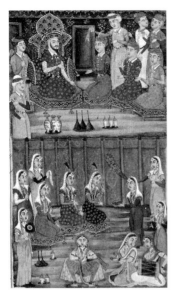

An illustration of the marriage of the three daughters of Sero, king of Yemen, from "Shahnameh" ("Book of Kings"), a sixteenth-century epic poem by Persian poet Firdausi. © The Art Archive/ Musée Condé Chantilly/Dagli Orti.

The Ottoman reign was dominated by the Hanafi school of law, which was not fundamentalist but tolerant. The empire had empowered its diverse religious communities to govern themselves internally and the Ottomans were instrumental in initiating a racial and ethnic blend throughout the empire. The real emphasis was on community and religious unity.

Islamic society had a healthy and well-developed attitude toward love and sex. Its laws and ethical system respected and protected the rights of all parties. This was reflected in the form of legal texts, medical treatises, *belles lettres*, erotica, and popular literature. Throughout the Middle East, regional variations existed but all of the Muslim societies extending across North Africa all the way to central Asia were bound together by common laws and social norms.

Within Middle Eastern Islamic culture, romantic courtships followed by **marriage** were not the norm. Family and community were central. Family was placed above the individual, therefore **love** marriages were extremely rare. Women were segregated and cloistered inside the home and contact with males from outside their immediate family was restricted. Marriages were usually arranged by the family, for economic and political reasons. Children were sometimes betrothed at an early age and their marriages were consummated when they reached puberty. First cousin marriages were especially prized. Islam allowed a man to marry up to four wives and permitted an unlimited number of **concubines**. Polygamous marriages were more common among the rich and the elites. However, in marriage a woman had the right to sexual satisfaction and a right to children. Contraception and **abortion** were accepted and practiced, but only with the wife's permission.

In Shia Islam, temporary marriages (*mut'a*) were permitted. These were marriages of convenience, and could be contracted for periods as short as an hour and the woman's compensation was fully fixed. *Mut'a* marriages were considered to provide an acceptable alternative to **prostitution**. They provided an outlet for sexual fulfillment, and protected both parties by fixing conditions, compensation, and responsibilities that were enforceable by law. However, these marriages were condemned by Sunni Islam.

Illegal activities flourished in large cities. Gambling and drinking were part of an underground economy, as was prostitution that provided for all types of sexual services. Drug use, especially the eating of hashish, had become popular in the larger cities and was associated with the lower strata of society. Hashish was believed to break down resistance to sexual advances and to contribute to effeminate behavior that led to passive **homosexuality**. In some quarters of Cairo, hashish eaters commonly stalked young boys and, in some cases, drugged them.

Within the courts or inner circles of the elite, large numbers of servants and retainers were trained to entertain. For the rest, however, enterprising businessmen and women in large cities ran businesses of varying kinds that catered to the fancies and carnal desires of all classes. **Brothels** and **harems** in cities such as Istanbul were filled with a dazzling array of beautiful women of all races and nationalities. Talented female and male slaves were trained to sing and dance, along with other skills, and they entertained and dallied with customers for a price. Public baths were often places where sexual favors could be purchased or places to rendezvous.

At the highest levels of the elite, female slaves were selected to serve as royal concubines to the sultan. Concubines became the preferred consorts because they were free of the political or family pressures and obligations entailed in marriages among the aristocracy. As a result, specially trained concubines became the favorites of the sultans and consequently bore their heirs.

Persia, which had long been politically dominated by different Turkish tribes, was conquered by the Safavids in the early sixteenth century. They were ethnically Turkish but culturally Persian, and had emerged out of eastern Anatolia. The Safavids and Ottomans frequently fought and remained in an extended state of hostilities. The Safavids espoused Shi'a Islam and established it as the state religion. Internally, this caused turmoil, which in turn sparked an exodus of Sunni Muslims, many of whom found sanctuary in Mughal India. At different times during this period, Tabriz, Qazvin, and Isfahan served as Persia's capital.

Besides political and religious changes, Persia experienced social change as well. The introduction of coffee and tobacco altered past social behavior. Coffeehouses proliferated in major cities, where men congregated and began smoking opium, which did not have the social stigma of alcohol or hashish. The proliferation of these establishments soon aggravated existing social ills and coffeehouses became equated with places of vice, where sexual favors could be purchased and/or exchanged. Court life in Safavid Persia was similar to that of the Ottomans. Harem life and sexual politics evolved in much the same way; however, opium and opium addiction took on a major role. Addiction and alcoholism among the courtly elites resulted in lives of dissipation and early death.

The Ottoman and Safavid dynasties maintained complex multicultural societies dominated by Islamic law and institutions. While moral laxity, dissipation, vice, and corruption as described above could be found, the majority of the populations adhered to strict moral codes. Belief in God, virtuous behavior, and the importance of family and community were sacred. To the east in central Asia, the Uzbek kingdom ruling from the cities of Samarqand and Bukhara, maintained similar cultural patterns, as did the Mughal Empire in India.

The early modern period ushered in increased social and economic changes and, increasingly, contacts with the West. Western imperialism would lead to a new world order that would come to marginalize the Middle East in centuries to come. *See also* Asia; Christianity; Judaism; Polygamy/Polyandry.

Further Reading: Afaf Lutfi al-sayyid Marsot, ed. *Society and the Sexes in Medieval Islam*. Malibu, CA: Undena Publications, 1979; Chebel, Malek. *Encyclopedie de l'amour en Islam, Erotisme, beautie et sexualite dans le monde arabe, en Perse et en Turqui*. Paris: Payot et Rivages, 1995; Giffen, Lois Anita. *Theory of Profane Love among the Arabs: The Development of the Genre*. New York: New York University Press, 1971; Musallam, Basim F. *Sex and Society in Islam: Birth Control before the 19th Century*. London: Cambridge University Press, 1983; Nafzawi, 'Umar ibn Muhammad. *The Glory of the Perfumed Garden: The Missing Flowers*. An English Translation of the Second and Hereto Unpublished Part of Shaykh Nafzawi's Perfumed Garden. London: Spearman, 1975.

Mark David Luce

MIDWIVES. A midwife was a person, usually a woman, who was in charge during the birthing process. In Europe, to assist in delivery, she had a knife, sponge, binders, herbal mixtures, and sometimes a collapsible birthing chair or stool. During childbirth, the midwife would put oil of lilies or almonds on her hands (the efficacy of washing hands was not yet known) and used the same oil to lubricate the pregnant woman.

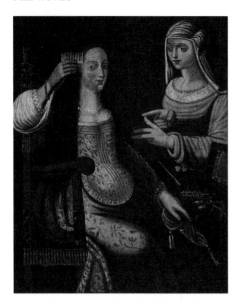

Sixteenth-century German illustration of a *Midwife's Instruction*. © The Art Archive/ Château de Gue-Pean/Dagli Orti.

She kept her nails trimmed. In the event of a difficult birth, other midwives or even a surgeon might be called in to assist.

Midwives worked formally and informally, and often under conditions that isolated them from other midwives. The midwives of Nuremberg and London, however, were well organized. Newer midwives trained with senior midwives for many years before practicing on their own. In London, most midwives were married or widows while, in Nuremburg, married women rarely became midwives. In Haarlem, in the Netherlands, only mothers could become midwives. Midwives held a middling position in society and were seen as honorable women, but they faced loss of social status and harsh penalties if they assisted in an **abortion**.

Midwives were paid in cash or kind according to the means of the woman. At the infant's baptism, godparents and others might also give the midwife some money or goods. Midwives could make a comfortable salary. A London midwife had the potential of earning enough to support a family at a respectable level.

Beginning in the fifteenth century, civil and ecclesiastical authorities began to license midwives. In England, licenses were not cheap, although there was no set fee. Not all midwives obtained licenses and those who did not could be excommunicated. Some were unable to obtain a license because of religious unorthodoxy. Others were too busy or too poor. Some saw no reason to do so. Besides religious orthodoxy, the authorities were concerned with the training and experience of candidates. In England, midwives proved their abilities through testimonials provided by satisfied clients or other midwives. In Schwarzburg, in Germany, midwives were examined by male physicians. Character was a third area that concerned authorities. A midwife had to be of impeccable repute because of the large amount of power she possessed.

Prior to the **Reformation**, it had been common for a midwife to perform an emergency baptism upon an infant in danger of death, which was necessary for salvation. With the advent of the Reformation, a variety of new beliefs about baptism emerged. In the Church of England, Elizabethan clergymen were divided on the issue. Those who believed baptism necessary for salvation supported the right of midwives to perform the rite when in dire circumstances. Others, who saw baptism as simply an entry rite to the earthly Christian community, saw no need for midwives to do so. Lutheranism did not allow second baptisms, and thus it was important that it be done correctly the first time, whether by a minister or midwife.

Midwives fulfilled a variety of other functions within the community and thus exercised a degree of power unusual for most women. They provided assistance in the treatment of female ailments. They examined the bodies of women in criminal cases to determine **pregnancy, rape**, or recent delivery. In England and Scotland, they were called upon to look for the devil's mark on those accused of witchcraft. They were thought to be able to ascertain whether a dead infant had received a soul yet, which was important because the killing of an ensouled infant was a serious crime.

In the early modern period, midwives were often required to obtain the name of the father of babies born to unwed mothers, even if this required the denial of assistance during labor until the desired information was provided. Such infants and their mothers were an economic drain on the local community and, the man named was required by law to provide financially for the child's upbringing.

Male midwives in England, anxious to usurp the position (and income) of female midwives, were well on their way to replacing women as providers of assistance in childbirth by the eighteenth century. Unlike in England, the male authorities and physicians in Schwarzburg disseminated information about anatomy and **medicine** to midwives. In Swiss Geneva, the majority of midwives were still women by the end of the century. *See also* Bastardy; Childbirth; Christianity; Remarriage/Widows; Witches.

Further Reading: Aiken, Judith P. "The Welfare of Pregnant and Birthing Women as a Concern for Male and Female Rulers: A Case Study." *Sixteenth Century Journal* 35 (Spring 2004): 9–41; Evenden, Doreen. *The Midwives of Seventeenth-Century London*. Cambridge: Cambridge University Press, 2000; Wiesner, Merry E. "The Midwives of South Germany and the Public/Private Dichotomy." In *The Art of Midwifery*, edited by Hilary Marland, 77–94. London: Routledge, 1993.

Tonya M. Lambert

MIKVEH. *Mikveh* (pl. *Mikva'ot*), "a place where [water] is being accumulated," is the Hebrew name for an artificial pool of water that practicing Jews utilize for purification purposes. The oldest known *mikva'ot* are from the period of the Second Temple (sixth century BCE–first century CE). New *mikva'ot* have been built ever since all over the world. Although a *mikveh* can serve various ritual purposes, its main and most crucial use, certainly after the destruction of the Second Temple in Jerusalem in 70 CE, is for women's purification ritual following **menstruation**.

According to Jewish law, following (evidently, not without modifications) Biblical law (especially Lev 15, Lev 18:19, and Lev 20:18), a woman is impure from the onset of her menstrual bleeding until her ritual immersion in water. This immersion must be performed after the completion of seven days following the end of her bleeding. Even if the bleeding period was shorter, the counting of seven days can not begin before the fifth day from the onset of the period. Therefore, for most women, the bath should take place around the twelfth day of the cycle. Until this ritual purification, the woman is considered to be *niddah*, often translated as "rejected" or "secluded," and she and her husband are prohibited from having intimate relations. Otherwise, they commit a major sin that is punishable, according to Jewish tradition, by death. Some domestic activities, considered by the rabbis as possible sources of intimacy, are also forbidden. According to some European traditions, mostly between the twelfth and seventeenth centuries, women who were *niddah* avoided entering synagogues as well.

Ritual immersion is generally performed in total nudity, and at night. It can take place in a natural body of water (lake, river, sea), but in cold countries, Jewish communities have generally built their own artificial *mikveh*, sometimes even before building a synagogue. Europe, the home of innumerable flourishing Jewish communities for hundreds of years, witnessed the construction of countless *mikva'ot*. Only a few of them have survived to this day.

The basic physical structure for ritual baths is determined by Jewish law. The water volume should consist of several hundred liters (the exact amount is a subject of debate). For a *mikveh* to be valid, its water, or at least a portion of it, must be accumulated in a "natural" way. For this reason, *mikva'ot* are typically located underground, in a place where water can be gathered naturally, often under or near synagogues. Today, the vast majority of modern *mikva'ot* are heated. Before the early-modern period, most *mikva'ot* did not have a built-in heating system.

A *mikveh* can also be used for other ritual purposes: to purify certain utensils produced by non-Jews; as a place for the necessary ritual immersion of converts to Judaism; and for the voluntary, but considered pious, ritual bath for men. Ritual baths for men had existed since early periods of Judaism, but it became common especially in the sixteenth to nineteenth centuries. *See also* Judaism; Menstruation.

Further Reading: Wasserfall, Rahel, ed. *Women and Water: Menstruation in Jewish Life and Law.* Waltham, MA: Brandeis University Press, 1999.

Evyatar Marienberg

MISTRESSES. A woman who has extramarital sexual relations with a man, regardless of the marital status of either party, is called his mistress. It is telling that men only can have or keep mistresses, while there is no corresponding male term except for the more gender-neutral "lover." The distinction between mistresses and **concubines** was culturally determined. Concubinage usually referred to longer-term arrangements than liaisons with mistresses, while in some cultures laws and customs defined the position of concubines.

In numerous early modern societies, the sexual rights of men and women were asymmetrical. Male sexual prowess was admired, and men were permitted more licence than women, from whom sexual restraint and/or **virginity** was more commonly required. This was partly because of the female childbearing capacity and the need to have undisputed paternity, and partly because of notions of honor. However, in some societies where maidenhead was no special virtue for nubile women, premarital sexual encounters between single and eligible men and women were tolerated, or even encouraged. However, sexual license has been more restricted for married persons than for singles in most societies, and fidelity is usually more required of married women than of their husbands.

The early modern Catholic, Protestant, and Orthodox churches perceived the distinction between marital and tolerated and non-marital and punishable sexual activity as relatively clear, with formalities normally required for true wedlock. Moreover, all forms of extramarital sexuality were often criminalized in secular law, and not simply punishable in ecclesiastical courts or the internal forum of the confessional. Canon law had classified voluntary extramarital heterosexual sex according to the marital status of the parties, and its definitions influenced medieval and early modern European secular laws. "Fornication" was defined to mean intercourse between two unmarried parties, while **adultery** involved one or two married parties (single or double adultery). In addition, sexual relationships could be incestuous (between relatives) or sacrilegious (either/both parties having taken vows). Secular society demonstrated a double morality, however, as women were more severely condemned and punished, and more frequently convicted, for the same sexual crimes.

This black-and-white attitude caused European explorers in general and missionaries and clerics in particular to condemn, for example, Polynesian and African sexual mores as lascivious and lewd. European explorers were often happy to take advantage of such customs, however, by initiating liaisons with native women, who were perceived as lustful and uninhibited. In seventeenth-century Central **Africa**, single and married men and women were reported to take many lovers without dishonor, which for Westerners was promiscuous and criminal.

In the colonies, Western men regularly took native and slave women as mistresses and concubines largely because of a scarcity of white women. In post-conquest Latin America, native women were to some extent offered to the Spanish as gifts and pledges of alliances, but the conquerors more often took the women they wanted. Matrimony between unbelievers and Christians was expressly forbidden. In the **Americas,** Colonial Africa, and **Asia,** interracial **marriage** between whites and native women was usually discouraged, whereas nonmarital relationships were tolerated, helping to integrate whites into the community and learn the local language, while the local women maintained the bachelors households and catered for their masters' and lovers' sexual needs. Nevertheless, the position of the children of such unions was precarious, and in some regions the half-breed offspring came to be perceived as an out-and-out menace.

In some early modern European countries, a royal mistress could obtain semi-official status, a position much sought after among the nobility. As the royal favorite, the principal official mistress (*maîtresse en titre*) could be powerful and influence royal policies, as in England under Charles II and France under Louis XIV. This semi-official "polygamy" has sometimes been compared to the harems of oriental potentates. Ambassadors of African and Asian rulers, themselves polygamous, even sent gifts both to the queen and "the other wife" of Louis XIV. Compared to the austere religiosity and strict morality of the era, sexual customs of early modern European courts were usually considerably more relaxed. Indeed, women serving at court were not expected to remain virtuous—or virginal. *See also* Christianity; Diane de Poitiers; Incest; La Malinche; Polygamy/Polyandry; Premarital Sex.

Further Reading: Gutiérrez, Ramón A. *When Jesus Came, the Corn Mothers Went Away: Marriage Sexuality, and Power in New Mexico, 1500–1846.* Stanford, CA: Stanford University Press, 1991; Harrington, Joel. *Reordering Marriage and Society in Reformation Germany.* Cambridge: Cambridge University Press, 1997; Sweet, James A. *Recreating Africa: Culture, Kinship, and Religion in the African-Portuguese World, 1441–1770.* Chapel Hill: University of North Carolina Press, 2003.

Mia Korpiola

MOTHERHOOD. Early modern mothers were deeply invested in their children. Because mothers were responsible in the family for the upbringing of children through infancy and early childhood, mothering was seen as the primary vocation of all women. More than this, motherhood was the primary metaphor for describing adult women's relationships and role in the world.

EXPECTATIONS. All of a woman's life led to her vocation in motherhood. Even celibate women, such as **Julian of Norwich,** employed the terminology of mothering to describe their relationships with others and their spiritual experiences of Christ. The most significant model for women in the Christian West, the Virgin Mary, was portrayed as the perfect mother, and she was accompanied by other godly mothers in early modern popular culture, including Monica, the mother of St. Augustine; St. Anne; and Birgitta of Sweden. The equation of **virginity** with female holiness remained a powerful ideal and ran counter to the promotion of motherhood. Some mothers felt that their love for their children drew them away from the perfection of religious contemplation and yearned for the carefree state of virginity. The **Reformation** challenged the preference given to **celibacy,** promoting an ideal of Christian motherhood that exalted childrearing as women's most important calling.

Martin **Luther** felt that "the entire female body was created for the purpose of nurturing children." One of the women characters in Niccolo Machiavelli's *Mandragola* put it thus: "Don't you see that a woman who has no children has no home?"

Most women came to motherhood through **pregnancy** and **childbirth**, important but daunting rites of passage given that maternal mortality struck down one in twenty and infant mortality took as many as one in seven in the first year of life. If the mother died, fathers often remarried in short order to provide a stepmother for his surviving children. Despite the risks, childbirth brought women into a closer community with their peers, a bond cemented through the women-only environment of the birthing. Moralists gave explicit directions as to how the mother should care for her newborn, preferring mothers to breastfeed and raise their own newborns. However, wealthier and urban mothers often resorted to wet nurses to nourish and care for their infants. In Thomas More's *Utopia*, women in Utopia were distinguished from what he felt was the common reality of sixteenth-century European elites in that "each woman nurses her own offspring unless prevented by either death or disease." The great theologian Erasmus of Rotterdam also derided the practice of wet-nursing, warning that this would disrupt the bonding of mother and child.

After infancy, mothers continued to direct their children's early lives through weaning, walking, and early education, although Erasmus noted that a mother's time with her sons was particularly limited as most boys came under their father's scope after the age of seven. Then, boys learned "harder lessons, which are the father's responsibility, rather than the mother's." In China, where Confucian philosophy put great emphasis on the family unit. the mother of the great classical Confucian disciple Mencius was praised for the care that she lavished on her young son and his environment in settling near a school so that he imitated the scholars in their tasks. Moralists warned against the common tendency of mothers to coddle their children, attributing such softness to women's pliant nature and loving attachment to their children. They urged fathers to intervene and ensure their children were being raised with discipline and vigilance. Mothers' authority to raise their young children as they saw fit was hemmed both by custom and law which gave the father free rein as head of the household, to direct child rearing against a mother's wishes.

Much was made of the physical care that mothers had to lavish on their children. Fathers were thought unfit to tend to delicate infants and were presumed to be busy with work of the world while mothers were charged with raising the children and protecting them from all the dangers of the workaday world. When children were sick, they were almost always under the care of their mothers, who nursed them as best they could with the limited range of herbal and folk remedies prescribed in contemporary handbooks. Spiritual dangers were also to be avoided through a careful education in the religious traditions under the watchful eye of the father who, as head of the household, maintained a strict control on the mother as well as the children.

EXPERIENCES. The physical and cultural passages of pregnancy and childbirth initiated women into the mysteries of maternity. For up to forty days after the birth, the new mother was sequestered in an enclosed room to recover from childbirth and nurture her newborn. Rarely did the new Christian mother attend her child's baptism, only rejoining the public community at her churching. As a mother, she would now be part of the community attendant upon other women in the community during their confinements, particularly those of her own daughters after they reached maturity.

Mothers were responsible for the vast majority of childcare, particularly in the aspects of routine care, feeding and early tutelage. The mother's role was critical in establishing the child's moral compass, and Renaissance humanists argued for the value of women's education in ensuring the health of the next generation. Reformation moralists agreed that mothers should at least have sufficient education to promote good religion in their offspring.

Even once their children reached adulthood, mothers exerted an authority second only to that of the father in most societies. In China, respect for parents was such a virtue that it was scandalous for a son to turn against his mother. A widow with property of her own was secure in her later years and expected the continuing obedience of her children in matters of **marriage** and business. Widowed mothers without provision had to rely on the goodwill of their children, which was sometimes wanting, even among the wealthiest, although the abandonment of aged mothers to public charity was widely condemned. At the end of life, the most common praise accorded a woman was to deem her a good wife and mother. *See also* Christianity.

Further Reading: Atkinson, Clarissa W. *The Oldest Vocation: Christian Motherhood in the Middle Ages*. Ithaca, NY: Cornell University Press, 1991; Fildes, Valerie, ed. *Women as Mothers in Pre-Industrial England*. London: Routledge, 1990.

Janice Liedl

MYSTICS. A mystic is a practitioner of mysticism, which can be defined as the pursuit of communion with or consciousness of God, spiritual truth, or some ultimate reality. Mystics pursue such an experience out of the belief that it is their destiny to do so or that the experience will provide them with valuable knowledge, understanding, or wisdom. Mystics have existed throughout history and are represented among the great religious traditions in both the West (including the Latin and Orthodox branches of **Christianity**) and the East (from the subcontinent of India throughout **Asia**).

Arguably one, in the Christian tradition for example, does not set out to become a mystic. In its ultimate reality, an individual seeks peace of mind and heart through deep prayer. Asceticism is the practice of meditation, prayer, fasting, and self-denial available to any human being—whether or not they live in a religious community. The ascetic sets out to live simply while practicing demanding spiritual exercises. Carried to the extreme, ascetics have sought separation from the world through denial of the flesh and often by engaging in self-imposed hardship. They may cross the line of pious self-discipline to the domain of morbid self-mutilation behavior. Theologians and psychologists have studied the presence of similarities and differences between the two sets of actions.

Many ancient, medieval, and modern believers would assert confidently that doing good works does not assure salvation. Nonetheless, doing what is good and useful to others—even if it means constantly praying for them practically every waking moment—may be part of the routine of the ascetic. What is the connection between the ascetic and the mystic? A true, though incomplete answer is that all mystics seem to be ascetics, but that not all ascetics seem to become mystics.

Mystics who have written about their experiences speak of three stages. The first stage is generally termed the *purgative way*, a period of mental, psychological, and spiritual review through which the mystic seeks to identify conscious and subconscious obstacles to contemplation. The second stage is the *illuminative way*, a phase characterized by God becoming present to the individual worshipper. It is similar to a glimpse of God's greatness to the finite heart, mind, and soul of that person. The third stage is

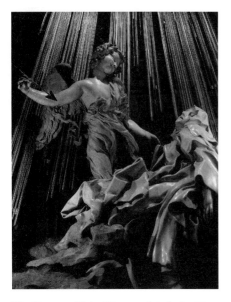

The Ecstasy of Saint Theresa of Avila, by Gian Lorenzo Bernini. © The Art Archive/Dagli Orti.

the *unitive way*. In it the individual is in a literal state of ecstasy (i.e., outside of the self) and in a completely indescribable union with the Deity (although the inspired prose and poetry of people who reach this state is nonetheless an attempt at description). It is God, or the One, who bestows such a grace of union on the individual soul through no merit of the individual soul itself.

Having achieved union with the divine, mystics write of the "dark night of the soul," which is a recurrent depression-like state, during which they long for union with God—often referred to as the Beloved—only to realize their minute place in the universe and the totality of the one-time divine presence. Nevertheless, mystics write of their union as having taken place outside of time as we perceive it. The dark night of the soul may be characterized by the aridity (dryness) of a total absence of prayer; it seems to be accompanied frequently by a total sense of rejection and unworthiness not unlike what mental health professionals find among the clinically depressed.

Spaniards John of the Cross (1542–1591), Teresa of Avila (1515–1582), and Ignatius of Loyola (1491–1556) are three of the foremost authors in the early modern Christian ascetic-mystical tradition. From the inception of the first house churches at the start of the Christian movement, through the Middle Ages and the Renaissance, Christian piety always impressed upon the faithful that the three enemies of humankind, ever to be avoided, were the devil, the flesh, and the world. These three assaulted saints and everyday people alike. Jacob Boehme (1575–1624) was a German Protestant mystic who led the life of a layperson. The Englishman George Fox (1624–1691) founded the Society of Friends (Quakers) and recorded his mystical experiences. Isaac ben Solomon Luria (1534–1572), a Palestinian, left records of the phenomena he lived through in the Jewish tradition. Kabir (1440–1518), an Indian poet and mystic, taught a syncretic (blended) form of **Islam** and **Hinduism** that was monotheistic. Abu Hamid al-Ghazali (d. 1111) was foremost among the Sufi mystic tradition of Islam. The Buddhist tradition is also rich in accounts of the state of mystic enlightenment. *See also* Buddhism; Judaism; Julian of Norwich.

Further Reading: On Al-Ghazali, see "Abu Hamid al-Ghazali (1058–1111 CE): Munkidh min al-Dalal (*Confessions*, or *Deliverance from Error*)." In *Medieval Sourcebook*, edited by Paul Halsall. See http://www.fordham.edu/halsall/basis/1100ghazali-truth.html; Boehme, Jacob (also Jakob). *The Way to Christ. The Fourth Book (in 3 parts): Of the SuperSensual Life, Of Heaven and Hell, The Way from Darkness to True Illumination, 1622*. See http://www.passtheword.org/DIALOGS-FROM-THE-PAST/waychrst.htm; Fox, George. *An Autobiography*. Edited by Rufus M. Jones. Christian Classics Ethereal Library. See http://www.ccel.org/ccel/fox_g/autobio.i.html?highlight=autobiography,george,fox; Idel, Moshe, and Bernard McGinn, eds. *Mystical Union in Judaism, Christianity, and Islam*. New York: Continuum, 1999; Kabir. *Songs of Kabir*. Translated by Rabindranath Tagore. New York: The Macmillan Company, 1915; Paper, Jordan. *The Mystic Experience: A Descriptive and Comparative Analysis*. Albany: State University of New York Press, 2004; Parrinder, Geoffrey. *Mysticism in the World's Religions*. London, 1976; "The Path of Allah." *Canada & the World Backgrounder* 72, no. 1 (2006); Saint Ignatius Loyola. *The Autobiography of St. Ignatius Loyola, with Related Documents*. Translated by Joseph O'Callaghan. n.p: Peter Smith,

1979; Saint John of the Cross. *Mystical Verse and Prose/Poesías y prosas místicas: A dual language book*. Translated and edited by Stanley Appelbaum. New York: Dover, 2006; Saint Teresa of Avila. *The Life of Saint Teresa of Avila by Herself*. Translated and edited by J. M. Cohen. New York: Penguin, 1957; Schoenberg, Shira. "Isaac ben Solomon Luria (1534–1572)." See http://www.meta-religion.com/World_Religions/Judaism/isaac_ben_solomon_luria.htm.

Nicolás Hernández, Jr.

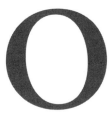

OBSTETRICAL MANUALS. Up until the seventeenth century, men were the primary, if not the only, authors of obstetrical manuals in western Europe. While some manuals were intended for a larger audience, many were specifically addressed to **midwives** who, unlike men, regularly participated in the birthing process. Due to a lack of practical experience, male authors tended to write manuals that were theoretical in nature. Difficult births were rarely discussed in detail, and no allusions to personal experience were ever included. Starting in the fifteenth century, more detailed descriptions of the birthing process began to emerge, and, in 1609, the first manual written by a woman was published. Unlike any of its predecessors, this manual was based on the author's personal experience as a midwife, and offered practical advice within a theoretical framework.

During the fifteenth and sixteenth centuries, few obstetrical manuals existed or were accessible to midwives seeking guidance on the safe delivery of children. Midwives, as well as others who assisted in the "birthing chamber," often relied on works like the classical work *Gynecology*, and the twelfth-century *Trotula*, until access to more modern works became possible.

Gynecology, the first known obstetrical manual, was believed to have been written in the second century by the Greek physician Soranus. Translated into Latin by the fifth century, it served as an authority on **childbirth** and women's health into the sixteenth century. Throughout the manual, Soranus offers detailed descriptions of women's anatomy. Among other topics, he discusses swelling of the uterus, difficult births, **menstruation**, and the removal of a dead fetus from the womb. He also offers guidance on selecting the best midwife and, if necessary, a wet nurse. Soranus embeds much of his advice within a fabric of anatomical and medical detail. He shows his extensive knowledge of women's health, offering advice and directives, but there is little evidence that his understanding is based on hands-on practice, and little information is given about the actual delivery of a child.

By the twelfth century, a second obstetrical manual, the *Trotula*, had begun to circulate in Europe. First thought to have been written by a woman, the book seems to have been written by at least three individuals, most likely men, corresponding to the three treatises of the work: *The Book on the Conditions of Women; Treatments for Women;* and *Women's Cosmetics*. The manual is addressed to midwives and other women. It covers an extremely wide array of topics, including conception, contraception, menstruation, adornments, and the whitening of teeth. As in *Gynecology*, however, a detailed description of the mechanics of giving birth is absent.

The first obstetrical handbook translated into English—its author and title unknown—was published during the fifteenth century. The manuscript, translated from Latin, discusses menstruation, unnatural and natural birth presentations, conception, and general maladies affecting women. Offering more detail about the birthing process than its predecessors, the manual seems to indicate that its author had some experience, secondhand or otherwise, with deliveries. Many herbal remedies are presented to help with women's gynecological problems. The handbook was first thought to be a reproduction of the *Trotula*, but the book contains sections on childbirth, as well as illustrations, which were not found with the *Trotula*'s original Latin text.

Published in 1513, *The Rose Garden for Pregnant Women and Midwives* (*Der Swangern frawen und he bammen roszgarten*) was one of the first obstetrical manuals written in the vernacular (German). At least one other manual, by Michele **Savoranola**, had been published in the vernacular (Italian) prior to that, during the mid-fifteenth century. Dedicated to the pregnant women and midwives of Ferrara, Savonarola's manual was similar to *The Rose Garden for Pregnant Women and Midwives*, but without illustrations.

It is said that the author of *The Rose Garden for Pregnant Women and Midwives*, Eucharius Rosslin, never attended an actual birth in his life. The manual seems to have been largely based on the work of Soranus, including the illustrations, which were primitive compared to other anatomical illustrations of the day. Rosslin's work was translated into Latin in 1532 and into English in 1540. It remained a standard textbook for midwives into the seventeenth century. More modern than its predecessors, it focused exclusively on **pregnancy**, childbirth, and the care of newborns. The book was so popular that it was reprinted fourteen times between 1513 and 1562.

First published in 1609, *Diverse Observations on Sterility, Miscarriages, Fertility, Childbirth, and Illnesses of Women and Newborn Children* (*Observations diverses sur la sterilite perte de fruit feocondite accouchements et Maladies des femmes et enfants nouveaux naiz*) emerged as the first obstetrical manual written by a woman. Its author, Louise Bourgeois, served as midwife to Marie de Medicis, queen of France, from 1601 to 1609. In total, Bourgeois wrote three books, all of which were intended to appeal to a wide audience, including physicians and surgeons as well as midwives. Bourgeois was well versed in medical theory, but had gained her skill as a midwife through an apprenticeship. Her writing stresses the importance of honing skills through experience, but also provides a foundation of knowledge regarding many gynecological conditions, including pregnancy.

Following in the footsteps of Bourgeois, other midwives, such as Justine Siegemund, Catharina Schrader, and Jane Sharp, began publishing their own obstetrical manuals in the seventeenth century. These women, even more so than Bourgeois, based their guidebooks on personal, hands-on experience. Their advice was almost exclusively focused on the actual delivery of a child, and they provided detailed instructions for specialized obstetrical techniques, such as the manual manipulation of a fetus during a difficult birth.

Further Reading: *Medieval Woman's Guide to Health: The First English Gynecological Handbook*. Translated with an introduction by Beryl Rowland. Kent, OH: Kent University Press, 1981; Perkins, Wendy. *Midwifery and Medicine in Early Modern Europe: Louise Bourgeois*. Exeter: University of Exeter Press, 1996; Rosslin, Eucharius. *When Midwifery Became the Male Physician's Province: The Sixteenth Century Handbook "The Rose Garden for Pregnant Women and Midwives."* Translated with an introduction by Wendy Arons. Jefferson, NC: McFarland & Company, Inc., 1994; Schrader, Catharina. "Mother and Child Were Saved." In *The Memoirs (1693–1740) of the Frisian Midwife Catharina Schrader*. Translated and annotated by Hillary Marland.

Amsterdam: Rodopi, 1987; Siegemund, Justine. *The Court Midwife*. Edited and translated by Lynne Tatlock. Chicago: University of Chicago Press, 2005; Soranus. *Gynecology*. Translated with an introduction by Owsei Temkin. Baltimore: Johns Hopkins, 1956; *The Trotula: An English Translation of the Medieval Compendium of Women's Medicine*. Edited and translated by Monica H. Green. Philadelphia: University of Pennsylvania Press, 2002.

Michelle Spinelli

ORAL SEX. In the early modern era, Western religious and political authorities viewed oral sex as one of many forms of unnatural sex and a sin against nature. In their eyes, natural sex was sexual intercourse between a husband and wife who performed the act in the so-called missionary position, with the female on her back and the man on top, facing her. The only legitimate purpose for sex was to beget offspring. Any behaviors that deviated from that ideal were aberrant and unacceptable, though not necessarily criminal. The Church discouraged oral sex and punished it in its own ecclesiastic courts, but we have no way of knowing the true extent of its frequency. In the early modern era, the Christian Church placed oral sex on par with contraception, one of the gravest sexual sins one could commit, and almost as serious as homicide. The sin of oral sex extended not merely to male homosexuals but also to married couples. Oral sex was a sin against nature because it violated the Christian Church's mandate that sex be had exclusively for purposes of procreation. In the early modern era, the Church condemned sex for pleasure even between married couples.

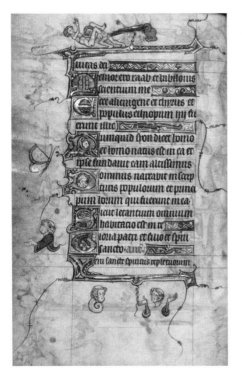

Man performing cunnilingus while a bird pecks at his rear end, from the fourteenth-century *French Book of Hours*. © The Pierpont Morgan Library/Art Resource, NY.

As a criminal act, few Western legal systems of the early modern era conflated oral sex with sodomy. Historically speaking, sex laws were defined in a more precise manner than they are today and legal authorities, to the extent that they would discuss the subject at all, held that sodomy referred exclusively to **anal sex** and to no other act. In canon and civil law, oral sex may be found under the designation *fellation*, from the Latin verb "to suck." It may be further broken down to *fellatio*, meaning "to suck," if performed on a man or *cunnilingus*, which means "vulva-licker," a phrase derived from the Latin *cunnus* meaning "vulva" and *lingere* meaning "to lick," when performed on a female.

In Eastern cultures for the same era there seems to have been a more liberal attitude toward ancillary sexual activities, especially for married couples. In India, the sex manual known as the **Kama Sutra** portrayed oral sex as a kind of love akin to a sexual addiction and attributed it with an eight-step process leading to orgasm. Chinese culture approved of fellatio so long as a man's procreative energies were not lost, and cunnilingus had even greater sanction as the Chinese thought it prepared the female to receive the male while, at the same time, enhancing the couple's sexual spirit. In cases of non-consensual sex, however, including **rape**, homosexual rape, and gang rape, Chinese authorities characterized oral sex as particularly offensive, because when done by force it was intended to humiliate. A sixteenth-century Chinese statute stipulated that anyone found guilty of "pouring foul material into the mouth of another person" would be punished with one hundred blows with a heavy bamboo cane. In Islamic culture, oral-genital sex was permissible between married couples, but only with the female's consent.

Eastern cultures tended to view sex as pleasurable for both males and females as well as procreative. They tended to emphasize the spiritual nature of pleasurable sex for the individuals involved and to value the spiritual union more than the merely biological, which they saw as crass and vulgar. For that reason, attitudes toward oral sex in Eastern cultures in the early modern era tended to be much more relaxed and respectful of the private side of consensual sex. This stood in stark contrast to Western cultures, where Church and state polities arrogated to themselves the right to control the sexual behaviors of those within their realms and determined that the only natural sex was that had for the purpose of begetting children. *See also* Christianity; Homosexuality; Islam; Marriage.

Further Reading: Bullough, Vern L. *Sexual Variance in Society and History*. New York: John Wiley & Sons, 1976; Sommer, Matthew H. "The Penetrated Male in Late Imperial China: Judicial Constructions and Social Stigma." *Modern China* 23, no. 2 (April 1997): 140–80; Tannahill, Reay. *Sex in History*. Revised and updated ed. New York: Scarborough Books, 1992.

Mary Block

ORPHANS. *See* Foundlings and Orphans

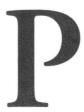

PEDERASTY. The term "pederasty" indicates the erotic and emotional bond between an adult male and a boy between the ages of twelve and eighteen. Pederastic relationships were temporary unions, bound to end by the time the younger partner entered adulthood. The age asymmetry between the two partners structured the relationship according to differentiated sexual roles, where the older was to take the active role, whilst the younger had the passive one. These distinct roles depended on specific cultural attitudes concerning male honor and virility. Adult males retained the pride of their own masculinity by refusing to be penetrated, while the boy, thought to be still lingering in a phase of sexual androgyny, could accept the passive role without compromising his future entrance into manhood.

It is often argued that pederasty was the prevalent mode of same-sex contact in early modern Europe, particularly in countries of the Mediterranean basin such as Italy and Spain. But, accounts of pederasty are not limited to southern Europe and the Maghreb in North **Africa**. Historical evidence indicates that it was extensively practiced also in England, France, the **Middle East**, Japan, and China.

Studies on boy-man love in the early modern period generally rely on fragmentary sources, such as short treatises, journals, and epigrams. Famous examples are *L'Alcibiade fanciullo a scuola*, an apology for pederasty that came out of seventeenth-century Florence, and *Shier Lou*, a short story that was written in sixteenth-century China. In times of harsh repression, judicial records from Inquisition offices provide significant insights into the specific dynamics through which pederasty was practiced and regulated.

In Florence between 1432 and 1542, special Inquisition offices and tribunals were created for the repression of sodomy and pederasty. Judicial records of the notorious Office of the Night reveal the distinctive features of boy-man love in Florence during these years, and provide the most extensive documentation on pederasty in the whole early modern period. Trial reports, registers, and confessions show, for instance, that adults who were sodomized by their younger partners were often ridiculed and punished with harsher sentences. Such judicial accounts generally provide detailed information about the sexual practices and roles performed by the boy and the adult during intercourse, but generally fail to give us insights concerning the emotional significance of many of these relationships for the subjects involved.

L'Alcibiade fanciullo a scuola, written by the Venetian priest Antonio Rocco, shows that in the seventeenth century there is a shift from the ancient pederastic ethos according to which the younger partner was not supposed to enjoy any sexual gratification during intercourse, a right that was generally retained by the older man. By the seventeenth century, ideas of erotic pleasure in pederastic unions seem to have changed markedly. Literary accounts that emphasize the duty of the older partner to gratify his younger companion are frequent and particularly rich with details about the best way for achieving mutual pleasure. *See also* Adultery; Anal Sex; Homosexuality.

Further Reading: Rooke, Michael. *Forbidden Friendships: Homosexuality and Male Culture in Renaissance Florence*. Oxford: Oxford University Press, 1996; Murray, Stephen O. *Homosexualities*. London: University of Chicago Press, 2000.

Sergio Rigoletto

PENITENTIAL PRACTICES. Catholic penitential practices, and especially the sacrament of penance or confession, were ubiquitous fixtures in the lives of Christians both in early modern Europe and in missionary territories opened up by European expansion overseas. Unlike in Central and Southern America, however, missionaries in East Asia did not operate within a framework of colonial dominance, but rather tried to accommodate local cultures and sociopolitical systems. In the early modern Chinese Christian communities, as was the case in Japan, awareness of sin and rituals to eliminate or control sins constituted one of the core religious offerings of **Christianity**. Missionaries built upon conceptions of sinfulness and confession that had already existed for centuries in **Daoism** and **Buddhism**, but they also introduced practices, such as auricular confession, which were new and controversial in the East Asian context.

Missionaries to China usually brought with them at least a treatise of casuistry or a confessional *summa*, and one of their first duties was to administer sacramental confession, memorizing confessional dialogues in Chinese even before they had reached sufficient fluency. Baptism was the initial ritual of "general confession" and absolution for catechumens. Early Jesuit *doctrinae* in Chinese dating from the late sixteenth and early seventeenth centuries described baptism as a way to cancel sins, keep at bay evil demons and ascend to paradise after death, as opposed to a scenario for the unbaptized dominated by Satan and leading to damnation in hell. Adult converts also placed great emphasis on baptism as a way to wash away past sins, rather than merely seeing it as a liminal ritual to join the Christian community, a fact reflected in written protestations of faith read on the day of baptism, acknowledging one's sins.

Chinese Christians were initiated to the sacrament of penance only gradually, as missionaries did not admit neophytes to confession and communion in the period immediately following baptism, fearing a possible relapse. Moreover, instruction up to the 1620s, especially in rural contexts and among commoners, was quickly accomplished during brief rural missions, and done orally or through very simple catechisms. Thus, sacramental confession remained a rare ritual, mainly performed annually, and depending on the presence of the few priests available.

Lay leaders imparted preliminary education on the sacrament mainly through texts cheaply and easily produced in the Chinese tradition of xylograph **printing**. Chinese-language texts on confession fell within four main categories, addressing both Christian and non-Christian publics: simple catechetical texts on confession for the vast majority of Christians; more sophisticated texts for Christian literati; apologetic texts in defense of the sacrament for non-Christians; and rare ritual manuals for Chinese priests. The exhaustive *Dizui zhenggui* (*Correct Rules to Wash away Sins*, 1627) and a more popular abridged version of it, both by the Italian Jesuit Giulio Aleni (1582–1649), are the foundational texts on sacramental penance in the China mission. These texts were inspired by contemporary Italian printed confessionals for penitents (such as *De* *sacramento poenitentiae* by Luca Pinelli S.J., 1613), which were no longer simple lists of sins in the late medieval tradition, but rather explanatory and devotional texts on the sacrament for lay readers. In their most simplified form, these texts became an outline of the penitential steps written in vernacular Chinese onto one single sheet of paper. These flyers were ideal for easy distribution by catechists preparing the local community for the visit of a confessor. They retained the essential elements of the penitential practice, and their simple language, often literally copied from Aleni's texts, was suited to a rural audience.

Catholic penitential rituals presented unique problems in the Chinese context. In Daoism and especially Buddhism, confession of sins was a public event, done by monks in front of their monastic communities, and did not entail close contact between priest and penitent as seen in the Catholic tradition. Even the so-called "ledgers of merit and demerit," texts popular among Confucian literati in the sixteenth and seventeenth centuries, and including what could be loosely called "examinations of conscience," never amounted to more than personal moral accounting. Overcoming shame, and revealing one's inner life to a foreigner, often considered a "barbarian" by society at large, presented formidable challenges in China. In particular, sins relating to one's sexual life (including **masturbation, homosexuality, adultery**, forbidden sexual practices, and **abortion**) were considered taboo topics in China, and questions found in confessional manuals must have sounded shocking to Chinese converts. The secrecy surrounding the rite was another problem. Chinese government officials, always suspicious of secret societies and heterodox religious groups, saw it as an indication of possible political subversion, a fact only worsened by the foreign connection of the missionaries. Given the strict segregation of sexes in late imperial China, moreover, the confession of women remained one of the most controversial aspects of Christian penitential rituals. Missionaries had therefore to exert particular caution while confessing female penitents, allowing an elder or a male member of the family to monitor the ritual from a distance. Buddhist monks were targeted in Chinese novels and plays as lecherous predators of female devotees visiting temples, or of innocent young nuns. Foreign missionaries were often seen as similarly preying upon their flocks. Especially during the period of prohibition of Christianity by imperial orders (1724–1844), cases of clerical solicitation for sexual favors during confession are indeed recorded in ecclesiastical archives. These cases show a breakdown in clergy discipline, and can be partly imputed to the conditions of clandestine proximity of the priests within the living quarters of their flocks during the period of anti-Christian campaigns. They also show, however, that unmarried rural women, sometimes vowed to religious celibacy for life, might have used their religious position within local Christian communities to create for themselves a social space outside the strictures of married life, including irregular relationships with foreign and Chinese priests. Confession represented a moment of rare intimacy, both spiritual and physical, that momentarily isolated priests and penitents from the dominant conventions of Chinese society, although it never substantially challenged the existing social hierarchy. Maybe for that reason, it was both accepted and coveted by Chinese Christians, and loathed by the Chinese government and the anti-Christian elites.

Further Reading: Delumeau, Jean. *L'aveu et le pardon: Les difficultés de la confession, XIII–XVIII siècle*. Paris: Fayard, 1990; Haliczer, Stephen. *Sexuality in the Confessional: A Sacrament Profaned*. Oxford: Oxford University Press, 1996; Standaert, Nicolas, and Ad Dudink, eds. *Forgive Us Our Sins: Confession in Late Ming and Early Qing China*. Sankt Augustin and Nettetal: Institut Monumenta Serica—Steyler Verlag, 2006; Waltner, Ann. "Demerits and Deadly Sins. Jesuit

Moral Tracts in Late Ming China." In *Implicit Understanding: Observing, Reporting, and Reflecting on the Encounters between Europeans and Other Peoples in the Early Modern Era*, edited by Stuart Schwartz, 422–48. Cambridge: Cambridge University Press, 1994; Wu, Pei-yi. "Self-Examination and Confession of Sins in Traditional China." *Harvard Journal of Asiatic Studies* 39, no. 1 (1979): 5–38.

Eugenio Menegon

THE PERFUMED GARDEN FOR THE SOUL'S DELECTATION (al-Nafzawi, Fifteenth Century). Written in the beginning of the fifteenth century by the North African Shaykh al-Imam Abu Abd-Allah al-Nafzawi, who was from the town of Nafzawa near Tunis, *The Perfumed Garden for the Soul's Delectation* is a titillating example of Arabic erotic literature.

The book is divided into twenty-one chapters, the last being the same approximate length as the first twenty combined. Topics covered include the traits of desirable men and women; factors that are and are not favorable to sexual intercourse; a list of names for both the male and female sexual organs; advice on bringing great pleasure to coition; a description of and treatment for the uterus of sterile women; causes and cures for **impotence**; prescriptions for increasing penis size; remedies for foul-smelling armpits and vaginas; signs of **pregnancy;** and indicators that may be used to determine the sex of an unborn child. The book presents in great detail the most lascivious and obscene material, describing erections, coitus, orgasms, sex positions, sexual movement, and sex acts, including kissing, hugging, licking, sucking, and sipping the mouth, cheeks, breast, neck, lips, waist, belly, navel, buttocks, thighs, penis, and vagina. Love, lust, lubricity, and libidinousness take center stage.

Explaining the origin of the book, the author relates that he had composed a shorter work, *The World's Illumination in the Secrets of Coition*, which came to the attention of the *wazir* (personal assistant) of Abd al-Aziz, master and ruler of Tunis. The *wazir* requested that al-Nafzawi expand the work to include additional material on a number of subjects such as cures and remedies, copulation, and pregnancy. Calling upon God's help, al-Nafzawi set out to write the book, to which he gave two different titles: *The Perfumed Garden for the Soul's Delectation*, and *The World's Illumination in the Knowledge of the Art of Copulation*.

Many of the stories contained within *The Perfumed Garden* exhibit typical traits of Arabic literature, which favors the implausible over the practical, the magical over the real, and the power of the imagination over the observable natural world. The book includes poetry, prose, rhymed prose, short stories, and a section on the interpretation of dreams. The book is a valuable resource for students of anthropology, ethnology, and linguistics, and provides insight into the customs, character, and lives of North African Arabs from the early 1400s. It is not known if the author, who was learned in medicine, pharmaceutics, law, literature, Arabic poetry, and the Koran, wrote any other books. The frequent mention of and praise for Allah as well as the author's call for God's assistance indicate that al-Nafzawi was a religious Muslim.

The Perfumed Garden for the Soul's Delectation, which begins with the author praising God for centering men and women's greatest pleasure and joy in each other's sexual organs, is a panegyric to sex and sexuality, passionate lasciviousness, and unbridled intercourse. The voluptuous delights of the flesh are enumerated, explored, appreciated and praised in *The Perfumed Garden*. Sir Richard Francis Burton, the Victorian explorer and Orientalist, translated *The Perfumed Garden* into English in the nineteenth century. *See also* Islam; *Kama Sutra*; Middle East.

Further Reading: al-Nafzawi Shaykh al-Imam Abu Abd-Allah. *The Illustrated Perfumed Garden: A Sensuous Paradise Where Erotic Love Grows and Blooms*. Edited by Jan Hutchinson et al. Translated by Sir Richard Burton. New York: HarperCollins, 1996; Dunn, Philip, ed. *The Performed Garden: Based on the Original Translation by Sir Richard Burton*. London: Hamlyn, 2004.

Ronna S. Feit

PLATONIC LOVE. Platonic love derives its name from its first and most famous proponent, the classical Greek philosopher Plato (428–348 BCE). The chronicler of the life and times of his teacher Socrates, Plato recorded thematic dialogues among Socrates and his disciples, including covering **love** and friendship. Plato distinguished sexual love, or **eros,** from higher more refined and spiritual forms of love that are best expressed in the love of men for virtues, for beauty, and for the practice of good government. For the most part, Plato and his followers, the Platonists and Neo-Platonists, valued this higher, more spiritual love over erotic, more physical love.

Although many of Plato's ideas influenced medieval thought in western Europe through the writings of St. Augustine, Plato's own writings were not translated into Latin from Greek until 1482. This translation, the work of Marsilio Ficino, was sponsored by Cosimo de' Medici. Both the translations and Ficino's own writings advocating Platonic philosophy as compatible with **Christianity** led to a revival of interest in Plato during the Renaissance, especially among humanists. Giovanni Pico della Mirandola (1463–1494), in particular, promoted Plato's philosophy in writings that circulated widely in Europe. As a result of the intellectual revival of his ideas, the Greek philosopher's notions of ideal love found their way into the art and literature of the Renaissance.

It was specifically Ficino, however, who formulated the beginnings of a modern notion of Platonic love based on Plato's works. For Ficino, the ideal loving relationship or friendship between humans should parallel the relationship between a person and God. As a Christian mystic within Ficino's Platonic system cultivates and is transformed by a relationship with God as the ultimate ideal, so could people also approach higher virtues by love and friendship. Ficino's idea of Platonic love was broader than the modern definition in that he did not reject sexual relationships as means for cultivating high ideals.

Ficino's notion of Platonic love influenced literature, philosophy, art, and behavior in Renaissance Italy. The idea that both romantic and friendly relationships between people could parallel the soul's aspirations toward God spread widely, especially in literate courtly circles. It also had an effect on the perception and definition of homosexual relationships between men. Whereas medieval philosophy stigmatized homosexual behavior simply as sinful acts, the notion of Platonic friendships between males provided a new and more positive vocabulary for framing homoerotic interactions.

Pietro Bembo (1470–1547) a Catholic cardinal and poet, stressed the need for humanity to cultivate a higher and more beneficial love than the sexual variety through the pursuit of learning and creative activities. He advocated the value of love for reading, writing, and gardening. He also stressed love as expressed in the virtuous conduct of government. This theme of ideal relationships as embodied in good government is common in art and literature of the period, including in the *Allegory of Good and Bad Government* by the Lorenzetti brothers. *See also* Art, European; Homoeroticism; Homosexuality.

Further Reading: Allen, Michael J. B. *Synoptic Art: Marsilio Ficino on the History of Platonic Interpretation*. Florence: Olschki, 1998; Allen, Michael J. B., and Valery Rees, eds. *Marsilio Ficino: His Theology, His Philosophy and His Legacy*. New York: E.J. Brill, 2002; Hankins, James. *Plato in the Italian Renaissance*. Columbia Studies in the Classic Tradition, Vol. 17. 2 vols. New York: E.J. Brill, 1994.

Rachel Goldman

POLYGAMY/POLYANDRY. Polygamy signifies simultaneous **marriage** to more than one spouse. There are two variations of polygamy: polygyny (several concurrent wives) and polyandry (several concurrent husbands). Polygyny involved contracting formal matrimony with the wives, while institutionalized polycoity permitted men to have **concubines** or **mistresses** as supplementary sexual partners. Most early modern cultures were sexually asymmetrical, polygyny and polycoity being male prerogatives.

While polygyny can be found in innumerable cultures in the early modern world, polyandry occurred in some societies in Polynesia, India, **Africa**, and Tibet, and perhaps also occasionally in Japan. Polyandrous relationships could involve a woman having several brothers or kinsmen as husbands. Not all polyandrous husbands were co-resident with the wife (e.g., a visiting-husband arrangement instead). Moreover, Orthodox Christians equated serial monogamy with simultaneous polygamy, calling both by the same word (*mnogoženstvo*). In Judaism, and in other societies, levirate, or obligatory marriage to one's brother's widow, accounts for some cases of polygyny.

The major advantage of polygyny was reproductive, enabling a man to have a potentially larger number of heirs. Economic factors could be important as multiple wives contributed their dowries and labor to the household. Polygamy was also a potent status symbol; people permitting polygamy were largely monogamous in practice, but rulers and the well-off showed their status and wealth by harems of wives and/or concubines (resource polygamy). This is as true of many early modern African tribes as of various Asian and American nations. Kings also used polygamy to cement political alliances and treaties. Male sexual gratification was another function.

Polygamous households could be riddled with rivalry and jealousy between wives and their offspring. Some societies reduced the risk of domestic factions by providing a separate house(hold) for each wife or by marrying kinswomen or sisters of the first wife (limited polygyny, cf. general polygyny with unrestricted male choice). The **harem** of the Ottoman sultans is the ultimate example of scheming and intrigue, partly because while sultans could have dozens of sons, their successors customarily dispatched their rivals through fratricide. Both the Ottoman one-son-per-mother policy and preference for slave concubines were adopted to minimize the claims of maternal lineages and loss of dynastic power and property. The Islamic Moghul rulers of India also practiced both polygamy—some scholars even suppose that they surpassed the number of co-wives permitted by Islamic law—and concubinage, but their wives were more frequently freeborn, and even occasionally widows. Marriages were political alliances, Rajput princesses, Persian families, and Pathan clans being amongst those favored. Among Hindus, rulers and the highest Brahmin caste were polygamous in the main.

The Islamic world from Africa to Indonesia observed the Koranic norm permitting men four legal wives in addition to concubines, provided he treated them equally. A fifth or consequent parallel marriage was, however, considered null and void (*batil*). All wives were entitled to dwellings separate from their co-wives, following Muhammed's example. Jews living in medieval Europe tended toward monogamy, resulting in an express ban on polygamy in many early modern Jewish communities. Jewish law could not annul polygamous marriages, however, and some rabbis allowed polygamy or concubinage in special circumstances. Polygamy was more frequent among Jews living under Muslim rule.

In Polynesia, polygyny was permitted everywhere, but resource polygamy was the trend. Rulers of various southern and southeastern Asian kingdoms, whether Hindu, Buddhist, or Muslim, practiced both polygamy and concubinage. The elite, emulating their monarchs, also took several wives. In China, polygamy was illegal—the emperor excepted—but concubines were commonplace among the upper classes. The harems of both Chinese emperors and Ottoman sultans were hierarchically arranged, the consorts and concubines being classified depending on the ruler's favor, the status of the union (concubinage/matrimony) and giving birth to children, especially sons.

In the **Americas**, the Aztec and Inca elites had both practiced polygamy and concubinage. The advent of **Christianity** ended polygamy, although the practice lingered in more remote regions of Latin America. Many North American native tribes accepted polygyny, more commonly among wealthy and prestigious seniors. Among some peoples, men married several sisters (sororal polygyny). *See also* Asia; Buddhism; Hinduism; Islam; Judaism; Middle East.

Further Reading: Ebrey, Patricia Buckley. *Women and the Family in Chinese History.* London: Routledge, 2003; Pierce, Leslie P. *The Imperial Harem: Women and Sovereignty in the Ottoman Empire.* Oxford: Oxford University Press, 1993; Quale, G. Robina. *A History of Marriage Systems.* Westport, CT: Greenwood Press, 1988; Tucker, Judith E. *In the House of the Law: Gender and Islamic Law in Ottoman Syria and Palestine.* Berkeley and Los Angeles: University of California Press, 1998.

Mia Korpiola

PORNOGRAPHY. The term "pornography," meaning literally writing about or by prostitutes, only dates from the nineteenth century. "Pornography" is a controversial, fighting word, often suggesting a debased, limited kind of writing, photography, or film intended merely to arouse the male masturbator. Some of this debate is relevant to the early modern period, but not all. Sexually explicit literature and art served many goals, and its motives were always mixed with satire, comedy, libertine philosophy, the carnivalesque inversion of norms, and the imitation of ancient Greek and Roman culture.

Salty references to the sexual organs and to the various positions and practices (notably oral and **anal sex**) were common in the Roman epigrams of Catullus and Martial, and therefore highly prized by Renaissance humanists (in private if not in public). Antonio Beccadelli of Palermo, for example, imagined his book of Latin poems *Hermaphroditus* (c. 1425) as a mischievous creature sporting the genital organs of both sexes. Although he addressed leading figures of the early Renaissance, his depiction of sex is low and grotesque. Many other poets tried this combination of sexual description and insult, first in elegant Latin, then in the various vernaculars. In English, John Donne, Thomas Nashe, and Thomas Carew wrote episodes that celebrated the sexual encounter directly, but placed it in a repulsive or punitive frame. In Donne's "To His Mistress Going to Bed," the white sheet suggests penitence as well as intimacy, and in Carew's "A Rapture," the vision of sexual Elysium dissolves when the poet calls his lover "Whore" in the final line—reducing her literally to porno-graphy. Nashe put some enthusiasm into his description of copulating with a favorite London **courtesan**, but the point turned out to be not fulfillment, but **impotence**; his alternative title, *Nashe's Dildo*, referred to the means she used to satisfy herself and to the poem itself as a kind of tool or supplement.

The most important sixteenth-century "porno-grapher" was Pietro **Aretino** (1492–1556), who declared in a famous letter that no taboo should attach to sex—the hands and mouth do shameful things, but the penis and vagina are natural and honorable, and should be displayed in public (as they were in ancient times). This was to justify the sonnets he had written to accompany a notorious set of prints showing sexual positions entitled *I Modi* [*The Ways*], which was designed by Giulio Romano and engraved by Marcantonio Raimondi in or about 1525. These images and their poems survive only in corrupt copies, but we can reconstruct enough to see that they involved heterosexual couples in positions that ran from the simple side-by-side to acrobatic balancing acts; the sonnets, however, often bring out the violent or absurd side of sex as much as the excitement. Other engravers soon produced their own erotic series, some crude but some highly sophisticated. In time all such prints became known as "Aretino's Figures" or "Postures," since he was believed to be the inventor of the positions, the images, and the verbal description. Meanwhile, other Renaissance artists, including Francesco Salviati, invented fantastic scenes in which enormous, detached genital organs took on a life of their own.

The real Aretino went on to write the *Ragionamenti* (1534–1536), which was soon translated as *Pornodidascalus*. In these vivid, foul-mouthed dialogues, a Roman prostitute shares her life experience. As in the contemporary tales of Rabelais, some episodes are highly sexual but others are satirical, and still others seem written for the sheer fun of linguistic experiment. The "purely" pornographic elements include spectacular numbers in which monks, nuns, and priests all copulate together using every available orifice, or passages in which an older woman instructs her daughter in bedroom techniques. These were soon codified (and plagiarized) in a little prose "Dialogue of Giulia and Madalena," which was falsely ascribed to Aretino and later called *La puttana errante* (*The Wandering Whore*). It was the first and most influential book to focus narrowly on the sex act in all its permutations. But in most of Aretino's work, and in the obscene poems written by his protegé Lorenzo Venier, violence and trickery prevail over pleasure, and current events intrude into pornotopia, including ugly scenes of gang-**rape**, and mock-heroic accounts of the "Whore-Errant" entering Rome, both of which evoke the atrocities visited on that city during the sack of 1527.

Alongside these openly prostitute-themed works, the private academies of Italy developed other discourses of sexuality intended for restricted, often homoerotic circulation. Antonio Vignali (1501–1559), founder of the Sienese Accademia degli Intronati (Academy of the Thunderstruck), wrote his dialogue *La Cazzaria* (*The Prickery*) in or about 1525. Here the speakers are not common whores but aristocratic young men, who explore a series of outrageous questions about sex, sometimes as an allegory of local politics, sometimes as an end in itself; "the excessively great pleasure of finding all the reasons and circumstances of fucking" turns out to be more compelling than real-life sex, and elite **homosexuality** more appealing than the hetero- version, even when lovers "find out the modes and secret ways." The sodomitic tradition continued in works that cash in on Vignali's own, such as the verse *Cazzaria del C. M.*, which celebrates "the trophies of prick in arse," and a prose continuation (in a Vatican manuscript) where the younger man, Sodo, recounts his life as a boy whore. (His clients include nineteen monks and a sacristan who invites him up to see "a most beautiful Book of little figures engraved in copper, which I know you would enjoy.") The most refined, and most explicit, homosexual narrative is Antonio Rocco's *L'Alcibiade fanciullo a scola* (*Alcibiades the Schoolboy*), which was written about 1625 as a "little carnival book" for another free-thinking Venetian academy, the Incogniti or Unrecognized.

The same academy produced the last and most sophisticated "whore" text, *La retorica delle puttane* (*The Whores' Rhetoric*) by Ferrante Pallavicino (born 1615 and executed by the papal authorities in 1644). In this work, sex is completely transformed into "art," as the high-class courtesan learns to hide all her mercenary desires behind a genteel facade (literally and metaphorically). Using the analogy of rhetoric, the older woman teaches both high-cultural accomplishments and refined sexual techniques (mostly anal) that appeal to men who really prefer boys. Her erotic art collection serves as a model for her simulated desire; ironically, the man believes he is truly, passionately loved while the woman remains unmoved and detached, enjoying her own "genius" as the author of this fiction.

By the mid-seventeenth century, the impetus to create sexual narrative had moved from Italy to France, and left behind the "porno-graphic" model entirely; the dialogue form continued, but now the older woman initiated the younger into pleasure for its own sake, inside and outside **marriage**. In England, in contrast, whore-themed political satire flourished in titles such as *Newes from the New Exchange, or the Commonwealth of Ladies* (London, 1650). Two texts in particular came to dominate the field for the next 150 years: the anonymous *L'Escole des filles, ou la Philosophie des dames* (*The Girls' School, or the Ladies' Philosophy*, burned by the public hangman in 1655)—in which Susanne instructs her little cousin in the facts of life and then trains her in the philosophy of pleasure once she has started an affair—and the vastly more sophisticated neo-Latin *Satyra Sotadica de Arcanis Amoris et Veneris* (*Sotadic Satire about the Secrets of Love and Venus*), composed by Nicolas Chorier between 1630 and 1665, and passed off as a work by the real-life Renaissance humanist Luisa Sigea.

In ancient Greece, the *porne*, a common prostitute, was counter-distinguished from the *hetairai*, who formed an educated and relatively liberated class: an exception to the general Greek contempt for women. The protagonists of explicitly sexual discourse evolved, during the early modern period, from the raunchy *puttane* of Aretino and *The Wandering Whore* to the aristocratic married women of Chorier's *Satyra Sotadica*. Chorier's "erudite" and self-determining female libertines (as they become after their long, drawn out wedding nights) could be called *hetairai* but not *pornai*, and when a young acolyte calls the private villas of their orgies "honorable brothels" (*honestae lupanares*) she is haughtily rebuked. So, the least "porno-graphic" text in the literal sense is the most pornographic according to the modern use of the term, since it moves systematically through all the perversions from the simplest to the most complicated, with the participants articulating their pleasure at each step. *See also* Masturbation; Prostitution.

Further Reading: Cossart, Michael de, trans. *Antonio Beccadelli and the Hermaphrodite.* Liverpool: Janus Press, 1984; Findlen, Paula. "Humanism, Politics and Pornography in Renaissance Italy." In *The Invention of Pornography: Obscenity and the Origins of Modernity, 1500–1800*, edited by Lynn Hunt. New York: Zone Books, 1993; Galderisi, Claudio, ed. *Il Piacevol Ragionamento de l'Aretino. Dialogo di Giulia e di Madalena.* Rome: Salerno, 1987; Pallavicino, Ferrante. *La Retorica delle puttane, composta conforme li precetti di Cipriano, dedicata alla Università delle Cortigiane più Celebri* (*The Whores' Rhetoric, Composed According to the Precepts of Cypriano [Soarez], Dedicated to the University of the Most Famous Courtesans*) (1642). Edited by Laura Coci. Parma: Ugo Guanda, 1992; Rosenthal, Raymond, trans. *Aretino's Dialogues.* Reissued with an Epilogue by Margaret Rosenthal. New York: Marsilio, [1971] 1994; Talvacchia, Bette. *Taking Positions: On the Erotic in Renaissance Culture.* Princeton, NJ: Princeton University Press, 1999; Turner, James Grantham. *Libertines and Radicals in Early Modern London: Sexuality, Politics and Literary Culture, 1630–1685.* Cambridge: Cambridge University Press, 2001, 2005; Turner, James Grantham. *Schooling Sex: Libertine Literature and Erotic Education in Italy, France, and England, 1534–1685.* Oxford: Oxford University Press, 2003; Turner, James Grantham. "Salviati's Phallic Triumph."

Print Quarterly 24 (2007); Venier, Lorenzo. *La Puttana errante . . . Littéralement traduit, text italien en regard.* Paris: Isidore Liseux, 1883; Vignali, Antonio. *La Cazzaria del Arsiccio Intronato (The Prickery, by "Burnt Thunderstruck").* Edited by Pasquale Stoppelli. Rome: L'Elefante, 1984.

James Grantham Turner

POZZO, MODESTA. *See* Fonte, Moderata

PREGNANCY. Women during the fifteenth and sixteenth centuries both feared and celebrated pregnancy. In this period, **childbirth** caused the death of many women and newborns, and, at the same time, offered hope for growing a population that had dwindled considerably due to disease and plague.

Pregnancy was inextricably tied to lineage, something paramount in European society. Only male heirs could carry on the family name. For this reason, boys were much preferred over girls. Affluent families wanted as many children as possible, especially boys, yet girls brought with them special needs, such as a **dowry**. In addition, families needed to ensure a daughter's **chastity** if she was to marry well.

Women of the higher social classes generally had more children than the poor because they had the means to hire wet nurses for feeding. This practice limited their own lactation and allowed them to conceive more quickly. Women who worked as wet nurses usually had lost their own babies or were not feeding their own babies. Breast feeding two infants from different families was forbidden. Intercourse during lactation was also strongly discouraged.

For couples who wanted to limit the size of their family, or for people who had relations outside of **marriage**, the main form of contraception was *coitus interruptus*. Sheaths of goatskin and other such material were sometimes used as condoms. These forms of contraception, aside from lactation, depended on the man's cooperation.

Conception usually occurred after or shortly before marriage. It was common for women to marry and start bearing children in their twenties. Women confirmed pregnancy only after they felt a baby kick, something referred to as "quickening." This usually occurred during the fifth month of pregnancy, and it was thought that quickening meant that God had imbued a fetus with a soul. **Abortion** past this point was not accepted. If a couple was not able to conceive a child, the causes for infertility were universally blamed on the woman.

To get pregnant, it was thought that both partners had to climax. Women were thought to have their own "seeds," and it was believed that both partners' seeds needed to be expelled at the same time for conception to occur. To facilitate conception, women sometimes used herbal potions.

Folklore and superstition surrounded pregnancy. For example, it was believed that wearing marten fur would facilitate an easy delivery. In addition, it was thought that women should not look at frightening or strange things during pregnancy and childbirth because it might result in the delivery of a monstrous child.

The prevalence of iconography around pregnancy and childbirth seems to indicate the cultural importance placed on bearing children in Renaissance society. Devotional scenes of a postpartum mother receiving guests or resting peacefully in her bed reassured women of the religious significance of motherhood. Poppy seeds and images of naked young boys symbolized fertility, and cheerful images of a birthing chamber were meant to soothe women's anxieties about childbirth. Symbolic scenes relating to childbirth could be found on wooden birth trays designed for carrying gifts to a new mother, as well as on ceramic wares, altarpieces, and marriage chests. Psychologically, pregnancy was hard on women because of its association with death, economy, and lineage. The writer Margery Kempe admitted to severe depression during and after childbirth.

During pregnancy, women of the upper classes generally dressed in fashionable, loose-fitting cloaks. Fur was often worn because it was thought to keep vermin away. Generally, pregnant women of means wore ornamented nightshirts. Fabric was colorful and fine, and many garments were lined with silk. Vests of wool became fashionable toward the late fifteenth century.

Obstetrical manuals, mostly written by men, instructed women and **midwives** on how to handle natural and unnatural birth presentations. More so, however, they served as general resources for issues concerning fertility, regular and irregular menstrual cycles, and a wide variety of female maladies. Pregnant women were specifically advised in manuals not to exert themselves. Light and easily digestible meals were recommended, including moderate amounts of wine and fish. Poultry, in particular, was prescribed for pregnant women, as well as for new mothers.

Childbirth itself took place in what was called a birthing chamber, an all-female space that was typically presided over by a midwife. During labor, a midwife would also administer herbal potions to try to alleviate labor pains. A male physician would be admitted only during a difficult birth, and even this was rare. The women in the birthing chamber were usually friends or family of the expectant mother. Attendants would typically be in the room as well.

The birthing process presented danger for both mother and child. A woman's body was especially taxed if she was older or had given birth many times before. Often, when a labor went on for too long or a more immediately critical emergency arose, a choice would have to be made between saving the mother or the child. Stillbirths were common. Many of the infants who died during childbirth were premature, especially in cases of twins, and the infant mortality rate was high in general. The days following delivery were dangerous for mother and child as well, as either could succumb to infection or other complications.

After a successful birth, wealthy women typically had a stream of female friends and family members visit them while they were in "confinement" at home. A woman of any means could be confined for religious or health reasons, such as **churching** or an illness. In elite homes, the confinement room, which had a bed in it for the new mother, was often elaborately decorated with colorful, fine linens, and it may or may not have been the room in which the woman gave birth. Visitors brought gifts of sweetmeats, silver spoons, goblets, and wine. Newborns were shown off in specially made clothing and cribs were often lined with taffeta and silk.

Infanticide, which was a sin as well as a crime, was used to hide illegitimate births, to economize in poor families, and to allow poor lactating women to serve as wet nurses for the elite. Often, the income from nursing prevented poor families from starving. *See also* Bastardy; Motherhood.

Further Reading: King, Margaret L. *Women of the Renaissance*. Chicago: University of Chicago Press, 1991; Klapisch-Zuber, Christiane. *Women, Family, and Ritual in Renaissance Italy*. Translated by Lydia G. Cochrane. Chicago: University of Chicago Press, 1985; Musacchio, Jacqueline Marie. *The Art and Ritual of Childbirth in Renaissance Italy*. New Haven, CT: Yale University Press, 1999; Ward, Jennifer. *Women in Medieval Europe, 1200–1500*. New York: Longman, 2002; Wiesner, Merry E. *Women and Gender in Early Modern Europe*. Cambridge: Cambridge University Press, 2000.

Michelle Spinelli

PREMARITAL SEX. In late medieval and early modern Europe, "premarital sex," or sex before or outside of **marriage**, was not easily defined in law and was even less clear in judicial practice. Compared with modern Western societies, conjugal unions in the early modern period was regulated by other rituals and frameworks, and justice was based on local custom and rules that held sway before the emergence of a centralized state. The way sex outside marriage was handled varied from time to time, country to country, and province to province. Although many differences emerged between Catholic and Protestant Europe in the seventeenth century, the treatment of premarital sex in northern, Protestant Europe in the sixteenth century was not completely dissimilar from what prevailed in Catholic countries.

In fifteenth and sixteenth-century Sweden, for instance, being husband and wife was defined by traditional agreements, rituals, and regulations that were confirmed by a *trolovning* (i.e., a betrothal). This practice included vows, the exchange of gifts, and, immediately or somewhat later, cohabitation. Premarital conceptions were usually accepted as long as the couple legitimized their relationship before the child was born. The Church insisted on a Christian wedding ceremony, but that was neither legally necessary nor a general practice. As late as the end of the sixteenth century, a Swedish archbishop traveled around the country using threats of corporal punishment and eternal condemnation to make couples marry within the Church.

Most archival references to premarital sex from early modern Sweden are related to the birth of an illegitimate child. Such a child had no rights to inherit from the father unless the parents were later betrothed to each other. A man who refused to live together with his child's mother diminished her chances for a later partnership. He had therefore committed *mökränkning* ("damage to a maid"). If he was convicted, part of the fine went to the maid's family as compensation for her damage and for the upbringing of the child. Single mothers were also socially stigmatized in several ways. After several relapses, a woman would be sentenced for committing *lönskaläge* ("sleeping together in secret"). This stigma seldom befell male fornicators.

The law was, on the other hand, very severe if one or both of the fornicating partners were already betrothed or married to someone else. Such deviances eroded the family as the primary social cornerstone and resulted in heavy fines or, occasionally, even death sentences for both offenders. Yet, men with enough social and economic capital could always find ways to entertain concubines and break sexual norms without serious consequences.

Generally, pragmatism, not moral considerations, was the guiding principle of most affairs in local courts until the beginning of the seventeenth century. The evolving Protestant **Reformation** did, however, lead to closer unions and mutual understanding between states and churches. The priests saw extramarital sex as a grave sin that must be prevented. As a concession to the Church, the Swedish state, by the middle of the seventeenth century, made fornication a secular crime punishable for both parties. That act signified the beginning of intensified stigmatization of generations of unfortunate women during the following centuries. *See also:* Adultery; Bastardy.

Further Reading: Ågren, Maria, and Amy Louise, Erickson, eds. *The Marital Economy in Scandinavia and Britain, 1400–1900.* Burlington, VT: Ashgate, 2005; Flaherty, David. "Law and the Enforcement of Morals in Early America." In *Law in American History. Perspectives in American History.* Vol. 5, edited by Donald Fleming and Bernard Bailyn. Cambridge, MA: Harvard University Press, 1971; Quaife, G. R. *Wanton Wenches and Wayward Wives: Peasants and Illicit Sex in Early Seventeenth Century England.* London: Croom Helm, 1979; Sharpe, James A. *Crime in Early Modern England 1550–1750.* London: Longman, 1984; Sundin, Jan. "Sinful Sex.

Legal Prosecution of Extramarital Sex in Preindustrial Sweden." *Social Science History* 16, no. 1 (Spring 1992): 99–128; Wrightson, Keith, and David, Levine. *Poverty and Piety in an English Village: Terling, 1520–1700*. New York: Academic, 1979.

Jan Sundin

PRINTING. The development of printing in Europe in the fifteenth century and even earlier in East Asia, made books about sex, whether practical, scientific, or erotic, widely available to early modern populations.

Mechanical reproduction of texts has been practiced in East Asia, in the form of woodblock printing, since at least the ninth century, when the earliest surviving books of this kind were produced. To print a book using this technique, letters were carved on a block of wood, and, after applying ink to the block, paper was placed over it and rubbed to obtain a copy. Experiments with movable types (separate characters that could be reused to compose different texts) were carried out in China in the eleventh century, and, by the fourteenth century, books could be printed in Korea using metal types arranged over a tray and fixed with wax. Nevertheless, until the nineteenth century, block printing was the more frequent and effective practice in China, Korea, and Japan, since the enormous number of ideographical characters needed to compose texts made the use of movable types a very expensive and demanding enterprise.

In Europe, the history of printing started in the mid-fifteenth century with Johann Gutenberg's hand press and commercial publishing. Although the use of woodblocks anteceded the press in the West by at least seventy years, and although printers continued to use them as one of the main processes for illustrating books, Gutenberg's technique became the main method of printing until the twentieth century. Printers using this technique would compose the text by choosing types, one at a time, and setting them on a *forme* (a flat surface on which the types were arranged on composing sticks). After that, the types were inked, the *forme* was put in place, and a sheet of paper was placed on the *platen* (the upper surface in the press), which was then lowered to apply pressure and produce a copy. Several pages were printed on one sheet that would later be folded, and, for this reason, the printer had to compose the pages with the folding in mind. For instance, a *folio* (a sheet that was folded only once) would have two pages printed on each side—the first and fourth pages on one side, and the second and third on the other.

This manner of organizing the texts was already employed by scribes to bind their codices, and, in fact, there were marked continuations between hand-copying and printing practices. In addition to imitating the form in which codices were assembled, printed books reproduced the script and the page layout of manuscripts. Thus, the ways in which a person would read and handle a book did not significantly change with the advent of printing. Nevertheless, the much larger scale on which books were reproduced and distributed had a strong cultural impact.

Although the lack of data and the fragmentary nature of some of the surviving *incunabula* (books made during the cradle years of printing; that is, before 1500) make it very difficult to calculate the number of books actually produced, Henri-Jean Martin, with the support of Lucien Febvre, estimated that between twelve and twenty million books were printed in Europe before 1500. In the sixteenth century, almost 200 million books would have come off of European presses. The large numbers and short time in which copies were obtained, as well as the lower cost per copy, made books accessible to early modern men and women across social, institutional, and economic boundaries.

The Latin works of ancient and humanist authors were made available to a wide audience across Europe, raising **literacy** rates. Moreover, the increasing number of books published in vernacular languages brought about a more inclusive conceptualization of literacy, one that valued the ability to read, write, and study in languages other than Latin, and therefore generated both a bigger market for the number of books that printers could now produce and a new learning space for lay intellectuals, merchants, craftsmen, and women.

The large quantities of vernacular texts that the press put into circulation also played a part in the formation of national identities. The languages of the emerging European nations started to be considered prestigious, literary languages—subject to the standardization of grammar, vocabulary, and spelling—and such standard languages overrode the various dialects in each region. The dynamics of the book trade were compatible with the ongoing processes of linguistic unification, since a book printed in a dominant dialect, instead of a minor one, reached the widest audience possible in a country. In turn, as Benedict Anderson argues in *Imagined Communities* (1983), this wide reach encouraged the individual reader to think of him or herself as part of a national community in which virtually every member could read the same text he or she was reading, while people in other territories would read it in a different language.

In addition to the formation of national languages and identities, the spread of the press influenced the formation of legal notions, such as the economic privileges and legal responsibilities of the author, the translator, and the printer. Systematic censorship was made possible by the fact that the censor granting a license would have to revise only one text that would be multiplied, instead of each of the individual copies that were made.

Following in the footsteps of Elizabeth Eisenstein, scholars have argued that printing was also a major agent of religious and intellectual change. The Christian Church was quick to hail the new printing technology as providential, and made early use of it in its campaign against the Turks, and in the printing of indulgences. The press was also a crucial instrument in the **Reformation** and Counter-Reformation movements, since, on the one hand, it made possible the massive distribution of Martin **Luther**'s 95 Theses throughout central Europe, and, on the other, it aided the distribution of Catholic writings and enabled the implementation of strong political and religious censorship (*see* **Index of Prohibited Books**). Eisenstein has also noted that the fixed nature of the printed text and the accumulation of scientific texts that printing made available to individual scholars, formed the basis for modern scientific thought. Other levels at which printing affected the development of scientific disciplines include the model that the increasing specialization of printers, regarding particular topics and languages offered for later classifications of fields of studies, as well as the encyclopedic scope that knowledge gained when a myriad of topics, from geographical descriptions to lovemaking handbooks, became accessible to a massive public.

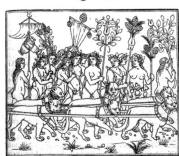

Francesco Colonna (?), *Hypnerotomachia Poliphili*. Aldus Manutius, Venice, 1499. [86.k.9]

Hypnerotomachia Poliphili, printed by Aldus Manutius, 1499. © The Art Archive.

The practice of sex was a frequent subject of early printed books, from catalogues of **courtesans** in Japan, to herbal, medical, and midwifery treatises in western Europe. **Love**, both in its erotic and in its allegorical dimensions, lay at the center of Renaissance literature. Ovid's *Epistolae heroidum* (fictional letters in which legendary heroines address the lovers that have abandoned them) was among the most frequently printed books in the incunabula period. Among vernacular texts, chivalric romances and their numerous translations became a highly successful enterprise for printers as early as the 1470s, in spite of persistent condemnation of their sensuality. Along a less popular line, Aldus Manutius' 1499 edition of the *Hypnerotomachia Poliphili* (*The Strife of Love in a Dream of Poliphilo*), in which the hero travels through a landscape filled with mythological allusions and iconographical play in search of his lover Polia, was also an early printing success. A testimony to the continued cultural centrality of classical and courtly love traditions, this work is regarded, in the words of Stephan Füssel, as "the most beautiful printed book of the Renaissance."

Further Reading: Anderson, Benedict. *Imagined Communities*. London: Verso, 1983; Eisenstein, Elizabeth L. *The Printing Revolution in Early Modern Europe*. 2nd ed. New York: Cambridge University Press, 2005; Febvre, Lucien, and Henri-Jean Martin. *The Coming of the Book: The Impact of Printing 1450–1800*. London: NLB, 1976; Füssel, Stephan. *Gutenberg and the Impact of Printing*. Aldershot: Ashgate, 2005; Park, Seong-Rae. "Six Perspectives in the History of Printing." *Gutenberg Jahrbuch* 73 (1998): 42–47.

Belén Bistué

PROSTITUTION. In the period between 1400 and 1600, western Europeans viewed prostitution not so much as a practice—the exchange of sex for money—but as a category of identity defining women whose unruly sexual behavior, in becoming public, revealed their nature as whores. As Ruth Mazo Karras points out, "prostitute" was used only occasionally and as a verb. "Common woman," "*meretrix*," "*femme publique*," "strumpet," and "*putain*," along with phrases like *femme de mauvaise vie*, or "woman of evil life," took precedence as ways of designating women whose sexual behavior threatened (but also defined) normative social and sexual order. Commercial prostitution nonetheless describes a cultural idea and material practice of sexuality that coincided with increasing urbanization and the growth of a commercial economy, particularly in western Europe and Shogunate Japan. It reflects the relative social anonymity, concentration of population, high demand for services, and simultaneous poverty and independence of single women and children characteristic of cities in this period.

Commercial prostitution can thus be contrasted with concubinage, a system with which it coexisted, in which continued sexual access is exchanged for long-term economic support. In large cities like London, Paris, Venice, and Seville, and in inns along thoroughfares, commercial prostitution was tacitly available to all men, except for Jews, although members of the clergy and married men were supposed to abstain and were sometimes fined. Similarly, in Shogunate Japan, commercial prostitution became concentrated in the cities of Kyoto, Edo, and Osaka, and was practiced in roadside tea houses. In colonial Latin America, commercial prostitution in urban centers like Mexico City and San Juan de Puerto Rico may well have been dominated by single women whose Iberian descent precluded them from performing other kinds of work, and who could demand payment for sexual services—in contrast to native and *mestizo* women, to whom sexual access was viewed as a colonial right.

Until the mid-sixteenth century, European city-dwellers, legislators, and even theologians, approached prostitution as a necessary evil. Like Augustine, they argued that prostitutes protected communities from **rape**, the deflowering of virgins, **adultery**, and sodomy (along with the commensurate decline in the birth rate that came with it) that men might commit with "honest" women (or men) if they had no other outlet. In this view, prostitutes needed to be tolerated but also contained and regulated because of the crime and disorder they would otherwise engender. City officials sought repeatedly and fruitlessly to confine prostitution to specific red-light districts, often outside of the city walls. Municipal and licensed brothels flourished in European towns until a mid-sixteenth-century change in attitudes toward sexuality.

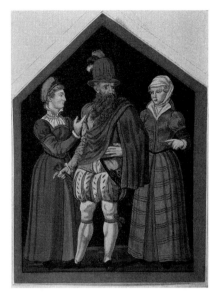

Sixteenth-century painting of a madam with a client and a prostitute in sixteenth-century Geneva, Switzerland. © The Art Archive/University Library Geneva/Dagli Orti.

The purported role that European prostitutes played in preserving sexual order was recognized, as Kathryn Norberg has noted, by invitations to participate in municipal processions and festivals in Lyons or to appear as wedding guests in Germany, and by the foundation of Magdalen houses or Repentes where prostitutes could repent and reform. Nonetheless, European prostitutes were often objects of shaming and violence, both official and unofficial. Once a woman became a sex worker in a municipal brothel, her movement in and out of the brothel was governed by rules, visits from family or friends were curtailed, and long-term relations with a man were prohibited. Within or outside of the brothel, venereal diseases and multiple partners limited the average prostitute's fertility, while any children she bore very likely became **foundlings**. Women convicted of being illegal whores or bawds could expect to have their heads shaved or hair cut, to have their hoods or outer garments taken away, to be forced to wear a defining mark such as a striped hood, to be paraded through the streets, to be pilloried, and, on subsequent infractions, and to be imprisoned or banished from the city. Prostitutes were subject to sumptuary laws requiring them to wear an identifying knot or arm band along with plain clothing. Men slashed the faces of women they perceived to be whores, urinated on them, dumped feces on them, and raped them, singly or in gangs. Regulations about whether a man could be prosecuted for raping a prostitute varied from place to place and over time, but men were not prosecuted for buying a prostitute's services. By the late sixteenth century, prostitutes lost all legal recourse.

The conservative estimate given by Leah Lydia Otis as to how many European women were involved in prostitution during this period is that there was one prostitute for every thousand people in European towns. The women who became casual or professional prostitutes did so out of constrained choice. In the sixteenth century, when the European population grew and unmarried women were excluded from trades, women who did not marry had only a few options for legitimate work: domestic service, brewing, laundering, and work in the textile trades. Women in the legitimate workforce sometimes supplemented their unreliable income with casual prostitution. Some women turned to prostitution after a sexual affair or rape rendered them unsuitable, in the eyes of employers, for legitimate work. Court records show that women and men sold girls and women, to whom they had promised good employment or whom they simply kidnapped, for rape to paying customers. Prostitution could be, in some cases, a family strategy with mothers, brothers, or husbands working as procurers for a younger woman. The women for whom prostitution became a sole profession were generally unmarried, unskilled, originally from another place than the town where they worked, and without the means to marry.

In the sixteenth century, legal documents, literary texts, and the remarkable status of a few **"courtesans"** laid the groundwork for enduring cultural associations of prostitution with illusion, theater, erotic education, the commodification of sexuality, profiteering, and urban decay. Works like Pietro **Aretino**'s *Ragionamente* (1534) cultivated an elite idea of the prostitute's tutelage in erotic arts. Popular motifs focused on the crafty old bawd who tricks an innocent young girl, and the prostitute who tries to pass as a fine lady, only to be unmasked. Scholars have recently begun to explore the lives, work, and contemporary images of women, like the published authors Veronica Franco and Tullia **d'Aragona**, who were recognized in Renaissance Italy for their writing, conversation, and artistic and musical skills, as well as their sex work. *See also* Brothels; Concubines.

Further Reading: d'Aragona, Tullia. *Dialogue on the Infinity of Love*. Edited and translated by Rinaldina Russell and Bruce Merry. The Other Voice in Early Modern Europe series. Chicago: University of Chicago Press, 1997; Karras, Ruth Mazo. *Common Women: Prostitution and Sexuality in Medieval England*. Oxford: Oxford University Press, 1996; Norberg, Kathryn. "Prostitutes." In *A History of Women in the West*. Vol. 3: *Renaissance and Enlightenment Paradoxes*, edited by Natalie Zemon Davis and Arlette Farge, 458–74. Cambridge, MA: Harvard University Press, 1993; Otis, Leah Lydia. *Prostitution in Medieval Society: The History of an Urban Institution in Languedoc*. Chicago: University of Chicago Press, 1985; Powers, Karen Vieira. *Women in the Crucible of Conquest: The Gendered Genesis of Spanish American Society, 1500–1600*. Albuquerque: University of New Mexico Press, 2005; Sone, Hiromi. "Prostitution and Public Authority in Early Modern Japan." In *Women and Class in Japanese History*, edited by Hitomi Tonomura, Anne Walthall, and Wakita Haruko, translated by Akiko Terashima and Anne Walthall, 169–85. Michigan Monograph Series in Japanese Studies, 25. Ann Arbor: The University of Michigan, 1999; Turner, James Grantham. *Schooling Sex: Literature and Erotic Education in Italy, France, and England 1534–1685*. Oxford: Oxford University Press, 2003.

Pamela Cheek

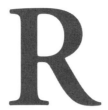

RALEIGH, SIR WALTER (1552–1618). An Elizabethan poet, courtier, soldier, and historian, Sir Walter Raleigh, although long a special favorite of English monarch **Elizabeth I**, fell into disgrace for seducing and secretly marrying one of the queen's maids of honor. Elizabeth's anger was born both of her own sexual attraction to Raleigh, a handsome, virile, and active man, and of her utter abhorrence of any sexual liaisons between her ladies and the men of her court, whose admiration and attention she preferred to have lavished on herself.

Born into a Devonshire gentry family, Raleigh (often spelled Ralegh) was educated at Oxford. In the late 1570s, he helped his half-brother Sir Humphrey Gilbert fight rebels in Ireland and outfit privateering expeditions against Spanish shipping. After 1581, he spent most of his time at court, where the queen knighted him in 1584 and appointed him captain of her guards in 1587. Between 1583 and 1589, he invested over £40,000 in six colonizing expeditions to North America, having received a grant from Elizabeth to plant colonies along the eastern coast of the continent. One such area Raleigh named Virginia, for Elizabeth, the "Virgin Queen." Although responsible for introducing potatoes and tobacco to England and Ireland, Raleigh's ventures were unsuccessful in establishing a permanent English colony in America. In 1595, Raleigh sailed on a fruitless search for the legendary land of El Dorado, which was supposedly to be found in Guyana, on the northern coast of South America.

Raleigh was part of the successful English attack on the Spanish port of Cadiz in 1596, and the unsuccessful Islands Expedition of 1597. He quarreled with the queen's favorite Robert Devereux, earl of Essex, in 1597, and thereafter was a consistent opponent of the earl's and much blamed for his eventual downfall. After Elizabeth's death in 1603, her successor, James I, persuaded by Raleigh's many enemies that he was a dangerous conspirator, had him arrested and tried for treason. From 1603 to 1616, Raleigh lay in the Tower of London, where he composed poetry and wrote his *History of the World*. Released to search for gold along the Orinoco River in South America, Raleigh found no gold but burned a Spanish settlement. He was rearrested upon his return on the insistence of the Spanish king, Phillip III, with whom James was attempting to negotiate a **marriage** for his son. Raleigh was executed on October 29, 1618.

Many probably apocryphal tales illustrate how successfully Raleigh engaged Elizabeth's attention and how large a role sexual attraction, if not actual sexual relations, played in their relationship. Besides the well-known story of Raleigh laying down his cloak so the queen could safely traverse a wet spot on the ground, there is the equally incredible tale of Raleigh and Elizabeth scratching couplets of poetry to each

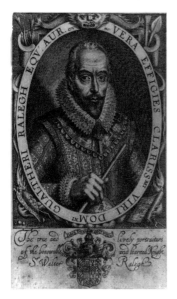

Undated portrait of Sir Walter Raleigh. Courtesy of the Library of Congress.

other on a windowpane. Certainly, Raleigh wrote poetry for the queen, including such innovative verses as "Farewell False Love," which circulated throughout the court during the early 1580s. The queen responded with many personal marks of her favor and affection, such as a small token depicting an anchor and a lady, which Raleigh ostentatiously displayed as evidence of the intimacy of his relationship with the queen.

Tall and dark-haired, with a well-proportioned body, refined features, and a passionate manner, Raleigh drew interest from many women, including, according to one account, an unnamed maid of honor with whom he was observed in engaging in intercourse against the trunk of a tree. He is also known to have been involved with Dorothy, the sister of the earl of Essex, a relationship that may have initiated the bad blood between the two men. Raleigh fathered at least one illegitimate child, a daughter by Alice Goold, an otherwise unknown woman he probably met while soldiering in Ireland.

In the early 1590s, Raleigh began a relationship with Elizabeth (Bess) Throckmorton, one of the queen's maids. Little is know of their courtship outside two poems, both addressed to "Serena," Raleigh's allegorical name for Bess, which are perhaps the most explicitly sexual verses Raleigh ever wrote.

> What shee and Youth and Forme perswade
> With Oppertunety, that's made
> As we could wish itt. Lett's then meete
> Often with amorous lippes, and greet
> Each other till our wantonne Kisses
> In number passe [the] dayes Ulisses
> Consum'd in travaile . . .

Like her queen, Bess was a strong-willed woman—her brother referred to her in his diary as "Morgan le fay." When she became pregnant in late 1591, she and Raleigh married in secret. Well aware of how deeply their marriage would offend the queen, the couple retired to Devon, where, on March 29, 1592, Bess gave birth to a son while Raleigh was at sea. Bess returned to court a month later, apparently hoping to keep her marriage and her **motherhood** secret. However, Elizabeth soon learned of both and in early June she placed both husband and wife in custody. The consummate courtier, Raleigh sought to win his way back into favor with lavish displays of devotion, including an exaggerated wrestling match with his keeper meant to show the queen, then sailing by in her barge, that he could only by restraint be kept from diving into the water to see her. Because the queen found these performances irritating and sorely lacking in contrition, she committed both Raleigh and Bess to the Tower of London in August.

Although still banished from court, both husband and wife were released from imprisonment by the end of 1592, possibly as a charitable reaction to the death of their infant son. Although eventually readmitted to favor—he returned to court in 1597—Raleigh never regained the special position he had previously held in the queen's affections. Bess, meanwhile, was never forgiven and, despite a determined attempt by her husband in 1601, never reinstated at court.

Further Reading: Coote, Stephen. *A Play of Passion: The Life of Sir Walter Raleigh*. London: Macmillan, 1993; Haynes, Alan. *Sex in Elizabethan England*. Stroud, England: Sutton Publishing,

1999; Lacey, Robert. *Sir Walter Ralegh*. New York: Atheneum, 1973; Trevelyan, Raleigh. *Sir Walter Raleigh*. New York: Henry Holt and Company, 2003; Williams, Norman Lloyd. *Sir Walter Raleigh*. London: Cassell, 1988; Winton, John. *Sir Walter Ralegh*. New York: Coward, McCann & Geohegan, 1975.

John A. Wagner

RAPE. Rape is a word generally used to describe coercive sexual intercourse. In reference to the early modern era, this definition can be refined to mean the extramarital, vaginal penetration of a woman by the use of explicit force. This being the legal definition of rape, historians more recently have broadened their view on the subject. Since Susan Brownmiller's highly influential study, perspectives on rape have, like many other sexual matters, undergone a cultural shift. Written in the context of the U.S. women's rights movement, Brownmiller's study focused mainly on twentieth-century topics, but also encompassed many premodern studies dealing with matters of sexual violence. Brownmiller has interpreted rape as "nothing more or less than a conscious process of intimidation by which all men keep all women in state of fear" (Brownmiller 1975, 15). Edward Shorter has refined this thesis, tracing it back to the early nineteenth century, but claiming other reasons (sexual frustration, repressive morals, late age of marriage) as being responsible for rape during the time span between the **Reformation** and the French Revolution. The tendency of both Brownmiller and Shorter to seek causes of rape—mostly in terms of more or less "structural violence"—while widely disregarding the victim's side as well as the perpetrator's personality and individual circumstances have raised recent criticisms of their works.

Rape has been penalized as a major crime throughout legal history. In the early modern era in central Europe, the reception of Roman law, which sentenced rapists to death, became most influential. In addition to that body of jurisprudence, many local differences, based on social class and other factors, can be traced regarding different views of both the victim and the perpetrator. For instance, often only reputable women and virgins were regarded as possible victims of rape while prostitutes or other women of dubitable reputation enjoyed less legal protection. Yet, from the sixteenth century onward, most legal codifications admitted women's own legal identity and did not assess rape as mainly a property offence toward the women's husband or father, as many medieval legal texts did. Normally, only vaginal penetration together with seminal emission qualified as a completed rape, while other forms of sexual violence, such as oral intercourse, did not violate the women's honor to the same degree and hence were followed by the less severe penalties imposed for attempted rape. As the latter was hard to substantiate, offenders were rarely prosecuted.

With the emergence of professional science in the seventeenth century, medical experts became increasingly important in rape trials. The theory that conception without positive female energy was impossible, therefore a woman impregnated by her attacker could not have been a rape victim because she obviously had not resisted the attacker wholeheartedly, existed until the late eighteenth century. Such concepts made the line between willing seduction and violent rape remarkably fluid. Only late eighteenth-century European legal codifications inspired by the ideas of the Enlightenment, such as the *Allgemeines Preußisches Landrecht* (1794), mark a turning point in the legal history of rape to a more modern conception of the crime.

Rape has mainly been considered to be an act done by men to adult women. Rapes of men were mostly heard as cases of forbidden homosexual practice (sodomy), while child rape did not become a publicly prominent problem until the second half of the eighteenth century, when the "emergence of child rape" (Vigarello 2001, 75) occasionally even overshadowed the rape of adult women as a public concern. *See also* Oral Sex; Pregnancy; Prostitution.

Further Reading: Brownmiller, Susan. *Against Our Will: Men, Women and Rape.* London: Secker & Warburg, 1975; Dane, Gesa. *"Zeter und Mordio." Vergewaltigung in Literatur und Recht.* Göttingen: Wallstein, 2005; Meyer-Knees, Anke. *Verführung und sexuelle Gewalt. Untersuchungen zum medizinischen und juristischen Diskurs im 18. Jahrhundert.* Probleme der Semiotik XII. Tübingen: Stauffenberg Verlag, 1992; Shorter, Edward. *The Making of the Modern Family.* New York: Basic Books, 1975; Smith, Sabine H. *Sexual Violence in German Culture. Rereading and Rewriting the Tradition.* Studien zum Theater, Film und Fernsehen XXVI. Bern: Peter Lang, 1998; Vigarello, Georges. *A History of Rape. Sexual Violence in France from the 16th to the 20th Century.* Translated by Jean Birrell. Cambridge: Polity Press, 2001.

Hiram Kümper

THE REFORMATION. The Protestant Reformation of the sixteenth century was a period of challenge, division, and renewal in the early modern Christian Church in **Europe**. In 1517, the Augustinian monk Martin **Luther** (1483–1546) made public a list —the 95 Theses—that summarized 95 objections that a faithful and reasonable Christian could levy against the inappropriate behaviors of some members of the clergy. Luther was reacting to the failure of the Fifth Lateran Council—Lateran V (1512–1517)—to follow the principle of *ecclesia semper reformanda* (the Church always reforming itself). His actions started a firestorm of debate that would see a fragmentation of Christian unity in the west, the creation of new sects and movements, significant changes in worship and culture, and bloody European wars over what constituted the belief of a proper Christian.

The 95 Theses were an expression of the great many concerns and criticisms Luther had over the practices of the Catholic Church, thoughts that were shared by many who were anxious to eliminate abuses and resolve doctrinal issues within the Church.

In addition to administrative issues of local, regional, and global mismanagement, key points in Luther's argument were:

1. the need to make the Bible readily available to all Christians in their vernacular languages, rather than in Latin alone;
2. the thorny debate over the question of Jesus' manifestation in the bread and wine that at his command and in whose remembrance become his Body and Blood (1 Cor 11: 23–26), known as the issue of transubstantiation;
3. the question of justification by God's grace alone, or through the living of a good life and good acts.

Theologically, the issues of transubstantiation and whether or not the attainment of grace is by God's forgiveness alone, regardless of the good works a Christian performs, were the most fraught. The transubstantiation debate, which still exists today, is over whether transubstantiation occurs, or if the real presence of Christ is in the consecrated elements (bread and wine, with a little bit of water) in the Eucharist, or communion. Transubstantiation is the belief that the bread and the wine literally become the body and blood of Christ (the Roman Catholic view), while belief in the real presence signifies that Christ is present in the bread and wine but both remain unchanged (the majority mainstream Protestant view).

The Reformation introduced a new order of service, as well as changes to the Catholic Mass. Among Protestant Christians, The Liturgy of the Word gained prominence and precedes the Eucharist in the liturgy. The Liturgy of the Word consists of a set of readings in the following order: one reading from the Old Testament and then two readings from the New Testament, first one of the letters by Paul the Apostle, or a passage from the Acts of the Apostles, and then the proclamation of a passage from the Gospel according to Matthew, Mark, Luke, or John. Before the start of the Reformation, readings were all done in Latin, with the priest speaking the vernacular only during the sermon that followed. The shape of the liturgy—known as the Order of the Mass—began to take its present state in the middle of the sixteenth century before, during, and following the Roman Catholic Council of **Trent** (1545–1547, 1551–1552, and 1562–1563).

Not unaware of the need for internal reform, the Catholic Church, in the face of extreme external pressures, began to re-examine its doctrines and practices, and to eliminate some abuses. The Council of Trent was the delayed Roman formulation of setting temporal affairs in order and marking the limits of what could be permitted within the approved doctrines. Trent resulted in a new Order of the Mass, the Tridentine Rite (or Mass), which continued as the blueprint for worship until the Second Vatican Council, known as Vatican II (1962–1965), modified it radically in the twentieth century. It was not until the conclusion of Vatican II that the mass was no longer said in Latin, but in the vernacular. Another significant Tridentine change was that the priest now faced the congregation at all times, rather than performing the Mass with his back to the people, or even behind a screen. The altar used for communion became free-standing in such a way that the people now could see the blessing invoked upon the gifts of bread and wine that would become the body and blood of Christ, which had been previously hidden.

Beyond the three major points raised above, there were any number of points of disagreement that remained between Protestant and Catholic thinkers. Luther saw the temporal ambitions of the papacy as particularly wrong, when at a time when popes such as Julius II (1503–1513) and Leo X (1503–1521), financed standing armies and began an unprecedented age of centralized architectural splendor. The selling of indulgences– a document, not unlike a modern bearer bond, that assured an individual that a deceased person would spend less time in purgatory than otherwise required— also infuriated Luther. Even the notion of purgatory itself, which is neither scriptural nor part of early Church teaching, but arose from medieval piety and lore and was comprehensively articulated by the Florentine humanist poet Dante Alighieri (1265–1321) in *The Divine Comedy* (1307–1321), was one that Luther demanded be re-examined.

The treatment of relics was a point of disagreement between Protestants, on the one hand, and Roman Catholics and the Orthodox Churches on the other, and continues to be so to this day. With serious concerns about avoiding the error of heretics going back to the Israelites at the foot of Mount Sinai (Ex 32: 1–35), Protestant **Christianity** strenuously objected to the role of the saints in liturgical life; moreover, the central importance of the Blessed Virgin Mary as mother of Jesus became the source of heated disagreement. Early in the councils of the Church (e.g., Ephesus in 431 and Chalcedon in 451), the role of Mary as *Theotokos*, God-bearer, was part of the Nicene Creed. Unfortunately, theology and actual religious practice do not always coincide; often, theology itself can be as ugly in its academic feuds as in any other field of knowledge (there is even a phrase for this, *odium theologicum*, "theological hatred"). Mainstream Christian thought today acknowledges the series of *latria*, which is the absolute worship of God the Father, Son, and Holy Ghost; *hyperdulia*, the special veneration of the Blessed Virgin Mary as the mother of Jesus, who marks the moment of God entering human history; and *dulia*, which is veneration or respect of the saints. The Protestant concern was that people might blur the line between praying for the intercession of the saints, including the Blessed Virgin, on their behalf to God and mistakenly begin adoring the saints instead of the mystery of God (The Most Blessed Trinity).

This concern led to conflict on the issue of Mariology, or how the Blessed Virgin Mary is seen in God's scheme for salvation. The image of the *Mater dolorosa*, the "suffering mother" (as in Michelangelo's *Pietà*) is a defining feature of Roman Catholicism, along with the image of the joyous mother who has recently given birth to Jesus. Protestant traditions that permit the Virgin Mary to be depicted tend to favor the younger mother rather than the suffering, middle-aged Blessed Virgin Mary, who was appealed to more to intercede with her Son. St. Elizabeth and her son St. John the Baptist remained acceptable to both traditions, but St. Elizabeth, Mary's cousin, was seen as more approachable. In the early modern period, Elizabeth was seen as someone whom every woman could relate to with reverence while avoiding a charge of meddling in matters of religion—or theology—which was still the exclusive domain of men (although two Roman Catholic nuns—St. Teresa of Avila and St. Catherine of Siena—would challenge that view). While devout women would readily accept the fact that Jesus was born of an unmarried (although engaged) young woman, it was likely easier for early modern women to identify with Elizabeth, whose son was conceived in the usual way.

How did the Reformation affect the lives of women, and did a new sense of self-determination come out of the reform movement? These questions are not easily answered. For both Catholics and Protestants, Eve continued to bear greater responsibility and guilt for the Fall than Adam. Neither Protestant nor Catholic reformers looked upon **divorce** as something acceptable to civil and to church law. Both sides prized **virginity** as an element of virtue and as a commodity for marriage. The patriarchal outlook of the Protestant Reformation could be as repressive for women as the Roman Catholic view.

How women fit into the social order outside of **marriage** was an issue that reformers on either side of the debate seemingly agreed on. A woman's main function was reproductive. Under most circumstances in western Europe, few women had the ability to own land, other tangible property, or control large amounts of capital, a circumstance that pertained both to the emerging bourgeoisie and to the lower and upper aristocracy. Poor women were seen as no more important than children. Dress, social gatherings, balls, and eventually literary salons became agents or means through which women could express class affiliation and religious outlook as well as display their intelligence and wit. Literature, circulated in manuscript form or published with the patronage of wealthy respected humanist men, was another mode of expression for some women. Female authors from the Republic of Venice, especially, illustrate this point. Perhaps the most famous of **courtesans**, Veronica Franco, was second to no male Venetian writer of her age. Protestant women soon gained access to direct reading of the Bible in their native language (if they were literate), whereas Catholic women were still prohibited from reading and studying directly the word of God.

The Reformation did have some harsh, unintended side effects for some women. In England, with the closing of monasteries and convents during the reign of **Henry VIII**, many nuns became homeless and destitute, and had to seek protection underground or flee to Europe.

IMPORTANT FIGURES OF THE REFORMATION. The German priest Philip Melanchthon (1497–1560), a colleague of Luther, was the systematic theologian who developed, mainly in the Confession of Augsburg (1530), the interpretive body of work that established the Evangelical Church, which later became known as the Lutheran Church in the United States. Luther and Melanchthon complemented each other in terms of rhetoric and diplomacy. John **Calvin** (1509–1564), a French priest, settled in Switzerland, establishing a Protestant movement that openly sought to break away from Rome. His major work is the *Institutes of the Christian Religion* (first edition 1536; final expanded version 1559). Ulrich Zwingli (1484–1531), a Swiss priest, separated himself from the Evangelical renewal movement begun by Luther because he came to view the Eucharist as a ceremonial action that lacked the real presence of Jesus Christ. John Knox (c. 1514–1572), also a former Roman priest, organized the Church of Scotland in the manner of Calvin as outlined in *The Book of Discipline* (drafted 1561; ratified 1567 when Mary Queen of Scots abdicated the Scottish throne); thus the Presbyterian Church became the established state religion in Scotland.

The leaders of the Reformation and the Catholic Counter-Reformation, the period of Catholic reform and revival that began after the Council of Trent, were learned men and women who wrote in Latin with the same ease that they wrote in their respective native languages. They represent an era of renewal of faith in God and in making the best possible use of the intellect that God had given them for the common good. They were, with few exceptions, humanists.

Desiderius Erasmus of Rotterdam (1466–1536) chose to reform the Roman Catholic Church from within, which required great diplomatic dexterity and common sense. Erasmus' *In Praise of Folly* (1511) satirized all European institutions at the start of the Spanish and Portuguese colonization of the New World. The original Latin title is a play of words on the name of his close friend Thomas More, *Moriae Encomium*. In 1516, More published *Utopia*, the other masterpiece that raised consciousness of the need for reform in the Church.

Many reformers were men of state, versed in the law (civil and canonical), the liberal arts, and theology. Others led their entire adult lives as members of religious orders. Sadly, among them martyrs became abundant on all sides. **Henry VIII** of England had his Lord Chancellor Thomas More beheaded because he would not sign the Act of Supremacy recognizing the king, rather than the pope, as head of the English Church. William Tyndale (1494–1536) was executed in Belgium for having translated into English the New Testament (a few copies of which found their way to England). Archbishop of Canterbury Thomas Cranmer (1489–1556), appointed by Henry VIII to head the hierarchy of the new Church of England, was later executed by order of Henry's Catholic daughter Mary I, who ascended the English throne in 1553. In 1549, Cranmer published the *Book of Common Prayer*, which set a new standard in grounding the liturgy on biblical scholarship. The *Book of Common Prayer* introduced the use of modern English prose as a literary language. John of the Cross (1542–1591), who co-founded the Discalced Carmelites with Teresa of Avila (1515–1582), suffered torture and imprisonment at the hands of the Spanish Inquisition.

On the Roman side, along with Erasmus and Saint Thomas More, there were four vigorous Spanish reformers. John of the Cross and Teresa of Avila have become Doctors of the Church, a recognition of their wisdom, knowledge of God's word, and ability to teach Christian doctrine to the learned and the common person alike. Teresa is the first woman so recognized. Saint Ignatius of Loyola founded the Society of Jesus, the Jesuits, in 1540, adopting the apostolate (mission) of education and evangelization. The Jesuits reformed the seminary system, normalizing the curriculum and spiritual preparation for the priesthood. The Society of Jesus, within its first generation, earned its way into the company of martyrs and joined the ranks of professors at leading universities. Cardinal Francisco Jiménez de Cisneros (1436–1517), a Franciscan friar, served six years, incarceration by order of the Archbishop of Toledo upon his return from studying in Rome. His monumental contribution to the Reformation was the publication of the six-volume *Polyglot Complutensian Bible* (1522). It consists of critically established texts in Hebrew, from the Greek Septuagint version and the Chaldean Targum versions of the Old Testament. It also includes new interlineal Latin translations—in addition to Jerome's Vulgate, for the Old and New Testaments—and the New Testament in new Greek and Latin editions. The sixth volume contains grammars and vocabularies of Hebrew, Chaldean, and Greek. Cisneros assembled and oversaw the team of scholar-translators, and personally financed the project at the University of Alcalá de Henares, which he had founded. *See also* Dowry; Elizabeth I, Queen of England; Mystics.

Further Reading: "Biblia Políglota Complutense." *Centro Virtual Cervantes. Instituto Cervantes.* 2003–2007: http://cvc.cervantes.es/actcult/ciudades/alcala_henares/indice/biblia.htm; "Jiménez de Cisneros, Francisco." *The Columbia Encyclopedia.* 6th ed. New York: Columbia University Press, 2001: www.bartleby.com/65/; "Ulrich Zwingli": http://www.wsu.edu/dee/REFORM/ZWINGLI.HTM; "William Tyndale's New Testament": http://www.bl.uk/onlinegallery/themes/landmarks/tyndale.html. *British Library Online Gallery;* Alighieri, Dante. *Purgatory.* Translated by Henry F. Cary. Chicago: Thompson & Thomas, 1901: http://www.gutenberg.org/files/8795/8795-h/8795-h.htm; Bellitto, Christopher M. *The General Councils: A History of the 21 Church Councils from Nicaea to Vatican II.* New York: Paulist, 2002; Calvin, John. *Institutes of the Christian Religion.* Translated by Bonham Norton. London: Hatfield, 1599: *Center for Reformed Theology and Apologetics.* http://www.reformed.org/master/index.html?mainframe=/books/institutes/; Cranmer, Thomas. 1662. *Book of Common Prayer.* [From a 1987 facsimile ed.]. Site maintained by Lynda M. Howell. http://www.eskimo.com/lhowell/bcp1662/; Erasmus, Desiderius. *In Praise of Folly.* Translated by John Wilson. 1516: *Modern History Sourcebook.* http://www.fordham.edu/halsall/mod/1509erasmus-folly.html; González, Justo L. *The Story of Christianity: The Reformation to the Present Day.* Vol. 2. New York: HarperCollins, 1985; Halsall, Paul, comp. Fordham University. *Internet Modern History Sourcebook:* http://www.fordham.edu/halsall/mod/modsbook.html; Ignatius of Loyola. *From the Spiritual Exercises of Ignatius Loyola.* Translated and edited by Elder Mullen. New York: Kennedy and Sons, 1914; *Medieval Sourcebook.* http://www.fordham.edu/halsall/source/loyola-spirex.html; John of the Cross. *Dark Night of the Soul.* Translated by Kieran Kavanaugh and Otilio Rodriguez. From Rev. Ed. *The Collected Works of St. John of the Cross.* Washington, DC: ICS Publications, 1991: *The Teresian Carmel.* http://www.karmel.at/ics/john/dn.html; Jones, Cheslyn, et al., eds. *The Study of Liturgy.* Rev. ed. New York: Oxford University Press, 1992; Knox, John. 1559. *A brief exhortation to England, for the speedy embracing of the Gospel heretofore by the tyranny of Mary suppressed and banished.* From *Selected Writings of John Knox: Public Epistles, Treatises, and Expositions to the Year 1559.* Kevin Reed, 1995: Presbyterian Heritage Publications. http://www.swrb.ab.ca/newslett/actualNLs/briefexh.htm; Livingstone, Elizabeth A. *The Concise Oxford Dictionary of the Christian Church.* New York: Oxford University Press, 1996; Luther, Martin. *95 Theses.* Translated by Bob Van Cleef. Project Guttenberg, 1992: http://www.fordham.edu/halsall/source/luther95.txt; Melanchthon, Philip. *The Augsburg Confession.* Concordia Historical Institute. 1530: http://chi.lcms.org/melanchthon/index.html#Augsburg; More, Thomas. *Utopia.* From *Ideal Commonwealths.* New York: P.F. Collier & Son, 1901: *Modern History Sourcebook.* http://www.fordham.edu/halsall/mod/thomasmore-utopia.html; Tanner, Norman P., et al. *Decrees of the Ecumenical Councils.* 2 vols. Washington, DC: Georgetown University Press, 1990; Teresa of Avila. *Interior Castle.* Translated by E. Allison Peers. Edited by Silverio de Santa Teresa. New York: Image Books, 1964: http://www.intratext.com/X/ENG0033.htm.

Nicolás Hernández, Jr.

REMARRIAGE/WIDOWS. In early modern Europe, the death of a husband could leave a newly widowed woman in a situation of complex and complicating transformation. Upon the death of her spouse, a woman's life was suddenly in flux, and the events and experiences that followed affected everything from her emotional state to her economic one. This change in status also affected such social institutions as the family and community. A few quantitative figures, based on the Florentine *catasto* (census) of 1427, help to situate our subject: 25 percent of the general population of adult women in Florence in 1427 were widows. Comparatively, only 4 percent of adult men were widowers. Thus, a significant percentage of the female population was widowed at any given time.

Upon widowhood, there were many expectations but just as many opportunities. Widowhood could last anywhere from one year to the remainder of a lifetime. In most parts of Europe, following the burial ceremony, women returned to live with their birth, or agnatic, families, at least for the requisite year of mourning. Other options included staying within the **marriage** household or rejecting the traditional household altogether, joining a convent or, in rare cases, even living independently. If they received an inheritance or gained control of their dowries, some widows found themselves in economically advantageous positions, resulting in financial security. Other widows might be forced to support themselves and their children; such circumstances could determine whether or not a widow was to remarry, a delicate negotiation that was usually decided by a male relative. Such arrangements could be problematic, especially if the widow had children, who then would be placed in a vulnerable and compromising position.

The consistently uncertain social, economic, and interfamilial mobility of widows in early modern Europe led to a substantial production of literature, from conduct books to sermons, governing the comportment of widows, particularly on the question of remarriage. This was a topic taken up by Juan Luis Vives, whose book, *A Very Fruitful and Pleasant Book Called the Instruction of a Christian Woman*, was the most influential women's conduct book of the sixteenth century. Because younger widows, especially, could remarry several times, commemorating the requisite year of mourning became a social and sometimes legal imperative.

The category of widow portraiture—depictions of the woman during and after her husband's funeral when she is recognized as his widow—can generally be characterized as follows: the widow is depicted in a three-quarter or bust-length pose; she is set in profile or frontally against a plain, dark background; she is depicted with a sober or severe expression; and, most importantly, she is simply veiled and dressed in dark colors. Such representations, commissioned by male family members, served as an official recognition of the mourning period and, subsequently, as a memorial to the deceased. This became especially important as widows frequently remarried and changed households. *See also* Dowry; Sati.

Further Reading: Bremmer, Jan, and Lourens van der Bosch, eds. *Between Poverty and the Pyre: Moments in the History of Widowhood*. London: Routledge, 1995; Calvi, Giulia. "Reconstructing the Family: Widowhood and Remarriage in Tuscany in the Early Modern Period." In *Marriage in Italy, 1300–1650*, edited by Trevor Dean and K.J.P. Lowe, 275–96. Cambridge: Cambridge University Press, 1998; Cavallo, Sandra, and Lyndan Warner, eds. *Widowhood in Medieval and Early Modern Europe*. London: Longman, 1999; Klapisch-Zuber, Christiane. "'The Cruel Mother': Maternity, Widowhood, and Dowry in Florence in the Fourteenth and Fifteenth Centuries." In *Women, Family, and Ritual in Renaissance Italy*, translated by Lydia Cochrane, 117–31. Chicago: University of Chicago Press, 1985; Klein, Joan Larsen, ed.

Daughters, Wives, and Widows: Writings by Men about Women and Marriage in England, 1500–1640. Urbana: University of Illinois Press, 1992; Levy, Allison, ed. *Widowhood and Visual Culture in Early Modern Europe*. Aldershot: Ashgate, 2003; Molho, Anthony. *Marriage Alliance in Late Medieval Florence*. Cambridge, MA: Harvard University Press, 1994.

Allison Levy

S

SATI. Known in the West as "suttee," *sati* is a traditional Indian funeral rite involving the voluntary self-immolation of a widow upon her husband's funeral pyre. Derived from the name of Satī, the virtuous consort of the god Shiva, who, in Hindu mythology, protested her father's disrespectful treatment of her husband by burning herself, the term "*sati*" refers also to any woman who distinguishes herself through her righteous and exemplary devotion to her spouse, especially by willingly following him into death. Although usually associated with Hindu society, *sati* was also practiced in various forms by cultures outside India, such as the Egyptians, Goths, and Scythians.

The first recorded instance of *sati* dates to around 510 CE, with the practice for long thereafter being a voluntary act confined largely to the wives of the Hindu warrior (*kshatriya*) **caste**. Although the exact origins of the rite of *sati* are unclear, the concept of eternal wifely devotion may be ancient. A series of double graves containing both male and female skeletons and dating from before 1500 BCE may indicate the existence at that time of a belief that wives should accompany their husbands from life into death. Over time, *sati* came to be viewed as the greatest act of selfless love, and both the act and those who undertook it became highly romanticized in Indian society. In 1303, Padmini, a princess of the Rajputs (i.e., descendents of Hindu warrior caste clans), led other Rajput wives in a *jauhur*, a mass *sati*, rather than submit to the invading king of Delhi. In 1587, when the Mogul emperor Akbar attacked the Rajput city of Chittor, dozens of women, including five queens, nine princesses, and numerous wives and daughters of military leaders, died in another *jauhur* as their husbands perished on the battlefield.

By the seventeenth and eighteenth centuries, as India fell slowly under British domination, *sati* had, through a hardening of tradition and community expectation, become less voluntary. Outliving one's husband was seen as a great disgrace, an indication that the wife had not properly nurtured her spouse. Widows who did not redeem themselves and their spouses through *sati*, which guaranteed salvation to the couple and to seven generations of their descendents, were expected to spend the rest of their lives doing penance and revering the memories of their dead husbands. **Remarriage** was strictly forbidden. In this social context, a widow's unwillingness to submit to *sati* was increasingly met with strong public pressure to act or with outright coercion. Although the frequency of *sati*, whether voluntary or involuntary, is uncertain, and the rite was rare or nonexistent in some localities, British authorities in India in the early nineteenth century recorded several hundred instances per year.

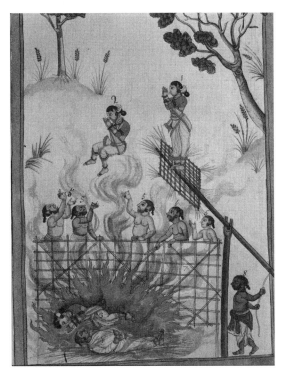

Funeral scene from the seventeenth-century manuscript, "The Book of the Mogul." © The Art Archive/ Biblioteca Nazionale Marciana Venice/Dagli Orti (A).

In 1829, the British governor-general, Lord William Bentinck, offended by what he saw as the barbarism of the rite, outlawed *sati* in all areas under direct British control. By 1846, all the independent Indian states had bowed to British pressure and also banned the rite. Although the practice continued despite these prohibitions, there was little open resistance until 1856, when the administration of another governor-general, Lord Charles John Canning, passed an act permitting widows to remarry. Suspecting a Christian attempt to subvert the Hindu religion, many Indians joined or supported the bloody but unsuccessful Sepoy Mutiny of 1857, while *sati* continued to be practiced into the twentieth century in remote parts of India.

Today, Indian law strictly prohibits *sati*, and even provides for sanctions against those who merely witness an act of *sati*, making no distinction between passive bystanders and those who actively promote the act. Other measures outlaw acts that glorify *sati* or its practitioners, and include laws that forbid the erection of shrines to dead widows, the encouragement of pilgrimages to *sati* sites, and any attempt to derive income from either. However, despite these laws and increasing societal pressure against the practice, *sati* still existed in the late twentieth century, the most famous case occurring in the state of Rajasthan in 1987, when an eighteen-year-old widow, acting with the encouragement of her family, voluntarily died upon her husband's funeral pyre. *See also* Hinduism; Marriage.

Further Reading: Fisch, Jörg. *Burning Women: A Global History of Widow Sacrifice from Ancient Times to the Present*. London: Seagull, 2006; Hawley, John Stratton, ed. *Sati, the Blessing and the Curse: The Burning of Wives in India*. New York: Oxford University Press, 1994; Mani, Lata. *Contentious Traditions: The Debate on Sati in Colonial India*. Berkeley and Los Angeles: University of California Press, 1998.

John A. Wagner

SAVONAROLA, MICHELE (1390–1462). Michele Savonarola was a university-trained physician born in Padua in 1390. He studied **medicine** at the University of Padua, where he later became a professor of medicine. In 1434 he was called to Ferrara to become personal physician to Nicolo III d'Este, Duke of Ferrara, and resided at the d'Este court. Beyond the wide recognition he received for his skill as a physician, he wrote many books and treatises on medically related topics. These include a recipe book, and a guidebook on the properties and merits of various Italian spas and thermal baths which was very popular in the **Middle East** and translated into both Persian and Arabic. He wrote several volumes of medical texts on gynecology and obstetrics in Latin, and was especially interested in instruments that could aid a difficult birth.

It was in his attitude toward the sexual roles especially that Savonarola showed that he was ahead of his time. In his handbook *Regimen for the Ladies of Ferrara*, written in 1460 in vernacular Italian and addressed to both midwives and laywomen, he stresses the importance of sexual satisfaction for both the male and the female participants in intercourse. At a time when most physicians and medical texts ignored the concept of a female orgasm, Savonarola advocated the importance of female orgasm in achieving conception. Thus he was a firm believer in foreplay, including fondling and rubbing both the male and female genitalia to arouse sexual desire and achieve orgasm. Some of his advice is written in a surprisingly jaunty and informal style, using such metaphors as "urging the gee-gee to make it to the post."

Because he wrote his book in the vernacular, it was available to a much wider audience than most of the medical texts of his day, which were written in Latin and therefore open only to the elite. Savonarola's handbook was one of a series of a large number of instructional manuals that became very popular in the Renaissance. Aimed at the educated middle class, these books were available at a reasonable price with the advent of the printing press. As most were written by male clerics, they reflect the patriarchal attitudes toward women that Renaissance society inherited. Against this tide of bias, Savonarola's book is more remarkable for its open attitude toward conjugal pleasure.

Savonarola was influential in the upbringing and education of his more famous grandson, the fiery friar Giralamo Savonarola, who before his cataclysmic decision to become a monk, was studying medicine and set to follow in his famous grandfather's footsteps. *See also* Childbirth.

Further Reading: O'Neill, Y. V. "Giovanni Michele Savonarola: An Atypical Renaissance Practitioner." *Clio Medica* 10, no. 2 (June 1975): 177–93.

Mary Hewlett

SCIENCE. Sexuality was studied and analyzed in many scientific traditions during the early modern period. Western early modern theories of sexuality differed between those that emphasized the similarities of the sexes, and those which emphasized their differences. The similarity school, drawing on Aristotelian and Galenic thought, believed women to be incomplete men, whose organs had not been fully pushed out due to insufficient heat. Thus the vagina was an inside-out penis, and the ovaries were often referred to as female testes. The similarity, or "one-sex," school emphasized the degree to which men's and women's organs were analogous—the male nipples to the female breasts, for example. The similarity school believed in the possibility of spontaneous sex changes caused by a sudden access of heat. Sex changes were believed to always be from female to male, as nature was always aiming at perfection, which was held to be the male. Some alleged cases of sexual transformation, such as the late sixteenth-century French girl-turned-boy Marie Germain, received extensive publicity. Another consequence of one-sex thinking was the emphasis placed on the female orgasm in conception. Since a man must climax to beget a child, a woman must also climax to conceive one.

The difference school, which had less ancient textual authority, conceived of men and women as radically different and complementary, at least in their sexual and reproductive roles. Difference thinkers minimized the importance of structural similarities and denied the possibility of spontaneous sex changes. The "two-sex" school also made a religious argument, claiming that since God created woman, and

God created all things perfect, women were equally perfect as men, although of an inferior kind. Sex changes were merely **hermaphrodites** whose male organs had been concealed, possibly women with enlarged clitorises, or simply frauds. The difference thinkers were an increasingly insistent presence in European anatomy beginning in the late sixteenth century.

The similarity approach was linked to an Aristotelian hierarchical cosmology. Women, exhibiting the qualities of coldness and moistness as opposed to the heat and dryness of men, were hierarchically subordinate to them. (Chinese medical science similarly identified heat and dryness with the male force of *yang* and cold and damp with the female force *yin*, although actual men and women participated in both forces.) Difference thinkers, however, often retained the categories of cold and heat to explain sexual difference, even though they were severed from the Aristotelian and Galenic context.

The most important change in Western scientific thinking about sexuality during the Renaissance was the rediscovery of the clitoris, ancient knowledge of which had been lost during the Middle Ages. Charles Estienne (c. 1505–1564), the first modern anatomist to describe it, associated the clitoris with urination. Estienne's description had no discernible influence, and priority in the "discovery" of the clitoris was keenly contested by two Italians. Gabriel Fallopio (1523–1562), best known for his discovery of the Fallopian tubes, described it in *Anatomical Observations*, a work written around 1550 but not published until 1561. Realdo Colombo (1510–1559) took advantage of the gap between Fallopio's writing and his publication to claim credit for the discovery in his *On Anatomy* (1559). Contemporaries generally judged Fallopio to have been the discoverer, but Colombo did innovate in his emphasis on the role of the clitoris in female sexual pleasure.

It took some time for the difference between the clitoris and the labia to become fully established in the medical literature. The establishment of the clitoris as a distinct organ of sexual pleasure tremendously affected the way male medical specialists thought about female sexuality, particularly in France. The clitoris's resemblance to the penis cast doubt on the "one-sex" approach to the vagina as an inside-out penis, but the clitoris had the greatest intellectual impact on the male scientific of sex between women. "Tribades" had been previously understood as anatomically normal women who performed sexually either by rubbing their genital regions together, or, much more shocking, using artificial instruments for penetration. Now women who penetrated other women were defined as monstrous, possessing freakishly enlarged clitorises. Clitoridectomy was recommended, and sometimes practiced, as a way of ending this behavior. *See also* Lesbianism; Medicine.

Further Reading: Furth, Charlotte. *A Flourishing Yin: Gender in China's Medical History, 960–1655*. Berkeley and Los Angeles: University of California Press, 1999; Laqueur, Thomas. *Making Sex: Body and Gender from the Greeks to Freud*. Cambridge, MA: Harvard University Press, 1990; Park, Katherine. "The Rediscovery of the Clitoris: French Medicine and the Tribade, 1570–1620." In *The Body in Parts: Fantasies of Corporeality in Early Modern Europe*, edited by David Hillman and Carla Mazzio, 170–93. New York: Routledge, 1997; Schleiner, Winfried. "Early Modern Controversies about the One-Sex Model." *Renaissance Quarterly* 53 (Spring, 2000): 180–91.

William E. Burns

SERAGLIO. *See* Harem/Seraglio

SHAKESPEARE, WILLIAM (1564–1616).

William Shakespeare was born in April 1654 in Stratford-upon-Avon, England. He married a pregnant Anne Hathaway on November 28, 1582, at the age of eighteen, but in spite of having three children together, the Shakespeares spent much of their married life apart—he in London, while she resided in Stratford. This distance, combined with the passionate intensity of his *Sonnets*, has lead to widespread speculation regarding his sexuality.

Shakespeare's *Sonnets*, published in 1609 and dedicated to the Earl of Southampton, bring the **homoeroticism** found in many of his plays to the foreground. Shakespeare's *Sonnets* appear to value the love of an unknown "fair youth" over the dangerous affections of a dark mistress. The indeterminacy of the beloved's gender in many of the sonnets exemplifies the opaqueness of sexuality in the early modern period. The *Sonnets* illustrate the extent to which love, or behavior, is not dictated by gender roles, an idea present in many plays.

In his late sixteenth-century comedy *A Midsummer Night's Dream*, the blurring of the line between love and sexuality forces Theseus to conclude that "the lunatic, the lover, and the poet / Are of imagination all compact" (4.2.7–8). Plays such as *The Merchant of Venice* are notable for the homoerotic bond between two of the central characters, and the Elizabethan-era prohibition against women acting on stage meant that female roles were performed by young apprentice boy actors, all of which contributed to the complex sexual dynamic in many of Shakespeare's plays. This blurring of gender lines became the basis for many of Shakespeare's comedies, including *As You Like It*, *Twelfth Night*, and *The Merchant of Venice*, in which female sexuality is often unleashed by cross-dressing. For example, in *As You Like It*, Rosalind, in disguise as Ganymede (itself a name that carries homoerotic undertones), insists that her beloved Orlando role-play and imagine her as Rosalind and molds him into the man she desires him to be.

In Shakespeare's tragedies, gendered desire becomes a more dangerous conceit. Demanding women, such as Goneril and Regan, become "unnatural hags" chasing their ambitious desires in *King Lear*, and Lady Macbeth asks spirits to "unsex me here" before plotting the murder of Duncan with her husband. The insistence of female desire within such plays as *Othello* and *Romeo and Juliet* often destabilizes the male character's perceptions of female chastity and obedience, resulting in chaos. Othello's immediate reaction to Iago's implicit suggestion of Desdemona's infidelity is to lament "that we can call these delicate creatures ours / And not their appetites!" (3.3.273–74), and later, as he prepares to strangle her, promises that "I will kill thee / And love thee after" (5.2.18–9). Most unsettling of all is Hamlet's horror of his mother's choice "to post / with such dexterity to incestuous sheets" (1.1.156–7) which inspires his rejection of Ophelia, and precipitates much of the play's tragic outcome. Shakespeare wrote his final play in 1613, before retiring to Stratford-Upon-Avon, where he died in April 1616. *See also* Actors; Ganymede; Theater.

Further Reading: Orgel, Stephen. *Impersonations: The Performance of Gender in Shakespeare's England*. Cambridge: Cambridge University Press, 1996; Smith, Bruce R. *Homosexual Desire in Shakespeare's England: A Cultural Poetics*. Chicago: University of Chicago Press, 1991; Traub, Valerie. *Desire and Anxiety: Circulations of Sexuality in Shakespearean Drama*. New York: Routledge, 1992.

Louise Geddes

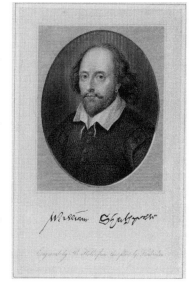

William Shakespeare. Courtesy of the Library of Congress.

SIKANDAR LODHI (d. 1517). Sikandar Lodhi (r. 1489–1517) was the second ruler of the Afghan dynasty, which was founded by his father, Behlol Lodhi. Sikandar was a most successful ruler who brought back the lost prestige of the Sultanate in northern India by completing the pacification of Jaunpur (1493), campaigning into Bihar, and founding the city of Agra (1504), which is today famous for the Taj Mahal, a royal tomb built in the city in the seventeenth century. In addition to his military skills, Sikandar became known for his religious fanaticism. Like his predecessors, Sikandar enforced the policy of Muslim occupation in India; he sought to replace the fabric of Hindu society and culture with a Muslim culture through the destruction of Indian religious language and places of knowledge. His punitive methods were described as "butchering" even by the partisan co-religionist Niamatullah in his chronicle *Tarikh-i-Khan Jahan Lodi*. Sikandar's counselors objected to his destruction of the Rajas symbolic Hindu temples and criticized his persecution of priests and intellectuals, including Kabir, the poet and mystic of the Bhakti tradition.

Little is known of Sikandar's private life and of the private lives of the Afghan rulers in general. Chroniclers mainly reported their military and religious campaigns. We do not know how many wives and **concubines** Sikandar had, or how many children they gave him. By custom, the imperial palace would host a multitude of women from diverse **castes** and religions. Because of the constant acquisition of territories, female slaves were abundant. **Marriage** alliances with neighboring states brought Sikandar princesses and entourages of servants. He rejected a marriage agreement with a powerful Rajput family when their alliance became unnecessary. Rajput princesses retained a privileged position in the palace and were allowed to keep their Hindu shrines; the influence of their families guaranteed them protection. Non-Islamic women eventually converted when not protected by strong political influence. Although women in India were more educated than women in the Muslim Ottoman empire, it is difficult to assess the educational level of the women in the Lodhi court. In later periods, women in the royal families were generally educated, patronizing the arts and writing in poetry. The ritualized and stylized character of Sufi poetry with the Persian lack of distinction between "he" and "she" makes it difficult to recognize any distinguished female voice.

In the seventeenth century, Princess Zebunnisa (1638–1702) was an example of a "hidden" female voice that we do know of. The eldest daughter of the Mughal Emperor Aurangzeb (1618–1707), Zebunnisa first lived in Agra and then held a separate court at Delhi, where she patronized arts and letters, becoming a major poet of her times. She was educated in Persian and Arabic, mathematics and astronomy, and built numerous astronomical observatories, schools, and sarais. Zebunnisa influenced her father politically and never married. Her verses were later compiled and published as *Diwan-i-Makhfi*, Diwan meaning the "hidden" or "invisible" one. *See also* Hinduism; Islam; Sufi Romances.

Further Reading: Lohdi Dynasty: http://www.indhistory.com/lodi-dynasty.html; Sikandar's Mausoleum: http://archnet.org/library/images/thumbnails.tcl?location_id=3599.

Lucia Bortoli

SLAVERY. Slavery is the ownership of one person by another, where the owned possess few or no rights, and are considered property under the law. They can be moved around or resold without their permission, and have limits, varying from society to society, on their ability to choose an occupation, their husbands and wives, or other sexual partners.

There are two types of slavery: domestic slavery, where individuals work in households or businesses; and productive slavery, in which slaves are employed in mines or in agricultural businesses. During the early modern period, individuals could become slaves if they were kidnapped by slavers or pirates; were born into slavery; if they were convicted or a crime, or were debtors; were sold by their families; or if they sold themselves into slavery to assuage a debt.

Slavery, and the slave trade, was ubiquitous throughout the early modern era, and there were few societies of the time that did not have, or did not permit, slavery. Most of the countries and societies in **Asia**, **Africa**, India, the **Americas**, and **Europe** permitted slavery under a wide variety of conditions. On religious grounds, slavery was permitted by Jewish, Muslim, and Christian societies, provided the enslaved individual was not a member of the owner's religion: a Christian was not to own a Christian, a Muslim not to own a Muslim, a Jew not a Jew. The Aztecs used slaves in rituals for religious sacrifice.

The early modern era saw the continuation and expansion of the international slave trade, by means of which millions of slaves were transferred far away from their homes and kinship networks to other parts of the world. African slaves were moved within Africa, from its west coast to the Americas and the Caribbean, and from its east coast up to Arabia, India, and China. Tatars, Slavs, Russians, Moors, Circassians, and Ethiopians were to be found in Italy, after moving down through slave-trading centers in Denmark and northern Europe or across the sea from Constantinople. Within Africa, women and children were the most desirable slaves, while male slaves were mostly sent to the Americas for hard labor on plantations. In Italy, female slaves under the age of eighteen were considered the most desirable, with their price increasing if they were virgins, and therefore considered to be of good moral character.

Certain vulnerable populations became the particular targets of slave cultures. The eastern Slavs were targeted by the Crimean Khanate after 1475, and almost completely obliterated or enslaved. This kind of targeting led other groups, like the Ndebu of Africa, to migrate long distances in an effort to avoid the predations of slave raids. The act of enslavement came with high casualties—the Khanate would kill two or more for every slave caught, while an average of 10–20 percent of the slaves on the ships that transported African slaves to the New World would die on the trip.

Slavery was considered economically and socially necessary for many slave-owning cultures. In many cultures, slave made up a significant portion of the population: in Zanzibar, a city-state and major slave trade hub on the eastern coast of Africa, upward of 90 percent of the population was made up of slaves, while over a third of the population of Senegambia was enslaved. Some states came to depend upon slaves socially and economically: the Ottoman Empire, for example, depended upon slaves for governmental administration, military protection in the form of the feared Janissaries, for many handicrafts, and for servants. The army of the Songhai Empire in what is now Mali was made up mostly of slaves, and the Empire had a high slave utilization rate throughout its economy and society. Although a very few slaves did manage to attain high positions in the societies they were in, as in China and among the Ottomans, slaves by and large were socially the lowest of the low, without honor or personal dignity, or anything except that which was given to them by their owners.

Normal human relationships were often impossible for slaves to maintain. In Islamic areas, slaves were permitted to marry with the permission of their owners, and sometimes owners would arrange marriages for their slaves. Amongst the slave owners of the American South, and Thai slave owners, there was no regard given to personal bonds amongst slaves. Slave families would be broken up, and members sold or parted from each other without a second thought on the part of the slave owner.

Female slaves in particular were subject to the desires of their owners around the world. Many slaves were sold into **prostitution**. Slave courtesans in the Ottoman Empire would be trained in the arts of entertainment; music, dancing, and singing; as well as being made available for sexual encounters. Many slaves were sold into harems, or made concubines in owner households. A male Muslim slave owner was entitled to sex with his slaves. (Muslim women were not.) Any resulting children were the owner's to control, and were slaves themselves. If the child was formally recognized, then it would be freed, and the mother given manumission upon the death of the father. In Italy, if a slave became pregnant by an individual other than her owner, the ownership of the child became an issue. A slave's value was diminished by pregnancy, and in Venice a man who impregnated another man's slave had to pay a fine to the owner equivalent to the slave's full value. Eventually, the problem of unauthorized sex with slaves in Italy remained grave enough that a man who slept with another man's slave was subject to a fine of 1,000 florins, or even be hanged. The crime was clearly an offense against property; the opinions or feelings of the slave, or even whether the encounter was consensual or a **rape**, were not relevant in a court of law.

One unintended result of the sexual encounters between slave owners and slaves was the mixing of races. As children of slaves became free and combined with the rest of the population, mixed-race individuals came to form a large percentage of the slave culture population. In North Africa, this combination of races was not problematic, and the positive word *mizaj*, or "mixture," was used to describe it. What mattered was cultural practice, rather than skin color. In other areas, there was extensive religious commentary on the subject, and interracial sex was considered transgressive and cause for community conflict in Spain. In central America, the mixing of native slave populations, through concubinage or overt rape, with Spanish settlers and conquistadors led to the creation of mestizo culture, while the mixed-race children of African and Carib slaves and European slave owners (mulattos) also came to make up a large percentage of the populations of those areas. The lives of many of these children remained harsh, even if freed, as the prevailing racism of the dominant European culture made it difficult, if not impossible, to move up the social ladder.

Slavery declined in Europe during the Renaissance, but continued unabated throughout the rest of the world. The 1500s saw the beginnings of the Atlantic slave trade, which brought millions of African slaves to the New World, and had deep and lasting repercussions for North American culture up to the present day. In Italy, and elsewhere in Europe, the widespread ownership of slaves declined after 1500 with the closing of the Black Sea trade to Italian merchants cut off supply and prices for human beings rose too high. However, slavery remained legal, and slaves continued to be bought as curiosities in the same way as exotic animals might have been during the Renaissance.

The inestimable human misery caused by slavery made it of the most despicable of human activities, and the human cost in destroyed cultures, family units, and lives made it one of the great tragedies of the early modern era. However, there was little outcry against the practice of slavery during the early modern period, with some exceptions. In Japan, in 1588, Toyotomi Hideyoshi abolished slavery, after a period of decline in the ownership of slaves in the country. Elsewhere, the Frenchman Jean Bodin (1530–1596) founded a school of anti-slavery thought, but his ideas, against the flow of early modern religious and social thought in Europe, did not catch on for many years. *See also* Concubines; Harem/Seraglio.

Further Reading: Collins, Robert O. *Problems in African History: The Precolonial Centuries.* Markus Weiner, 2005; Davidson, Basil. *Africa in History: Themes and Outlines.* Collier Books, 1991; Davis, Natalie Zemon. *Trickster Travels: A Sixteenth-Century Muslim Between Worlds.* New York: Hill and Wang, 2006; Mvuyekure, Pierre-Damien, ed. *World Eras.* Vol. 10: *West African Kingdoms 500-1590.* Farmington Hills, MI: Thomson Gale, 2003; Origo, Iris. "The Domestic Enemy: The Eastern Slaves in Tuscany in the Fourteenth and Fifteenth Centuries." *Speculum* XXX, no. 3 (July 1955): 321–66; "Slavery." *Encyclopaedia Britannica Online.* 20 Aug. 2007. http://www.britannica.com/eb/article-9109538.

Kristen Pederson Chew

SODOMY. *See* Anal Sex

"THE STORY OF LAYLA AND MAJNUN" (Ganjavi). "The Story of Layla and Majnun" appears at the center of the *Khamsa*, or "the Five Poems," a collection of narratives written by the greatest romantic epic poet in Persian literature, Nizami Ganjani (1141–1209). The story is based upon a well-known Bedouin romance of the seventh century that survived in several folk versions. Nizami collected a number of them and shaped them into a single poem of 4,000 stanzas.

The poem narrates the tale of madness and death of Qays, nicknamed Majnun (madman), who makes the fatal mistake of professing his love for Layla publicly and causing the anger of her family. Qays has all it takes to become a powerful tribe leader until he falls prey to **love sickness**, an actual mental and physical disease in the medical manuals of the times (this form of insanity is still considered today a cause of suicide among the youth). Majnun loses his mind and escapes into the mountain wilderness, where he spends his time singing the praises of his beloved. The overpowering intensity of the experience becomes the reason of his being; he transforms his love for the unattainable Layla into a religious search for purity and beauty, reaching a state of spiritual ecstasies (described as a Sufi experience, by some). The poem offers Majnun's sickness as the necessary medium for the hero's eloquent outpouring of poetic creativity.

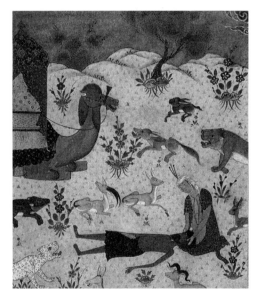

Layla Comforting Majnun, a miniature from the sixteenth-century Turkish manuscript, "Majalis al-Ushshaq by Sultan Husayn Mirza" (MS. Ouseley Add 24 folio 66v). © The Art Archive/Bodleian Library Oxford.

Although suffering from equal emotional deprivation, Layla remains quite commonsensical; with dignity she safeguards the honor of her family, and at the same time devises to remain faithful to Majnun. In Nizami's version she marries but refuses to consummate the marriage; in other versions, she submits to her marital obligations and has children. Her story provides the reader with a reliable portrait of the living conditions of Muslim women in the twelfth century. Forced to live in *purdah*, Layla denounces her imprisonment in her father's tent and her inability to act upon or to express her emotions publicly. In Nizami's narrative, she comes across as an ambivalent character: on one hand she is praised for accepting her society's rules with dignity, but on the other she is indirectly accused of cruelty. Nizami's portrayal of Layla's husband hopelessly waiting for acceptance at her door is heart breaking.

"The Story of Layla and Majnun" was well known in Europe and it influenced many expressions of contrasted love in the Middle Ages and the Renaissance. Among them are the troubadours' celebration of the inaccessible and beautiful lady, Dante's transformation of his earthly love for Beatrice into a spiritual search for God, and William **Shakespeare**'s rendering of Romeo and Juliet's purity and vulnerability.

Further Reading: Ganjavi, Nizami. *The Fire of Love, The Love Story of Layla and Majnun.* Translated by Louis Roger. New York: Writers Club Press, 2002.

Lucia Bortoli

SUCCUBI. *See* Incubi/Succubi

SUFI ROMANCES. Islamic mystical poetry is multifaceted, but at its heart it addresses the eternal **love** between man and God. Sufiism, or Islamic mysticism, has had a major influence on the literature of Muslim societies. This manifested itself in a plethora of narrative and didactic mystical works in Arabic, Persian, Turkish, and the local vernaculars of the Indian subcontinent. Typically, these romances were written as poetry rather than prose, which were usually reserved for manuals and hagiographies; however, there are a number of prose Sufi allegories. Persian practitioners developed the *mathnawï* form of poetry, and its use of rhyming couplets made it extremely suitable for epics, narratives, and didactic works. Because it was rhymed, these *mathnawï* works lent themselves easily to memorization, which was a great advantage for those who were illiterate.

The *mathnawï*'s characteristics caused it to become the preferred narrative story telling form. This form frequently inserted frame stories, parables, and allegories into these lengthy *mathnawï*'s. Such Sufi masters as Ùakïm Sana'ï, Farid al-Dïn 'Attär and Jalaluddin Rumi perfected the *mathnawï*'s use in this genre. While these mystics did not necessarily write separate *mathnawï*'s focusing solely on a story of a Sufi romance, the form allowed them to insert numerous Sufi romantic themes throughout their works. The Sufi romances took their characters from a wide cast of famous and not-so-famous lovers, usually associated with the Arabs, Byzantines, Egyptians, Persians, and Turks. As **Islam** and Sufiism expanded outside their original confines of the **Middle East**, North **Africa**, and central and south **Asia**, and with the additional proliferation of literatures in local vernaculars, new Sufi romances emerged. This occurred most notably on the Indian subcontinent with the emergence of Urdu, Hindi, Punjabi, Bengali, and other new written vernaculars.

These romances are far from uniform and include a wide variety of lovers. Perhaps, the most famous lovers are Majnun and Layla. Their story emerged from the pre-Islamic desert poetry of the Arabian Peninsula, where it introduced the concept of unrequited love (*ùubb al-udhrï*). Majnun was forbidden from marrying his beloved Layla and as a result became crazy and demented from his incessant love. Ultimately he wasted away to nothing. The Arabic original was a story of secular love. Nizami Ganjavi's (1141–1209) Persian *mathnawï* "Majnun and Layli" is perhaps one of the most famous of the "Sufi Romances." However, Nizami wrote that the story could be interpreted as a tale of earthly love as well as a parable of mystical love. Numerous other Persian and Turkish *mathnawi*s about Majnun and Layla have been written, notably, one by the mystic Jami (1414–1492).

A few more additional characters, who became the subjects of these allegories of divine love, are Yusuf and Zulaykha (Joseph and Potiphar's wife), Farhad and Shirin, Salämän and Absäl, Gul and Nawruz and Mahmud and Ayaz. All of them highlight a loss of reasoning, which is totally overpowered and consumed by the love of God, but all are different. Yusuf and Zulaykha came from the Torah and the Koran. Farhad was a humble stonecutter, while Shirin was a princess. Salämän was a prince and Absäl was his nurse, twenty years his senior. Gul and Nawruz were completely fictional while Mahmud was a sultan and Ayaz was his serving boy. *See also* Love Sickness.

Further Reading: De Bruijn, J.T.P. *Persian Sufi Poetry, an Introduction to the Mystical Use of Classical Poems*. London: Curzon Press, 1997; Schimmel, Annemarie. *Mystical Dimensions of Islam*. Chapel Hill: University of North Carolina Press, 1975.

Mark David Luce

SUTTEE. *See Sati*

T

TAOISM. *See* Daoism

THEATER. The European Renaissance saw a major shift from the writing and performance of exclusively sacred to secular theater. The English theater tradition of Christopher **Marlowe** and William **Shakespeare** grew out of medieval morality plays, a communal, primarily amateur tradition that presented short didactic or liturgical plays with the primary aim of offering religious instruction. The break with the morality tradition saw English theaters locate themselves in "the Liberties," an area beyond the walls of the City of London, and beyond the jurisdiction of the city fathers. Many playwrights thrived in this gritty urban environment, including Christopher Marlowe, who was alleged to have noted that "they that love not tobacco and boys are fools," and who presented a heretic, a tyrant, and an openly homosexual king on stage, before being killed in a bar brawl at the age of twenty-nine.

Spain employed a tradition, similar to that of the English morality and miracle plays, known as *autos sacramentales*. Literally "sacramental acts," *autos* were often heavily allegorical and presented alongside secular plays throughout Spain. Unlike the English morality tradition, *autos* flourished well into the seventeenth century, becoming more elaborate and lavish. Different genres thrived together during what is now known as Spain's Golden Age, and many playwrights, such as Pedro Calderon de la Barca, were adept at writing both *autos* and full-length plays. The popularity of these plays transferred across the Atlantic to the Spanish colonies—Sor Juana Inès de la Cruz was a Mexican nun who wrote *autos* as well as popular secular plays during the seventeenth century. The most prolific playwright to come from Spain was Lope de Vega, thought to have written over two thousand dramas and *autos* in his lifetime. De Vega fathered at least sixteen children with many different women (many of whom are thought to have inspired the strong female characters in his work), despite taking clerical orders in 1614. Throughout his career, he managed to balance a devotion to the church with a complicated personal life.

Theater flourished in other areas around the globe during the early modern era, but remained deeply connected to its ancient origins. In **Africa**, performance existed alongside oral storytelling traditions, integrating traditional dance, spoken text, and religious ritual. In **India**, theater continued to be viewed as a form of performed poetry, looking back to the Golden Age of Sanskrit drama in the second and third centuries. As a direct response to the writings of Zeami, Japanese Nôh theater flourished during the fifteenth and sixteenth centuries as an aristocratic form of entertainment, using elements of traditional Japanese dance to narrate tales. The Nôh tradition was highly stylized, sung by men in masks and accompanied by music. During the seventeenth century, civil strife in Japan destabilized Nôh's popularity, and it was eventually overtaken by Kabuki as the dominant mode of Japanese theater. *See also* Actors.

Further Reading: Banham, Martin. *A History of Theatre in Africa*. Cambridge: Cambridge University Press, 2004; Goldberg, Jonathan. *Sodometries: Renaissance Texts, Modern Sexualities*. Stanford, CA: Stanford University Press, 1992; Stoll, Anita K., and Leslie R. Smith. *Gender, Identity and Representation in Spain's Golden Age*. Lewisburg, PA: Bucknell University Press, 2000.

Louise Geddes

***THE TRAVELS OF SIR JOHN MANDEVILLE* (c. 1366).** Noted for its unusually explicit commentary on both Western and non-Western sexuality, *The Travels of Sir John Mandeville*, a late medieval travel narrative probably written between 1365 and 1371, was immensely popular during the early modern period. By 1500, it had been translated into almost every major European language, and it survives today in over three hundred manuscripts. Although the text was once taken as autobiographical, it actually combines elements from multiple previous narratives into a plausible, coherent whole. The narrator of the *Travels* describes his fantastic voyage through the lands of **Africa**, **Asia**, and the **Middle East**, often pausing to digress on the economic, political, and moral characteristics of the lands through which he journeyed. Claiming that "I have compiled this book and written it, as it came into my mind, in the year of Our Lord Jesus Christ 1366, that is to say in the thirty-fourth year after I left this land and took my way to those parts" (Moseley, 189), the *Travels*'s multifaceted textual legacy as pilgrimage guide, travel manual, personal memoir, and proto-anthropological record fueled its consistent popularity through the seventeenth century, preconditioning accounts of travel to exotic locales from Christopher Columbus to *Othello*. However, in the early modern age of exploration, the fantastic content of the *Travels* caused it to fall out of use as a serious book, although it retained some popularity as a fantastic, allegorical travel story.

One of the many unusual aspects of the *Travels* is the narrator's unusually frank (for the period) pseudo-anthropological commentary on sex. The narrator typically employs a Western standard of sexual morality by which to measure foreign sexual practice. Throughout the text, he attributes sexual excess to foreign others, and reports on the legal or moral precedents for sexual and marital activity in these societies. He often records punishments for **adultery**, spends time describing the Indian practice of suttee (*see* **Sati**), habitually notes the presence or absence of **incest**, and repeatedly characterizes the "Saracens" as a polygamous culture who imagine paradise full of "beautiful damsels, and [a man] shall lie with them whenever he wishes, and he will always find them virgins" (Moseley, 104). This hypersexualized view of the foreign other is by no means restricted to the Islamic East, but manifested throughout the text as a primary attribute of the exotic non-Western other.

The narrator's adherence to Western sexual norms, however, sometimes becomes relative to his larger moral judgment on the culture in question. Reporting, for example, that the naturally innocent and somewhat naive inhabitants of the isle of Lamory "go completely naked and they are not ashamed to show themselves as God made them," he elsewhere notes that in countries influenced by Saturn, such as India and Ethiopia, the residents are habitually lazy, and because of the heat "women . . . are not ashamed if men see them naked. Much ugliness can be seen there" (Moseley, 120, 127).

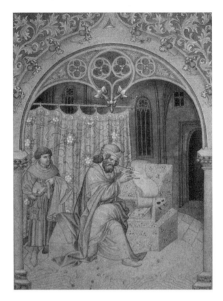

Sir John Mandeville in his study, fifteenth century. © HIP/Art Resource, NY.

Throughout the text, the narrator alternates between such practical rationales for non-Western behavior and conventionally pejorative moral critique as an observational model. This containment of potentially subversive appreciation of different cultural practices provides continuous tension throughout the text.

Even more remarkably, the titular Mandeville often uses reports of foreign attitudes toward sex as an opportunity to comment on the hypocrisy of Western sexuality. Reporting that Saracens "say Christian men are wicked and evil because they do not keep the Commandment of the Gospel, with Jesus Christ ordained for them" allows the narrator to comment at length on the abuses of the clergy and the hypocrisy of the Church in Europe; likewise, his observations that the people of Calamay "suffer so much pain and mortification of their bodies for love of [their] idol that hardly would any Christian man suffer the half—nay, not a tenth—for love of Our Lord Jesus Christ" allows him to praise the dedication of these virtuous pagans while criticizing the general cynicism that pervaded Western Christendom (Moseley, 107, 126).

Although he often characterizes non-Western sex and sexuality as dangerous, deceitful, and, frequently, ugly, the narrator makes no attempt to deny that sexuality is everywhere a part of culture, occasionally the focus of culture, and always a powerful force in human societies. *See also* Christianity; Islam.

Further Reading: Bassnett, Susan. "Travelling and Translating." *World Literature Written in English* 40, no. 2 (2004): 66–76; Camargo, Martin. "The Book of John Mandeville and the Geography of Identity." In *Marvels, Monsters, and Miracles: Studies in the Medieval and Early Modern Imaginations*, edited by Timothy S. Jones and David A. Sprunger, 67–87. Kalamazoo, MI: Western Michigan University, 2002; Fleck, Andrew. "Here, There, and In Between: Representing Difference in the Travels of Sir John Mandeville." *Studies in Philology* 97, no. 4 (2000): 379–400; Higgins, Iain. "Imagining Christendom from Jerusalem to Paradise: Asia in Mandeville's Travels." In *Discovering New Worlds: Essays on Medieval Exploration and Imagination*, edited by Scott D. Westrem, 91–114. New York: Garland, 1991; Higgins, Iain Macleod. *Writing East: The "Travels" of Sir John Mandeville*. Philadelphia: Philadelphia University Press, 1997; Lomperis, Linda. "Medieval Travel Writing and the Question of Race." *Journal of Medieval and Early Modern Studies* 31, no. 1 (2001): 147–64; Moseley, C.W.R.D., ed. *The Travels of Sir John Mandeville*. New York: Penguin Books, 1983; Salih, Sarah. "Idols and Simulacra: Paganity, Hybridity and Representation in Mandeville's Travels." In *The Monstrous Middle Ages*, edited by Bettina Bildhauer and Robert Mills, 113–33. Cardiff: University of Wales Press, 2003; Sobecki, Sebastian I. "Mandeville's Thought of the Limit: The Discourse of Similarity and Difference in the Travels of Sir John Mandeville." *Review of English Studies* 53, no. 211 (2002): 329–43.

Barbara Zimbalist

TRENT, COUNCIL OF (1545–1563). Convoked by Pope Paul III (r. 1534–1549) in 1545, the Council of Trent, an assembly of bishops and theologians that met intermittently until 1563 in the Italian city of Trent, was the nineteenth ecumenical council of the Roman Catholic Church. Because it responded to the doctrinal attacks of Protestant reformers, such as Martin **Luther**, and addressed both Protestant and Catholic demands for institutional reform, the Council of Trent was instrumental in defining the future shape and direction of the Catholic Church. Among the many issues addressed by the council during its three main periods of activity (1545–1547, 1551–1552, and 1562–1563) was the question concerning the sacrament of matrimony, the Catholic view of which had been strongly challenged by Protestant reformers.

Calls for a council, initiated in hopes of reconciling the Protestants with Rome, were first issued in the early 1520s, with Charles V, the Holy Roman emperor and king of Spain, being the chief royal proponent of such a meeting. However, political and military factors, such as the ongoing war between the Empire and France, and clerical resistance, particularly on the part of popes who feared conciliar limitations on their authority, delayed the opening of the council until well past the time when divisions between Protestants and Catholics could have been healed. These tensions continued even after the council convened, and help to explain its length, its intermittent sessions, its lack of a clear agenda, and its acrimonious debates. Political and ecclesiastical conflicts also explain the council's fluctuating attendance; only thirty-one prelates were present for the opening session, and no more than 200 were present at any time during the council's existence. Also, none of the five popes who reigned between 1545 and 1563 ever attended a session at Trent, with Paul IV (r. 1555–1559), who believed that he could reform the Church more swiftly and appropriately on his own authority, flatly refusing to reconvene the assembly.

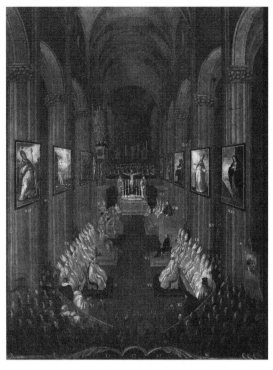

Council of Trent Inaugural Session, by Nicolo Dorigati. © The Art Archive/Museo Tridentino Arte Sacra Trento/ Dagli Orti (A).

The council made no attempt to devise a complete statement of Catholic belief, but sought instead to address the chief criticisms of Protestants and to reform the most egregious clerical abuses. In 1546, the council responded to Luther's emphasis on scripture as the sole basis for teaching and belief by declaring that apostolic tradition must also be considered. By accepting the Vulgate, the traditional Latin text of the Bible, and by retaining Latin as the liturgical language, the council implicitly rejected the Protestant demand for publication of vernacular Bibles to encourage the reading of scripture by the laity, a practice that the Church continued to regard as dangerous to the faith. Responding to Luther's doctrine of justification through faith alone, the council decreed that while salvation came indeed through grace, the efficacy of good works could not be dismissed. Finally, in a rejection of Protestant attempts to reduce the number to two—baptism and the Eucharist—the council reconfirmed the existence of seven sacraments, including matrimony.

Although all attempts to reform the papacy or to produce a statement of papal supremacy failed, the council enacted significant reforms of the episcopacy and the parish clergy. The council decreed that bishops had to be resident in their dioceses and could not hold more than one ecclesiastical office at a time. Bishops were also to hold regular synods with their diocesan clergy, were to promote more and better preaching and were to preach regularly themselves, and were to more strictly oversee the selection of candidates for the priesthood and the qualifications of confessors. Each diocese was also required to establish a seminary for the training of poor boys for the priesthood, a practice that over time became the accepted method of training all priests.

On November 11, 1563, as part of the decrees resulting from its twenty-fourth session, the council issued its pronouncements regarding **marriage**. In response to contrary Protestant beliefs, the council upheld the inclusion of matrimony among the sacraments of the Church and reconfirmed the Church's ban on clerical marriage. Matrimonial cases remained the province of ecclesiastical judges and the prohibition against weddings taking place during certain times of the year (e.g., Advent, Lent), which Protestants derided as superstition, was maintained. The council also declared that, to be valid, all marriages had to be performed by a priest in the presence of two or three witnesses, and that no valid marriage could be made through force or abduction. All parish priests were enjoined to keep a book in which all marriages held in the parish were registered. Finally, besides clarifying the technical impediments to marriage and the reasons for which marriages could be considered invalid and therefore dissolvable, the council reaffirmed, against Protestant belief, that **virginity** and **celibacy** were more blessed states than marriage. *See also* The Reformation.

Further Reading: Bulman, Raymond F., and Frederick J. Parrella, eds. *From Trent to Vatican II: Historical and Theological Investigations*. Oxford: Oxford University Press, 2006; Jedin, Hubert. *Crisis and Closure of the Council of Trent*. Translated by N. D. Smith. London: Sheed & Ward, 1967; Jedin, Hubert. *A History of the Council of Trent*. Translated by Ernest Graf. St. Louis: B. Herder Book Company, 1957–1960; Tanner, Norman P., ed. *Decrees of the Ecumenical Councils*. Vol. 2: *Trent to Vatican II*, 655–799. Washington, DC: Georgetown University Press, 1990. 655–799.

John A. Wagner

TWO-SPIRITED PEOPLE. *See* Berdache

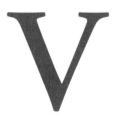

VENEREAL DISEASE. "Venereal disease" (Lat., *morbus venereus*, *lues venerea*) is the most widespread synonym given to the "French disease" or "French pox" (Lat., *morbus Gallicus*) in early modern Europe. The adjective *venereus/a* stresses the direct relationship between this disease and the pleasures of Venus or, in other words, its close bond to individual sexual behavior. The Latin noun *lues* was applied from antiquity to any condition that liquefied flesh, but also emphasizes the early modern perception of venereal disease as a contagious and calamitous scourge from both physical and moral viewpoints.

Over the sixteenth century, the designation "venereal disease" was mostly used in France, where it became increasingly widespread not only in the medical academic world but also at popular levels, not least because the French rejected a name implying that this disease came originally from France and was even natural to them. Yet, during the seventeenth century, the designation "venereal disease" (*morbus venereus* as well as *lues venerea*) was adopted all over Europe, sharing an *ex aequo* leadership with that of "French pox," whose use declined dramatically in eighteenth-century Europe at the expenses of the former.

When the French pox broke out epidemically in Europe in the mid-1490s, contemporary evidence concurred in perceiving it as a new, unheard-of disease included among the numerous calamities (floods, earthquakes, epidemics, famines, wars) that befell Europeans—Italians, in particular—at the end of that century. The first news about it went back to Italy in late 1495 and early 1496. Apparently, it spread following the itinerary covered by the French army of King Charles VIII during its overland retreat from the kingdom of Naples, and its rapid diffusion throughout Europe has been traditionally related to the breaking up of a mercenary army of disparate origins. At all events, the notoriety the designation "French pox" soon achieved all over Italy was closely associated with the tragic consequences of this French invasion for the fragile Italian political equilibrium. Additionally, as at the turn of the sixteenth century, Spaniards replaced the French as the new *barbari stranieri* who were devastating Italy, and Italians were prompt to accept that the new disease also originally came from the New World. The great prestige and cultural hegemony of Renaissance Italy throughout Europe were highly instrumental in ensuring the rapid popularization of both theories into a single and integrated narrative in early modern Europe.

Medical practitioners described the French pox as a loathsome and incurable disease consisting of sores usually beginning in the genitals but eventually covering the whole body, and of severe aches in the bones. This lingering and disfiguring condition was initially related to a range of various kinds of causes (divine punishment, corrupt air, harmful star constellations, and bad life regime, among others), which could be at work either collectively or separately. Yet, from the late 1490s, some doctors began to claim that a specific external cause transmissible through contagion by contact—sexual, mostly—could also be involved in the spread of the French pox. Attention to its venereal transmission did not stop growing as time went by, although the ways through which the new disease was linked to sex were as plural, open, and equivocal as the views about disease causality owing to Latin Galenism—the medical system dominant among university practitioners in Renaissance Europe. Until the mid eighteenth century, the unity of the venereal disease on the basis of a unique and specific *virus venereum* was unanimously defended by European academic doctors, whether they were ascribed to Galenism, to chemical **medicine**, or to any other medical school.

The designation "venereal disease" as synonymous with "French pox" does not appear to have been first recorded as the title of a medical work until 1527, when the French doctor Jacques de Béthencourt published in Paris *Nova poenitentialis quadragesima, necnon purgatorium in morbum Gallicum sive venereum* [*New Penitential Lent and Also a Purgatory for the French or Venereal Disease*]. Béthencourt, who was then practicing medicine in Rouen, widely used the language and imagery of religion to support his medical views, so that both the title and contents of his printed work evoke the climate of religious exaltation and of moral rearmament present in **Reformation** Europe.

Like plague and other infectious diseases, venereal disease damaged all social strata and ravaged the most humble people, although its wide diffusion among courts and urban patriciate—along with the quantity and expressiveness of surviving historical sources referring to these elites—promoted its perception as a condition typical of the privileged social strata. At the turn of the sixteenth century, medical practitioners debated each other whether courtiers were, or were not, more likely victims of venereal disease than the common people by arguing from alleged differences between those who were well-off people and the poor in terms of complexion, regime, social life, and sexual behavior. Sometimes their views implied a criticism of life at court by contrast to life at the countryside, which was allegedly considered to be healthier both morally and physically. Yet, according to the theologian Erasmus of Rotterdam's complaints, venereal disease had become so typical in sixteenth-century Europe that it had turned people entirely to pleasure, instead of being considered as a scourge sent by God to correct and make humankind think about chastity and moderation. He wrote, "[a]mong courtiers, who see themselves as beautiful and funny people, anybody free from the French Pox [*scabiem Gallicam*] is at risk of being considered plebeian and rustic" (Allen & Allen: VIII [1934], 383). *See also* Abortion and Contraception; Brothels; Henry VIII, King of England.

Further Reading: Allen, Peter Lewis. *The Wages of Sin: Sex, and Disease, Past and Present.* Chicago: University of Chicago Press, 2000; Allen, P. S., and H. M. Allen. *Opus epistolarum Des. Erasmi Roterdami.* 12 vols. Oxford: Clarendon Press, 1906–1958; Arrizabalaga, Jon, John Henderson, and Roger French. *The Great Pox: The French Disease in Renaissance Europe.* New Haven, CT: Yale University Press, 1997; Siena, Kevin. *Venereal Disease, Hospitals and the Urban Poor: London's "Foul Wards," 1600–1800.* Rochester, NY: University of Rochester Press, 2004; Siena, Kevin, ed. *Sins of the Flesh: Responding to Sexual Disease in Early Modern Europe.* Toronto: Victoria University in the University of Toronto, 2005; Stein, Claudia. *Die Behandlung der Franzosenkrankheit in der Frühen Neuzeit am Beispiel Augsburgs.* Stuttgart: Medizin, Gesellschaft und Geschichte [Beihefte, 19], 2003; Temkin, Oswei. "On the History of "Morality and Syphilis." In *The Double Face of Janus and Other Essays in the History of Medicine,* edited by Oswei Temkin, 472–84 Baltimore: Johns Hopkins University Press, 1977.

Jon Arrizabalaga

VILLON, FRANÇOIS (1431–c. 1463). François Villon, considered the greatest French medieval poet, was born François de Montcorbier, or des Loges, to a poor Parisian family originally from Bourbon. After the death of his father, his mother put him under the guidance of a scholar of canon law, Guillaume de Villon, whose name the poet eventually took. Villon was a student, first, of liberal arts and then of law and received his *licence* and *maîtrise* in 1452 when he was twenty-one. Both his writings and Parisian legal records document his preference for gambling, drinking and carousing in the midst of his studies. Parisian students of this time were, in general, raucous and reflected French society's preference for frivolity in the wake of the strain and austerity imposed by the only recently concluded Hundred Years War. In 1455, Villon killed a priest during a brawl and fled the city. He was later pardoned by King Charles VII, thanks to the intervention of Guillaume de Villon and to the victim's admission before dying that Villon was provoked.

On Christmas night of the following year he was caught with four others robbing the school of Navarre of 500 gold pieces but escaped to Angers. There is evidence that he spent time with the abbess of Pourras, or Port-Royal, known at that time for its dissolute lifestyle. He also appeared at the courts of two poetry enthusiasts, the Dukes of Bourbon and Orléans. In this period Villon wrote his first well-known poem, *Lais,* as well as flattering poems for members of the court of Orléans. By 1461 he was imprisoned in Meung-sur-Loire for having performed, despite his status as scholar, with acrobats and fair performers. The new king, Louis XI, passing through Meung, declared Villon and other prisoners free. Returning to Paris, Villon was soon arrested for robbery and imprisoned in Châtelet but then released. Discovered in yet another brawl, he was re-arrested, tortured and sentenced to be hanged. Parliament subsequently nullified the sentence and Villon was banished from Paris for ten years. There is no record of Villon after this point. Pierre Levet published the first edition of Villon's poetry in 1489 and subsequent editions followed regularly with nine appearing between 1520 and 1530. The most notable collection, edited by Clément Marot, appeared in 1533. Villon's persona as bon-vivant appeared as celebrated as his poetry. Rabelais featured Villon as a ribald jokester in *Pantagruel* (1532) and the *Quart Livre* (1552).

Villon's poetry is notable for its diversity of themes, tone, and style, ranging from a wistful and devout tribute to the Virgin Mary to satirical diatribes against the injustices of the legal system. His wittier verses date from before 1461 and are marked by a mocking tone, with multiple vulgar colloquialisms and contemporary references, which are obscure for modern readers. He offers vivid portraits of city life in which he details the need, the power, and the effects of money on the rich and the poor alike, establishing a level of realistic imagery previously not seen in French poetry. He evokes both with fondness, and ridicules the prostitutes, moneylenders, and beggars whom he frequents.

Villon's more profound and somber works, notably *Débat du Coeur et du corps, Ballade des pendus*, and *Ballade des Dames du Temps Jadis*, were composed in the aftermath of his brutal imprisonments. This latter work evokes famous women, from the beautiful and learned—Heloise—to the devout and brave—**Joan of Arc**—in offering his bittersweet reflections on the passage of Time. Its refrain, "Mais où sont les neiges d'antan?", is Villon's, and arguably French poetry's, most memorable and celebrated verse. The theme of death, presented by means of an austere style and vocabulary, dominates his later compositions. He writes of his own anticipated execution as well as of the common destiny of all humans. Villon's emphatic expression of love for humanity and the world in the face of suffering and his call for mercy and forgiveness reveal his essential Christian perspective. At the same time, Villon's emphasis on his own experiences and regrets anticipates Montaigne's secularized self-study over a century later in the *Essais*. *See also* Christianity; Prostitution.

Further Reading: Fein, David A. *François Villon Revisited*. New York: Twayne Publishers, 1997; Sargent-Baur, Barbara N. *François Villon: Complete Poems*. Toronto: University of Toronto Press, 1994.

Margaret Harp

VIRGINITY. Broadly characterized as a status in which an individual (especially a female) has never experienced sexual activity with another person, virginity's precise nature and significance have always been controversial. At any time, multiple overlapping definitions of virginity typically exist.

During the early modern era, much received wisdom concerning virginity was challenged or overturned. Virginity was at issue in multiple realms, including **medicine**, religion, law, and folk culture. These discourses often shared a behavioral baseline defining virginity as a condition pertaining to a female whose vagina had never been penetrated, particularly by a penis. Correspondingly, virginity was commonly considered destroyed the first time a vagina was penetrated. However, early modern virginity was not as simple a matter as this definition might suggest.

MEDICAL VIRGINITY. Medical definition of virginity was complicated by changing understandings of female genitalia. The existence of an anatomical telltale of lost virginity had been under debate since at least the second century. Eleventh-century Persian physician Avicenna proposed that a web or veil of tissue lay within the virginal vagina and was torn upon penetration, causing bleeding. His theory was popular among Latin and Arab physicians but was not universally accepted.

This theoretical web or veil only gradually acquired a distinctive name. It was not until 1461 that Michele **Savonarola** uses the term "hymen" (Greek, "membrane") to identify "a subtle membrane" that covers the cervix (the hymen is actually found at the entrance to the vagina). The relation of "hymen" to virginity rapidly became standardized: Thomas Elyot's 1538 *Dictionary* defines "hymen" as a "skinne in the secrete place of a maiden, which whanne she is defloured is broken."

Concern for the hymen predated confirmation of its existence. The hymen was not located in dissection until 1544, when anatomist Andreas Vesalius located it in two dissections at the University of Pisa. Vesalius did not publish his discovery until 1546, when a brief unillustrated description was published within an unrelated text, the *Letter on the China Root*.

After Vesalius, numerous conflicting and often quackish medical texts, including Severin Pineau's influential 1597 *De virginitatis et corruptionis virginum notis*, claimed to identify the true nature of the hymen as well as the nature of its relation to virginity. An anatomically accurate drawing of the hymen, however, was not published until Danish scholar Thomas Bartholin's 1668 *Anatomy*. (The nature of the hymen's relationship to virginity, if any, has yet to be definitively ascertained.)

The *morbus virginaeus* or sickness of virgins, also called "greensickness," was the preeminent gynecological disorder of the era, first defined in German physician Johannes Lang's *Medicinalium epistolarum miscellanea* (1554). The symptoms, including amenorrhea, a pale or greenish complexion, lack of appetite, and sometimes derangement and death, were believed curable through the loss of virginity.

VIRGINITY IN RELIGION. While major world religions accepted a basic behavioral definition for virginity, virginity dogmas and doctrines varied. This was particularly true within early modern **Christianity**. Catholicism had long posited virginity as the pinnacle of human existence, teaching that only virgins received heaven's full reward. Protestantism rejected such claims and stated unequivocally that paradise was equally accessible to all true believers. The Council of **Trent** proclaimed this Lutheran dogma heretical.

Attitudes about virginity were emblematic of the Christian schism. Despite Protestant denial of virginity as the state of supreme holiness, Protestantism continued to uphold the importance of chastity and monogamy in all stages of life. It has been suggested that after Trent, a conceptual split arose in the West in which "**chastity**," applicable to all states of life, was viewed as a Protestant virtue while the more specific "virginity" acquired specifically Catholic overtones.

SOCIAL AND LEGAL VIRGINITY. Socially, virginity was a matter of partnered sexual activity, but also an issue of age and marital status. The strength of this association is reflected linguistically: many languages use words for "virgin" interchangeably to indicate unmarried young women, e.g., English *maiden*, German *Jungfrau*.

Female virginity was typically considered prerequisite for **marriage**, and loss of virginity considered a critical legal aspect of solemnizing marriage. Unconsummated marriages were quickly annulled or otherwise stricken from the record. Because the legal and social event of marriage was to a large degree conceived of as being coterminous with first intercourse, unmarried women who were raped were sometimes forced to marry their rapists to legitimize lost virginity. Women who consensually lost their virginity prior to marriage (or were believed to have done so) might face substantial punishments: fines, shunning, and beatings were common across cultures and geographic regions. Death was less common but also occurred as punishment. Unmarried nonvirgins were likely to remain unmarried and were thus often destitute.

In **rape** cases generally, punishments for rapists were often lighter or cases dismissed entirely if victims could be established as having been already non-virgin at the time of the rape.

TESTING AND COUNTERFEITING VIRGINITY. Virginity tests of varying sorts were common in the early modern era. Wholly unreliable, they included genital examination performed by **midwives** or physicians, the use of inhalants and fumigants which were believed to trigger uncontrollable urination in non-virgin women, visual examination of women's urination and urine, and careful measurement of the neck on the principle that as intercourse was believed to widen the "neck of the womb," it would sympathetically broaden the throat. These methods, many of them centuries old, were transmitted both orally and in gynecological texts; regional and generational variants are common. The same is true of methods for counterfeiting virginity, which included applying irritant or astringent douches and ointments, inserting bladders or sponges filled with blood into the vagina, or making small cuts to the vaginal entrance in advance of the wedding night. *See also* Celibacy; Chastity.

Further Reading: Blank, Hanne. *Virgin: The Untouched History*. New York: Bloomsbury, 2007; Kelly, Kathleen Coyne. *Performing Virginity and Testing Chastity in the Middle Ages*. New York: Routledge, 2000; Jankowski, Theodora. *Pure Resistance: Queer Virginity in Early Modern English Drama*. Philadelphia: University of Pennsylvania Press, 2000; Loughlin, Marie H. *Hymeneutics: Interpreting Virginity on the Early Modern Stage*. Lewisburg, PA: Bucknell University Press, 1997.

Hanne Blank

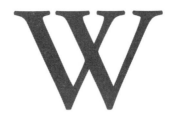

WIDOWS. *See* Remarriage/Widows

WITCHES. Witchcraft was strongly linked with sex, whether actual or theoretical. Witches were portrayed as having power over sexuality. Among many other areas, witches afflicted men with impotence, a very common form of evil magic, and performed love-magic, a common service of professional witches.

Witches in Christian Europe, where witch hunting was most prevalent during the Renaissance period, procured impotence by using the ligature, a magical device that worked in its simplest form by tying a knot in a lace, preferably at the wedding ceremony. (Magical impotence was not always blamed on witches, however.) Heinrich Kramer's ***The Malleus Maleficarum*** (1486), the most misogynist of demonological texts, held that it was within the power of witches, and also their frequent practice, to remove penises from men entirely, although this never became mainstream demonological opinion. Kramer acknowledged that such acts were illusions, but portrayed them in highly realistic language. Belief in witch-caused impotence was much more common in continental Europe than in the British Isles, where witchcraft was much less sexualized.

Love-magic has been found in many cultures, and particularly in Mediterranean Europe was the province of an active class of professional witches, whose power was religiously suspect but who were not usually charged with being directly in league with Satan. Numerous magical formulae and practices existed to attract the attention of a lover or determine the identity of a future spouse.

Although the full-fledged concept of the witch was not commonly found in Islamic cultures, the very popular concept of the "evil eye" had many similarities to belief in the power of evil witches, and persons with the evil eye—a form of involuntary but malevolent magic—were frequently suspected of magic that interfered with sex and reproduction such as procuring impotence or drying up mother's milk. Belief in the evil eye had spread from its original home in the **Middle East** to Europe and India, and in the sixteenth century it spread to the Americas with the Spanish conquest.

Sex between humans and demons played a large role in both demonological theory and actual witch trials in Europe. It was the ultimate form of physical interaction between the witch and the devil, whether Satan himself or a lesser demon, **incubus**, or succubus. Demonic sex played a smaller role in spontaneous confessions by European witches than in demonological theory, and when it appeared it was often described in banal terms. Sex was frequently associated with the satanic pact, the devil expressed his new power over the witch, and the witch her subordination. Ordinary people, who thought of devils as material anyway, had less difficulty with the idea that devils could have bodily intercourse with humans.

Although many European demonologists discussed sex, Kramer was particularly obsessed with women's sexual connections with Satan and other devils. (Kramer saw sex as the root of all sin, and that for which Adam and Eve originally fell.) He ascribed women's greater likelihood to become witches to their insatiable sexual lusts, a departure from the demonological mainstream that ascribed the phenomenon to women's greater weakness overall. He also suspected that the reluctance of many great ones in the land to persecute witches was caused by their reception of demonic sexual favors.

One question that vexed demonologists was whether sexual intercourse with demons brought pleasure to female witches (no one seems to have questioned that it brought pleasure to males), and whether it was lesser or greater than sex with a human male. The tendency as debate developed was to place more emphasis on the painful and degrading nature of demonic intercourse. (Demonologists and magistrates may have feared that emphasizing pleasure made being a witch too attractive to women. There

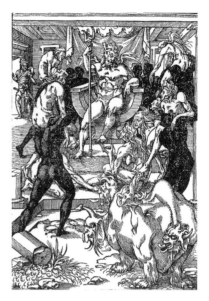

Satan holding court for newly appointed witches. From Gerard d'Euphrates's *Livre de l'historie & ancienne cronique*, printed in Paris, 1549. Courtesy of the Dover Pictorial Archives.

are some cases where women described the devil as a better lover than their husbands, although the reverse was more common.) Descriptions of the devil's penis grew increasingly grotesque over the course of the witch hunts, emphasizing its incredible size, bizarre conformation and the icy coldness of both penis and ejaculate. The early seventeenth-century French witch-hunter Pierre de Lancre claimed that the devil's penis was three-pronged, to simultaneously enter the vagina, anus, and mouth. The idea that the devil took animal form to have sex with female witches became more common. Children were also more frequently charged with having had sex with the devil.

Human/demon sex usually played a smaller role the farther north in Europe the witch hunt extended. In England, the belief that witches often had "familiar spirits," taking animal form, who nursed at an extra nipple known as the "witch's mark" in a demonic parody of motherhood fulfilled some of the same functions as demonic sexuality in establishing the physical connection of witch and demon. Witches and demons also interacted through kissing. Depictions of sabbats, the periodic gathering of witches, demons and the Devil, often featured witches kissing the devil, sometimes in animal form, on the anus or buttocks, as well as promiscuous sex, whether human/demon or human/human.

One curious aspect of human/demon sex as envisioned in early modern Europe was that it was hardly ever same-sex. Kramer and other early demonologists even emphasized the horror demons felt at the unnatural vice of "sodomy." Although there are scattered incidents of men confessing to having been sodomized by the devil, it never became a common theme in witch hunting. Not all sex engaged in or affected by witchcraft was demonic. Female witches were sometimes described as promiscuous, and in some regions witchcraft and sexual promiscuity were strongly linked in popular stereotype. In Sweden, for example, brothels were called "witch-houses." *See also* Anal Sex; Christianity.

Further Reading: Briggs, Robin. *Witches and Neighbours: The Social and Cultural Context of European Witchcraft.* 2nd ed. Oxford: Blackwell, 2002; Dundes, Alan, ed. *The Evil Eye: A Folklore Casebook.* New York and London: Garland, 1981. Robbins, Kevin C. "Magical Emasculation, Popular Anticlericalism, and the Limits of the Reformation in Western France circa 1590." *Journal of Social History* 31 (1997): 61–83; Stephens, Walter. *Demon Lovers: Witchcraft, Sex, and the Crisis of Belief.* Chicago and London: University of Chicago Press, 2002.

William E. Burns

THE WITCHES' HAMMER. See *The Malleus Maleficarum*

Z

ZINÄ. *Zinä*, the Muslim term used for unlawful sexual intercourse, can be defined as meaning **adultery** or fornication. Adultery is defined as sexual intercourse between a man and a woman who are not lawfully married or within a legal master/slave relationship. In Islamic law, both Sunnis and Shi'ites upheld stoning as the same punishment for adulterers, who were free adult Muslims. Generally, for those who were unmarried and free or considered minors or non-Muslim, the punishment was 100 lashes and banishment for a year. In the case of slaves, the punishment was fifty lashes and six months banishment.

Originally, the punishment for women prescribed in the Koran (IV: 15) was confinement within their homes. However, due to a number of complexities and several other verses in the Koran (XXIV: 2–3), non-Koranic punishments were established. Stoning was adopted as a punishment based on religious tradition (*ùadith/hadith*). Offenses could not be considered adultery or fornication, if the act(s) was performed because of force or compulsion.

A confession or the testimony of four eyewitnesses was necessary before punishment could be meted out. The witnesses were required to testify that they had seen the accused *in flagrante*. Four male eyewitnesses had to testify to this, but among the Shiites one male could testify with six women. False accusations of adultery or fornication were punishable by eighty lashes (Koran XXIV: 4). Confessions were only allowed if they were repeated four times in court, but it was possible to retract a confession. Only the Mäliki school of law allowed circumstantial evidence, such as the **pregnancy** of an unmarried girl. A husband was permitted to kill his wife and her lover on the spot, if he discovered them. If both of the accused were sentenced to be stoned, the male was first stoned by the witnesses, then by the judge, and then by the onlookers. In the case of a woman, she was first buried up to her waist.

When the husband accused his wife of adultery but could produce no witnesses, he was required by the Koran to swear four times that he told the truth and then swear once to God to curse him, if he lied. The wife could avert punishment by swearing four times that her husband was a liar and once to God to curse her, if her husband told the truth (Koran XXIV: 6–9). If both husband and wife swore, then there was no punishment, but the **marriage** was ended and the woman was not allowed to marry again.

Homosexual acts (*liwät*) were treated differently between the Sunni law schools and the Shi'ites. Some schools upheld the same requirements, conditions, and punishments as those for heterosexual fornication, except that only the active partner would be stoned and the passive partner flogged and then banished, but this was not uniform.

Shi'ite doctrine varied in that it considered sodomy with both men and women (outside of a lawful marriage), as well as lesbian relations, as fornication, but it also considered the accused's situation, such as the circumstances of their lawful partner and whether such a person was imprisoned or traveling for an extended period of time. Additionally, the Shi'ites sentenced offenders to death in cases of **incest, rape**, or when a non-Muslim man had relations with a Muslim woman. In cases of homosexual penetration, the judge made the final decision on the type of execution. The condemned man could either be decapitated by sword, stoned to death, thrown down from an elevated location, or burned to death. In cases where there was no penetration or concerning lesbian acts, the punishment was one hundred lashes.

Islamic law was extremely well developed and fully capable of addressing all contingencies within a complex society. However, in remote and isolated areas where judges or courts were not present, or in tribal areas or different sectarian groups, local practices, or "folk Islam," were frequently practiced. *See also* Homosexuality; Islam; Lesbianism; Middle East.

Further Reading: Peters, R. "Zinä." In *Encyclopaedia of Islam*, edited by P. Bearman, Th. Bianquis, C. E. Bosworth, E. van Donzel, and W. P. Heinrichs. Leiden: Brill, 2007; Roberts, Robert. *The Social Laws of the Qoran*. London: Curzon Press, 1990.

Mark David Luce

Selected Bibliography

The following bibliography contains a selection of important general or primary materials not cited within individual entry bibliographies. For information on a particular topic, please check both this bibliography and the "Further Reading" listings at the ends of relevant entries.

Ahmed, Leila. *Women and Gender in Islam*. New Haven, CT: Yale University Press, 1992.
Binns, J. "Women or Transvestites on the Elizabethan State: An Oxford Controversy." *Sixteenth-Century Journal* 5 (1974): 95–120.
Brown, J. *Immodest Acts: the Life of a Lesbian Nun in Renaissance Italy*. New York: Oxford University Press, 1986.
Burnett, Charles, and Anna Contadini, eds. *Islam and the Italian Renaissance*. London: Warburg Institute, 1999.
Chartier, Roger. *A History of Private Life*, vol. 4: *Passions of the Renaissance*. Translated by Arthur Goldhammer. General eds. Phillipe Aries and Georges Duby. Cambridge, MA and London: The Belknap Press of Harvard University Press, 1989.
Cohen, Elizabeth S., and Thomas V. Cohen. *Daily Life in Renaissance Italy*. Westport, CT: Greenwood Press, 2001.
Davis, Natalie Zemon. *The Return of Martin Guerre*. Cambridge, MA: Harvard University Press, 1984.
de Erauso, Catalina, et al. *Lieutenant Nun: Memoirs of a Basque Transvestite in the New World*. Boston: Beacon Press.
Edwardes, A. *The Jewel in the Lotus: A Historical Survey of the Sexual Culture of the East*. New York: Julian Press, 1959.
Fagioli, Marco. *Shunga: The Erotic Art of Japan*. New York: Universe Publishing, 1998.
Gerard, K., and G. Hekma, eds. *The Pursuit of Sodomy: Male Homosexuality in the Renaissance and Enlightenment*. New York: Harrington Park, 1989.
Goffman, Daniel. *The Ottoman Empire and Early Modern Europe*. Cambridge: Cambridge University Press, 2002.
Gutierrez, Ramon. *When Jesus Came, the Corn Mothers Went Away: Marriage, Sexuality, and Power in New Mexico, 1500–1846*. Stanford, CA: Stanford University Press, 1991.
Hinsch, B. *Passions of the Cut Sleeve*. Berkeley and Los Angeles: University of California Press, 1990.
Levathes, Louise. *When China Rule the Seas*. New York: Simon and Schuster, 1994.
Machiavelli, Niccolo. *The Prince*. Washington: Dante University of America Press, 2003.
Mann, Charles C. *1491: New Revelations of the Americas Before Columbus*. New York: Alfred A. Knopf, 2006.
Marmon, Shaun, ed. *Slavery in the Islamic Middle East*. Princeton, NJ: Markus Wiener Publishers, 1999.

SELECTED BIBLIOGRAPHY

Muir, Edward, and Guide Ruggiero, eds. *Sex and Gender in Historical Perspective*. Baltimore: Johns Hopkins University Press, 1990.

Murray, J., and K. Eisenbichler, eds. *Desire and Discipline: Sex and Sexuality in the Premodern West*. Toronto: University of Toronto Press, 1996.

Neret, Gilles. *Erotica Universalis*. vol. 2. Cologne, Germany: Tachen, 1994.

Ozment, Stephen. *Burgermeister's Daughter; Scandal in a Sixteenth-Century German Town*. New York: Harper, 1997.

Ruggiero, Guido. *Binding Passions: Tales of Magic, Marriage, and Power and the End of the Renaissance*. Oxford: Oxford University Press, 1993.

Salgado, Gamini. *The Elizabethan Underworld*. Phoenix Mills, UK: Wrens Park Publishing, 1977. (Originally published by J.M. Dent & Sons.)

Sautman, Fracesca Canadé, and P. Sheingorn, eds. *Same Sex Love and Desire among Women in the Middle Ages*. London: Palgrave Macmillan, 2001.

Tannahill, Reay. *Sex in History*. Briarcliff Manor, NY: Scarborough Books, 1982.

Tavacchia, Bette. *Taking Positions: On the Erotic in Renaissance Culture*. Princeton, NJ: Princeton University Press, 1999.

Taylor, C. "Homosexuality in Precolumbian and Colonial Mexico." In *Male Homosexuality in Central and South America*, edited by S. Murray, 4–21. New York: Gai Saber, 1987.

Wiesner-Hanks, Merry. *Christianity and Sexuality in the Early Modern World*. London: Routledge, 1999.

Wilson, Katerina, ed. *Women Writers of the Renaissance and Reformation*. Athens: University of Georgia Press, 1987.

Winkler, J. *The Spirit and the Flesh: Sexual Diversity in American Indian Culture*. Boston: Beacon Press, 1986. (Reprint ed. with a new introduction, 1992.)

Index

Boldfaced page numbers indicate main entries.

Abortion and contraception, **3–5**, 48, 162
Actors, **5–6**
Adolescents, **6–8**
Adultery, **8–10**. *See also* Mistresses; *Zinā*
Afghan dynasty, 212
Africa, **10–12**
Akbar Namar, 122, 123
Americas (North and South), **12–16**, 43
Anal sex, **16–17**, 111–12
Annulment, **17–19**
Anteros, 79–80
Architecture, European, **19–20**
Aretino, Pietro, **21–22**, 187
Art, European, **22–24**
Asia, **24–26**

Baptism, 168
Barnfield, Richard, 110–11
Bastardy, **27–28**
Bembo, Pietro, 184
Berdache, **28–29**
Bestiality, 15–16, **30**
Betrothal, **31–32**
Bloodletting, 164
Boleyn, Anne. *See* Henry VIII
Book of the Courtier, The (Castiglione), **32–33**
Borgia, Lucrezia, **33–35**
Brothels, **35–36**
Bucer, Martin, 72
Buddhism, 25, **36–37**, 42. *See also* Tantric Buddhism

Calvin, John, **38**, 71
Caste, **39–40**
Castiglione, Baldassare. *See Book of the Courtier, The*
Castillo, Bernal Díaz del. *See* Díaz del Castillo, Bernal
Castration, **40–41**. *See also* Eunuchs
Celibacy, **41–43**. *See also* Elizabeth I, Queen of England
Censorship. *See Index of Prohibited Books*
Chastity, **43–44**. *See also* Elizabeth I, Queen of England; Virginity
Child abandonment, **47–48**. *See also* Foundlings and orphans
Childbirth, **45–46**, 47. *See also* Churching; Midwives; Pregnancy
Childhood, **46–49**
Child-murder. *See* Infanticide
Children: circulation of, 48; religious dimensions of, 48–49; uniqueness of the West regarding, 49. *See also* Foundlings and orphans; Motherhood
China, 25, 74, 120, 178; celibacy in, 42; concubines in, 56–57; masculinity and, 160; penitential practices in, 181–82. *See also* Confucianism; Footbinding
Chinese literature, 60, 67
Chinese treasure fleets, **49–50**
Christianity, 42, 48, **51–54**, 55; love and, 144. *See also* Calvin, John; Luther, Martin; Penitential practices; Reformation; *specific topics*
Churching, 55
Concubines, **56–57**, 101, 167, 170
Confucianism, **57–61**, 160
Contraception. *See* Abortion and contraception
Cortés, Hernán, 135
Council of Trent. *See* Trent, Council of
Courtesans, **61–63**. *See also* D'Aragona, Tullia
Courtier, The. See Book of the Courtier, The
Cross-dressing, **63–64**, 112. *See also* Berdache
Cupid. *See* Eros

Daoism, 25, **65–67**
D'Aragona, Tullia, **68–69**
Demons, sex with, 228–29. *See also* Incubi/succubi
Diana (Roman hunting goddess), 22, 70
Diane de Poitiers, **69–70**
Díaz del Castillo, Bernal, **70–71**
Divorce, 9, **71–72**. *See also* Annulment
Domestic violence, **72–73**
Dona Marina. *See* La Malinche
Dowry, **73–74**
Dudley, Robert, 77–78

INDEX

Eastern Orthodox Churches, 52
Edward II (Marlowe), 156
Eisenstein, Elizabeth, 193
Elizabeth I, Queen of England, 76–78, 197–98
Eros, 78–80
Eunuchs, 40, 41, 80–81. *See also* Castration
Europe, 81–84. *See also* Architecture, European; Art, European; Exploration and colonization, European; Literature, European
Exploration and colonization, European, 84–88

Family, 143–44
Fatherhood, 89–90
Ferrand, Jacques, 146–47
Ficino, Marsilio, 184
First Blast of the Trumpet Against the Monstrous Regiment of Women, The (Knox), 90–91
Fonte, Moderata, 92
Footbinding, 92–94
Fornication. *See* Premarital sex; *Zina*
Forteguerri, Laudomia, 94–95
Foundlings and orphans, 95–96

Ganjavi, 215–16
Ganymede, 97–98
Gerson, Jean, 161
Gilles de Rais, 98–100
Gynecology, 176. *See also* Medicine; Science

Harem/seraglio, 101–2, 123, 214
Henry II, King of France, 69–70
Henry III, King of France, 103–4
Henry VIII, King of England, 18, 104–6, 111–12
Heresy. *See* Index of Prohibited Books
Hermaphrodites, 106–7, 210
Hinduism, 24–25, 107–10. *See also* Caste
Homoeroticism, 97, 110–11, 121, 156–57, 211
Homosexuality, 111–12; Buddhism and, 37; Confucianism and, 59; 'ishq and, 121; Islam and, 231–32; in North America, 15. *See also* Berdache; Lesbianism; Pederasty
"Homosociality," 110
Honor, 143–44
Household structure, 47
Humanists, 48

Il Cortegiano. *See Book of the Courtier, The*
Illegitimacy. *See* Bastardy
Impotence, 114–15
Incest, 115–16
Incubi/succubi, 116–17. *See also* Demons, sex with
Index of Prohibited Books, 117–18
Infanticide, 47, 118–20, 190
'Ishq, 121
Islam, 121–25; adultery and, 9–10; concubines and, 56, 101, 167; harems and, 101, 123; in India, 24; polygamy and, 56, 101, 123, 185; Shia, 124, 232; slavery and, 213, 214. *See also* Middle East; Sufism; *Zina*

Japan, 26, 42
Jeanne d'Arc. *See* Joan of Arc
Joan of Arc, 126–28
Judaism, 10, 128–31, 185–86
Julian of Norwich, 131–32

Kali, 107, 109
Kama Sutra, 133–34
Knox, John, 90–91
Krishna, 107–8

La Malinche, 135–36
Lesbianism, 15, 136–38, 161. *See also* Forteguerri, Laudomia
Literacy, 60, 138–39, 193
Literature, Chinese, 60, 67
Literature, European, 139–41. *See also Index of Prohibited Books*; Printing
Love, 121, 142–45; Eros and, 78–79; Platonic, 184; premodern, 142–43; religion and, 144. *See also* Magic, love, and sex
Love sickness, 146–47, 163, 215
Love songs, 147–49
Luther, Martin, 71–72, 149–50, 200

Madrigals, 148
Magic, love, and sex, 152–53, 228
Malinal. *See* La Malinche
Malleus Maleficarum, The (Kramer), 153–54
Mandeville, Sir John. *See Travels of Sir John Mandeville, The*
Marguerite de Navarre, 154–56
Marlowe, Christopher, 156–57
Marriage, 56, 157–59; in Africa, 11–12; Council of Trent and, 222; Jewish, 129–30. *See also* Dowry
Mary, Blessed Virgin, 201–2
Masculinity, 159–60
Masturbation, 161
Medical virginity, 226
Medicine, 162–63, 164. *See also* Obstetrical manuals; Science
Menstruation, 163–65
Middle East, 165–67
Midwives, 46, 47, 167–69
Mikveh, 169–70
Ming dynasty, 59–61, 67
Mistresses, 170–71
Mogul Empire, 122–24, 185
Mohammed, 121–23
Motherhood, 171–73; expectations, 171–72; experiences, 172–73. *See also* Childbirth; Pregnancy
Mystics, 173–74

Nafzawi, Shaykh al-Imam Abu Abd-Allah al-, 183
North America. *See* Americas

Obstetrical manuals, 176–77, 190
Oral sex, 178–79
Orphans. *See* Foundlings and orphans
Ottoman Empire, 124–25, 165–67, 185

"Pearl Sewn Shirt, The" (Feng), 60
Pedagogues, 48
Pederasty, 180–81
Penitential practices, 181–82
Perfumed Garden for the Soul's Delectation, The (al-Nafzawi), 183
Persia, 167
Plato, 184

Platonic love, **184**
Polygamy/polyandry, 56, 101, 123, 130, 171, **185–86**
Pornography, **186–88**
Pozzo, Modesta. *See* Fonte, Moderata
Pregnancy, **189–90**. *See also* Childbirth; Midwives
Premarital sex, 11, **191**. *See also* Chastity; Virginity
Priests, 53
Printing, 138, **192–94**
Prostitution, **194–96**, 214. *See also* Brothels; Courtesans; Pornography
Purgation, 164, 173

Radha, 108
Raleigh, Sir Walter, **197–98**
Rape, **199–200**, 214
Reformation, 53, **200–204**; important figures in, 202–4 (*see also specific figures*); and marriage, 158–59; Scottish, 91
Remarriage/widows, **205**
Renaissance, 61–63, 112, 139–41

Sacraments. *See* Penitential practices
Safavids, 167
Sati, **207–8**
Savonarola, Michele, **208–9**
Science, **209–10**. *See also* Medicine
Seraglio. *See* Harem/seraglio
Shakespeare, William, 110–12, 140, **211**
Shi'ites/Shia Islam, 124, 232. *See also* Islam
Shiva, 108–9
Shulhan Arukh, 129–31
Sibling sex, 115
Sikandar Lodhi, **212**
Slavery, **212–15**. *See also* Concubines
Sodomy, 178. *See also* Anal sex
Songs. *See* Love songs
South America. *See* Americas
Spain, 218
Spanish colonizers, 12–14
"Story of Layla and Majnun, The" (Ganjavi), **215–16**
Succubi. *See* Incubi/succubi
Sufi romances, **216–17**
Sufism, 121, 165

Tantric Buddhism, 37, 152–53
Taoism. *See* Daoism
Theater, **218–19**. *See also* Shakespeare, William
Throckmorton, Elizabeth (Bess), 198
Travels of Sir John Mandeville, The, **219–20**
Trent, Council of, **220–22**

Venereal disease, **223–24**
Villon, François, **225–26**
Virginity, **226–27**; medical, 226; in religion, 226–27; social and legal, 227; testing and counterfeiting, 227. *See also* Chastity; Elizabeth I, Queen of England

Wang Yangming, 59, 60
Widows. *See* Remarriage/widows
Witches, 114, 153–54, **228–30**
"Woman marriage," 12

Yoga, sexual, 66, 67. *See also* Tantric Buddhism

Zheng He (Cheng Ho), 49–50
Zinä, **231–32**
Zoophilia, 15–16. *See also* Bestiality

About the Editors and Contributors

Jon Arrizabalaga
IMF-CSIC
Barcelona, Spain

Balaka Basu
The Graduate Center
City University of New York
New York, New York

Belén Bistué
University of California, Davis
Davis, California

Hanne Blank
Independent Scholar
Baltimore, Maryland

Mary Block
Department of History
Valdosta State University
Valdosta, Georgia

Lucia Bortoli
Comparative Studies Department
The Ohio State University
Columbus, Ohio

Hans Peter Broedel
Department of History
University of North Dakota
Grand Forks, North Dakota

Brooke Bryant
The City University of New York
New York, New York

William E. Burns
Independent Scholar
Washington, DC

David Cast
Bryn Mawr College
Bryn Mawr, Pennsylvania

Pamela Cheek
Department of Foreign Languages
  and Literatures
University of New Mexico
Albuquerque, New Mexico

Kristen Pederson Chew
Independent Scholar
Toronto, Ontario, Canada

Thomas Cohen
Department of History
York University
Toronto, Ontario, Canada

Katherine R. Cooper
North Greenville University
Greenville, South Carolina

Emily Detmer-Goebel
Department of Literature and Language
Northern Kentucky University
Highland Heights, Kentucky

Sally Ann Drucker
Department of English
Nassau Community College
Garden City, New York

ABOUT THE EDITORS AND CONTRIBUTORS

Konrad Eisenbichler
Victoria College
University of Toronto
Toronto, Ontario, Canada

Ronna S. Feit
Department of Foreign Languages
Nassau Community College
State University of New York
Garden City, New York

David J. Fine
The Graduate Center
City University of New York
New York, New York

Louise Geddes
The Graduate Center
City University of New York
New York, New York

Rachel Goldman
The Graduate Center
City University of New York
New York, New York

Cherrie Ann Gottsleben
Liberty University
Lynchburg, Virginia

Margaret Harp
University of Nevada, Las Vegas
Las Vegas, Nevada

Nicolás Hernández, Jr.
Russell Sage College
Troy, New York

Mary Hewlett
Centre for Renaissance and
Reformation Studies
University of Toronto
Toronto, Ontario, Canada

Reginald Hyatte
University of Tulsa
Tulsa, Oklahoma

Margaret L. King
Broeklundian Professor
Brooklyn College
Brooklyn, New York
Professor of History, the Graduate Center
City University of New York
New York, New York

George Klawitter
Department of English
St. Edward's University
Austin, Texas

Mia Korpiola
Faculty of Law
University of Helsinki
Helsinki, Finland

Adele Kudish
New York University
New York, New York

Hiram Kümper
Historisches Institut
Ruhr-Universität Bochum
Bochum, Germany

Tonya M. Lambert
University of Alberta
Edmonton, Alberta, Canada

Allison Levy
Wheaton College
Norton, Massachusetts

Janice Liedl
Department of History
Laurentian University
Sudbury, Ontario, Canada

Maritere López
Department of History
California State University, Fresno
Fresno, California

Mark David Luce
University of Chicago
Chicago, Illinois

Evyatar Marienberg
Erasmus Institute
University of Notre Dame
South Bend, Indiana

ABOUT THE EDITORS AND CONTRIBUTORS

Pamela McVay
Ursuline College
Pepper Pike, Ohio

Eugenio Menegon
Boston University
Boston, Massachusetts

Andrew Meyer
Brooklyn College
Brooklyn, New York

Victoria L. Mondelli
Department of History
The Graduate Center
City University of New York
New York, New York

Patricia Nardi
Graduate Center
City University of New York
New York, New York

Christopher J. Nygren
Department of the History of Art
The Johns Hopkins University
Baltimore, Maryland

Todd H. J. Pettigrew
Department of Languages and Letters
Cape Breton University
Sydney, Nova Scotia, Canada

Roderick Phillips
Department of History
Carleton University
Ottawa, Ontario, Canada

Karen Swallow Prior
Liberty University
Lynchburg, Virginia

Sergio Rigoletto
Department of Italian Studies
University of Reading
Reading, England, United Kingdom

Lynn Robson
Regent's Park College
Oxford, England, United Kingdom

William John Silverman, Jr.
Department of English
Florida State University
Tallahassee, Florida

Michelle Spinelli
Independent Scholar
Brooklyn, New York

Jan Sundin
Linköping University
Linköping, Sweden

Julie Sutherland
Pacific Theatre
Vancouver, British Columbia, Canada

Nicholas Terpstra
Department of History
University of Toronto
Toronto, Ontario, Canada

Georgia Tres
Oakland University
Rochester, Michigan

James Grantham Turner
University of California, Berkeley
Berkeley, California

Sharmain van Blommestein
SUNY Potsdam
Potsdam, New York

John A. Wagner
Independent Scholar
Scottsdale, Arizona

Andrew J. Waskey
Division of Social Sciences
Dalton State College
Dalton, Georgia

Barbara Zimbalist
Department of English
University of California, Davis
Davis, California